PSYCHOGASTROENTEROLOGY

Editor

LAURIE KEEFER

GASTROENTEROLOGY CLINICS OF NORTH AMERICA

www.gastro.theclinics.com

Consulting Editor
ALAN L. BUCHMAN

December 2022 • Volume 51 • Number 4

ELSEVIER

1600 John F. Kennedy Boulevard • Suite 1800 • Philadelphia, Pennsylvania, 19103-2899
http://www.theclinics.com

GASTROENTEROLOGY CLINICS OF NORTH AMERICA Volume 51, Number 4
December 2022 ISSN 0889-8553, ISBN-13: 978-0-323-98721-9

Editor: Kerry Holland
Developmental Editor: Hannah Almira Lopez

Gastroenterology Clinics of North America (ISSN 0889-8553) is published quarterly by Elsevier Inc., 360 Park Avenue South, New York, NY 10010-1710. Months of issue are March, June, September, and December. Business and Editorial Offices: 1600 John F. Kennedy Blvd., Suite 1800, Philadelphia, PA 19103-2899. Customer Service Office: 6277 Sea Harbor Drive, Orlando, FL 32887-4800. Periodicals postage paid at New York, NY and additional mailing offices. Subscription prices are $368.00 per year (US individuals), $100.00 per year (US students), $973.00 per year (US institutions), $395.00 per year (Canadian individuals), $100.00 per year (Canadian students), $1002.00 per year (Canadian institutions), $468.00 per year (international individuals), $220.00 per year (international students), and $1002.00 per year (international institutions). Foreign air speed delivery is included in all *Clinics* subscription prices. All prices are subject to change without notice. **POSTMASTER**: Send address changes to *Gastroenterology Clinics of North America*, Elsevier Health Sciences Division, Subscription Customer Service, 3251 Riverport Lane, Maryland Heights, MO 63043. **Telephone: 1-800-654-2452 (U.S. and Canada); 314-447-8871 (outside U.S. and Canada). Fax: 314-447-8029. E-mail: journalscustomerservice-usa@elsevier.com (for print support); journalsonlinesupport-usa@elsevier.com (for online support).**

Reprints. For copies of 100 or more, of articles in this publication, please contact the Commercial Reprints Department, Elsevier Inc., 360 Part Avenue South, New York, New York 10010-1710. Tel. 212-633-3874, Fax: 212-633-3820, E-mail: reprints@elsevier.com.

Gastroenterology Clinics of North America is also published in Italian by Il Pensiero Scientifico Editore, Rome, Italy; and in Portuguese by Interlivros Edicoes Ltda., Rua Commandante Coelho 1085, 21250 Cordovil, Rio de Janeiro, Brazil.

Gastroenterology Clinics of North America is covered in *MEDLINE/PubMed (Index Medicus), Excerpta Medica, Current Contents/Clinical Medicine, Science Citation Index, ISI/BIOMED,* and *BIOSIS.*

Contributors

CONSULTING EDITOR

ALAN L. BUCHMAN, MD, MSPH, FACP, FACN, FACG, AGAF
Professor of Clinical Surgery, Medical Director, Intestinal Rehabilitation and Transplant Center, The University of Illinois at Chicago/UI Health, Chicago, Illinois, USA

EDITOR

LAURIE KEEFER, PhD
Professor of Medicine and Psychiatry, Division of Gastroenterology, Icahn School of Medicine at Mount Sinai, New York, New York, USA

AUTHORS

SARA AHOLA KOHUT, PhD, CPSYCH
Department of Gastroenterology, Hepatology, and Nutrition, Hospital for Sick Children, Department of Psychiatry, University of Toronto, Child Health Evaluative Sciences, SickKids Research Institute, Toronto, Canada

TINA ASWANI-OMPRAKASH, BS, BA
Mount Sinai Icahn School of Medicine, South Asian IBD Alliance, New York, New York, USA

SARAH BALLOU, PhD
Division of Gastroenterology, Beth Israel Deaconess Medical Center, Boston, Massachusetts, USA

ALYSE BEDELL, PhD
Department of Psychiatry & Behavioral Neuroscience, The University of Chicago, Chicago, Illinois, USA

HELEN BURTON MURRAY, PhD
Assistant Professor of Psychology (Psychiatry), Division of Gastroenterology, Massachusetts General Hospital, Harvard Medical School, Department of Psychiatry, Massachusetts General Hospital, Boston, Massachusetts, USA

SAMANTHA CALABRESE, CNP
Division of Gastroenterology, Massachusetts General Hospital, Boston, Massachusetts, USA

SHAYNA COBURN, PhD
Assistant Professor, Division of Gastroenterology, Children's National Hospital, The George Washington University School of Medicine, Washington, DC, USA

JORDYN H. FEINGOLD, MD, MSCR, MAPP
Department of Psychiatry, Icahn School of Medicine at Mount Sinai, New York, New York, USA

ALANA FRIEDLANDER, MA
Department of Psychiatry & Behavioral Neuroscience, The University of Chicago, Department of Psychology, Roosevelt University, Chicago, Illinois, USA

MONIQUE GERMONE, PhD
Associate Professor, Departments of Psychiatry and Pediatrics, University of Colorado Anschutz Medical Campus, Aurora, Colorado, USA

RUBY GREYWOODE, MD, MS
Assistant Professor of Medicine, Division of Gastroenterology, Einstein-Montefiore Medical Center, Bronx, New York, USA

KIMBERLY N. HARER, MD, ScM
Clinical Lecturer, Division of Gastroenterology and Hepatology, University of Michigan/ Michigan Medicine, Ann Arbor, Michigan, USA

CHRISTINA H. JAGIELSKI, PhD, MPH
Clinical Instructor, Division of Gastroenterology and Hepatology, University of Michigan/ Michigan Medicine, Ann Arbor, Michigan, USA

SARAH W. KINSINGER, PhD, ABPP
Associate Professor of Medicine, Division of Gastroenterology and Nutrition, Loyola University Medical Center, Maywood, Illinois, USA

BRJÁNN LJÓTSSON, PhD,
Professor, Department of Clinical Neuroscience, Division of Psychology, Karolinska Institutet, Solna, Stockholm, Sweden

SARA HOFFMAN MARCHESE, PhD
Postdoctoral Fellow, Department of Psychiatry & Behavioral Sciences, Section of Bariatric & Outpatient Psychotherapy, Rush University Medical Center, Chicago, Illinois, USA

JOSIE MCGARVA, BS
Division of Gastroenterology and Hepatology, Northwestern University Feinberg School of Medicine, Chicago, Illinois, USA

A. NATISHA NABBIJOHN, BSC, MA
Department of Psychology, University of Guelph, Guelph, Ontario, Canada

BROOKE PALMER, PhD
Assistant Professor, Department of Medicine, Division of General Internal Medicine, Assistant Professor, University of Minnesota Medical School, Minneapolis, Minnesota, USA

ANJALI U. PANDIT, PhD, MPH
Assistant Professor of Medicine, Division of Gastroenterology and Hepatology & Psychiatry, Northwestern University Feinberg School of Medicine, Chicago, Illinois, USA

MEGAN PETRIK, PhD
Assistant Professor, Department of Medicine, Division of General Internal Medicine, Assistant Professor, University of Minnesota Medical School, Minneapolis, Minnesota, USA

JOHANNAH RUDDY, MEd
Chief Operating Officer, The Rome Foundation, Doctoral Candidate, Campbell University, School of Pharmacy and Health Sciences, Raleigh, North Carolina, USA

JESSICA K. SALWEN-DEREMER, PhD, DBSM
Assistant Professor of Psychiatry & Medicine, Section of Gastroenterology, The Geisel School of Medicine at Dartmouth, Staff Psychologist, Dartmouth-Hitchcock Medical Center, One Medical Center Drive, Lebanon, New Hampshire, USA

NEHA D. SHAH, MPH, RD, CNSC, CHES
Colitis and Crohn's Disease Center, University of California, San Francisco, San Francisco, California, USA; South Asian IBD Alliance, New York, New York, USA; Neha Shah Nutrition, San Francisco, California, USA

MICHAEL SUN, PhD
Postdoctoral Fellow, Department of Psychological and Brain Sciences, Dartmouth College, Hanover, New Hampshire, USA

EVA SZIGETHY, MD, PhD
Professor of Psychiatry, Pediatrics, and Medicine, University of Pittsburgh, Pittsburgh, Pennsylvania, USA

TIFFANY TAFT, PsyD, MIS
Research Associate Professor, Division of Gastroenterology and Hepatology, Northwestern University Feinberg School of Medicine, Chicago, Illinois, USA

Contents

Stigma is a centuries-old phenomenon that pervades chronic digestive diseases, regardless of classification. Patients with gastrointestinal (GI) illness perceive others hold stigmatizing beliefs about them and their illness, including from medical professionals, and may go on to internalize or believe these negative stereotypes as true. These perceptions seem to be based on the thought that the public views GI diseases negatively. The effects of GI stigma are substantial and influence quality of life, psychological distress, treatment adherence, disease severity, and health-care utilization. These realities underscore the need for stigma to be addressed by the GI community and measures taken to mitigate its impacts.

In this review article, we show that stress and resilience play an integral role in the brain–gut axis and are critical to symptom expression across all digestive disorders. The relationship between stress, coping, and resilience provides a mechanistic basis for brain–gut behavior therapies. Psychogastroenterology is the field best equipped to translate and mitigate these constructs as part of patient care across all digestive disorders.

Integrated models of care for chronic digestive conditions, such as irritable bowel syndrome (IBS) and inflammatory bowel disease (IBD), are becoming the standard of care and require patients to have access to brain–gut behavior therapies. Further progress is needed to implement this approach across GI practice settings and will require gastroenterologists to build collaborative relationships with GI Psychologists. This review provides guidance on practical steps for integrating brain–gut behavior therapy into a GI practice, including guidance on assessing patients for their appropriateness for referral, effective communication strategies to recommend brain–gut behavior therapy, and tips on how to develop a referral pathway and successful collaboration with a GI Psychologist.

With growing evidence to support their efficacy, brain–gut behavior therapies are increasingly viewed as a key component to integrated care management of disorders of gut–brain interaction. However, the types of brain–gut behavior therapies differ in how and for whom they purportedly work. We provide a conceptual review of these brain–gut behavior therapies, with an emphasis on describing how (ie, mechanisms) and for whom (ie, moderators) they work as hypothesized and/or supported by evidence. Based on evidence to date, we recommend that brain–gut behavior therapies prioritize gastrointestinal-specific targets, such as gastrointestinal-specific anxiety.

Behavioral digital therapeutics represents a diverse range of health technology tools that can offer beneficial options for patients with gastrointestinal disorders, particularly with the shortage of mental health providers. Challenges to the uptake of behavioral digital interventions exist and can be addressed with mobile device applications, improved interoperability of technology platforms, and flexible integration into clinical practice.

Several chronic digestive conditions are physiologically based on food intolerance, including celiac disease, nonceliac gluten sensitivity, and eosinophilic esophagitis. Patients are expected to follow medically prescribed diets to eliminate identified food triggers to control symptoms. However, the psychological impacts of these dietary approaches are largely unaddressed in clinical practice. Hypervigilance and anxiety regarding food and symptoms, and disordered eating, may emerge and negatively affect outcomes. Clinicians working with pediatric and adult populations with food intolerances should be aware of these psychological comorbidities, and equally emphasize effective ways to help patients manage the mental and physical aspects of their condition.

Eating disorders are characterized by cognitions (eg, fear of gastrointestinal symptoms around eating, overvaluation of body shape/weight) and behaviors (eg, dietary restriction, binge eating) associated with medical (eg, weight loss), and/or psychosocial impairments (eg, high distress around eating). With growing evidence for bidirectional relationships between eating disorders and gastrointestinal disorders, gastroenterology providers' awareness of historical, concurrent, and potential risk for eating disorders is imperative. In this conceptual review, we highlight risk and maintenance pathways in the eating disorder—gastrointestinal disorder intersection, delineate different types of eating disorders, and provide recommendations for the gastroenterology provider in assessing and preventing eating disorder symptoms.

Obesity is a prevalent progressive and relapsing disease for which there are several levels of intervention, including metabolic and bariatric surgery (MBS) and now endoscopic bariatric and metabolic therapies (EBMTs). Preoperative psychological assessment focused on cognitive status, psychiatric symptoms, eating disorders, social support, and substance use is useful in optimizing patient outcomes and minimizing risks in MBS. Very little is known about the psychosocial needs of patients seeking EBMTs, though these investigations will be forthcoming if these therapies become more widespread. As MBS and EBMT inherently alter the gastrointestinal (GI) tract, considerations for the longer-term GI functioning of the patient are relevant and should be considered and monitored.

Chronic pancreatitis is a chronic digestive disorder that greatly diminishes the quality of life and is associated with significant psychological distress. A best practice recommendation in treating chronic pancreatitis is offering care in a multidisciplinary model that includes access to a behavioral health provider among other medical professionals. Behavioral interventions for patients with chronic pancreatitis have promise to improve the management of pain, comorbid psychiatric symptoms, and quality of life. If surgical interventions such as a total pancreatectomy islet autotransplant are considered, evaluating and mitigating psychosocial risk factors may aid the selection of appropriate candidates.

Patients with gastrointestinal (GI) disorders are at increased risk of sexual dysfunction (SD) due to a combination of biomedical, psychological, social, and interpersonal factors. While most patients desire information on the impact of their GI disorder on sexual function, few providers initiate this conversation. GI providers should routinely assess their patients for SD, validate these concerns, and provide brief education and a referral for evaluation and/or treatment. Treatment of sexual concerns is often multidisciplinary and may involve a sexual medicine physician, pelvic floor physical therapists, and sex therapists.

Sleep is an essential physiologic process, and unfortunately, people with gastrointestinal (GI) conditions are more likely than people in the general population to experience poor sleep quality, sleep disorders, and fatigue. Herein, we present information on common sleep disorders, fatigue, and data on these problems in various GI populations. We also discuss several treatments for sleep concerns and emerging research on the use of these treatments in GI populations. Cases that illustrate the GI/sleep relationship are presented, in addition to guidance for your own practice and cultural considerations.

Chronic gastrointestinal disorders are prevalent in youth worldwide. The chronicity of these conditions often results in their persistence into adulthood. Challenges typically faced by young people transitioning to adulthood are often exacerbated in those with chronic gastrointestinal disease. Increased awareness of these challenges among health care professionals and appropriate policies and procedures for health care transition are critical. This article summarizes research on the challenges faced by emerging adults with the gastrointestinal disease during the transition to adult care. Barriers to optimal transitional care and current guidelines are discussed and used to offer practical recommendations for health care professionals working with this population.

Patients with gastrointestinal (GI) complaints report high rates of previous psychological trauma such as physical, emotional abuse and neglect, sexual trauma, and other traumatic experiences. History of trauma is considered a risk factor for the development of disorders of gut–brain interaction, including irritable bowel syndrome. This article discusses key points for providers in understanding how various aspects of trauma can affect patients' physical and mental health and medical interactions, as well as trauma-informed strategies providers can use to increase patient comfort, improve communication, and improve effectiveness of treatment.

The prevalence of inflammatory bowel disease (IBD) is increasing substantially in non-White races and ethnicities in the United States. As a part of promoting quality of life in patients with IBD, the optimization of food-related quality of life (FRQoL) is also indicated. It is known that the practices of food avoidance and restrictive eating are associated with a reduced FRQoL in IBD. Gaining insight into sociocultural influences on FRQoL will aid in the provision of culturally competent interventions to improve FRQoL in patients with IBD.

GASTROENTEROLOGY CLINICS OF NORTH AMERICA

FORTHCOMING ISSUES

March 2023
COVID-19 and Gastroenterology
Mitchell S. Cappell, *Editor*

June 2023
Management of Obesity, Part I: Overview and Basic Mechanisms
Lee M. Kaplan, *Editor*

September 2023
Management of Obesity, Part 2: Treatment Strategies
Lee M. Kaplan, *Editor*

RECENT ISSUES

September 2022
Diagnosis and Treatment of Gastrointestinal Cancers
Marta L. Davila and Raquel E. Davila, *Editors*

June 2022
Medical and Surgical Management of Crohn's Disease
Sunanda V. Kane, *Editor*

March 2022
Pelvic Floor Disorder
Darren M. Brenner, *Editor*

SERIES OF RELATED INTEREST

Clinics in Liver Disease
(Available at: http://www.liver.theclinics.com/)
Gastrointestinal Endoscopy Clinics of North America
(Available at: http://www.www.giendo.theclinics.com/)

THE CLINICS ARE AVAILABLE ONLINE!
Access your subscription at:
www.theclinics.com

Foreword

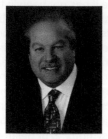

Alan L. Buchman, MD, MSPH
Consulting Editor

Many clinicians probably wonder how much of their patient's disease is psychological. It is well known that trauma and other events may manifest itself in gastrointestinal disorders. The converse is just as important; that being, how much of the psychosocial issues patients may experience is caused or triggered by their underlying disease. One might even wonder about how these issues affect the treating gastroenterologist! One might even wonder how the perception of what the patient thinks the doctor thinks of them may shape their own view of their disease and symptoms. The big question is, how do we as clinicians uncover these issues and address them appropriately?

Nowhere in medicine is there a stronger concern for the mind-body interaction than in gastroenterology. Even in individuals with no gastrointestinal issues, the thought of them evokes concern and fear. I once did a story on CNN on capsule endoscopy, and when we finished the full day of filming, I queried as to whether they'd want to do a story on intestinal failure and short bowel syndrome, which most people are completely unaware of. The response was one of disgust once the media folks found these patients had lots of diarrhea; their audience doesn't want to hear about that they told me. GI disease is a stigma. Nobody brags about their belly pain, their indigestion, their diarrhea, and even one of my kids, who was once so proud of himself as a youngster that he could pass wind on demand, found that was no longer socially acceptable and he began to abstain.

Behavioral medicine is an often overlooked and underutilized tool in the management of gastrointestinal disease; certainly, irritable bowel syndrome, but also inflammatory bowel disease, celiac disease and food intolerances, obesity management, pancreatitis (both acute and chronic), transplant, and others as described in this issue of *Gastroenterology Clinics of North America*. Many of the issues are rhetorical: how do stress and other behavioral issues cause, contribute to, or magnify gastrointestinal complaint; even cause or worsen inflammation, and how do the gastrointestinal issues themselves worsen stress, other behavioral issues, or even organic psychiatric disease? Perhaps the lack of consideration of the mind-gut axis explains some of the limits of even advanced biological therapies on remission rates in inflammatory bowel

Gastroenterol Clin N Am 51 (2022) xiii–xiv
https://doi.org/10.1016/j.gtc.2022.08.001
0889-8553/22/© 2022 Published by Elsevier Inc.

disease. Adherence and compliance also enter into the equation. These are all pieces of the psychogastroenterology puzzle.

The field of psychogastroenterology is complex. It is not well known; it even gets a red underline in Word as I type this Foreword, perhaps because it has not been in the running for "Word of the Year" in *Websters*. It is important that no space be left between psycho and gastroenterology; psychogastroenterologists are not "psycho." Dr Keefer and many of her esteemed colleagues have provided a terrific introduction to the understanding of the role of psychogastroenterology in the diagnosis, treatment, and ultimate prognosis of patients with gastrointestinal disorders as they seek to unravel a more exacting role in patient management. The future is wide open for exploration with regard to effects on medication effectiveness, pain control, inflammation, and a host of other issues; there may even be genetic predispositions and gene mutations that predispose to altered perceptions or symptoms of gastrointestinal disease. Perhaps at some point we'll need to have our psychogastroenterologist on speed dial.

Alan L. Buchman, MD, MSPH
Intestinal Rehabilitation and Transplant Center
University of Illinois at Chicago
840 South Wood Street
Suite 402 (MC958)
Chicago, IL 60612, USA

E-mail address:
Buchman@uic.edu

Preface

The Three Faces of Psychogastroenterology: Science, Practice, and the Patient

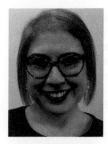

Laurie Keefer, PhD
Editor

Psychogastroenterology, the application of psychological science and practice to gastrointestinal (GI) health and illness, leverages the best practices and scientific tools from the fields of behavioral intervention science, cognitive science, neuroscience, experimental psychology, and psychophysiology. At its core is the biopsychosocial model of disease, which recognizes that the mind, body, and spirit cannot be disentangled when caring for an individual living with a chronic digestive condition. Integrated GI care has become best practice in areas such as bariatrics, irritable bowel syndrome, and inflammatory bowel disease, and gastropsychologists, usually clinical or health psychologists with a special interest and training in gastroenterology, are now embedded in gastroenterology practices around the world.

Each article in this special issue is grounded by Drs Ballou and Feingold's article relating to how the science of stress, resilience, and the gut-brain axis applies across the spectrum of digestive disorders. Drs Brjann Ljotsson and Helen Murray expand on these principles of stress and resilience and remind us of the mediators, moderators, and context of behavior change as we refine our brain-gut behavior therapies. We attempt to address the significant lack of access to experts providing gastropsychology services through Drs Ruby Greywoode and Eva Szigethy's article relating to the future of digital GI behavior therapeutics.

Two additional themes permeate this special issue. First, psychogastroenterology is patient centered. We start and end the issue with the voices of patient advocates. In the first article, patient advocate Johannah Ruddy partners with renowned stigma researcher Dr Tiffany Taft. In the final article, Tina Aswani-Omprakash partners with Neha Shah, RD to share her story and considerations around disparities, culture, and food-related quality of life.

Gastroenterol Clin N Am 51 (2022) xv–xvi
https://doi.org/10.1016/j.gtc.2022.07.010
0889-8553/22/© 2022 Published by Elsevier Inc.

The second theme reflects the diverse role of the practicing gastropsychologist. In addition to a practical article by Dr Sarah Kinsinger on how to work with a gastropsychologist with varying levels of resources, you will see articles on how a gastropsychologist might approach disorders such as Celiac disease, eosinophilic esophagitis, chronic pancreatitis, inflammatory bowel disease, celiac disease, and obesity. You will see the gastropsychology approach to common extraintestinal symptoms seen across digestive disorders, including sexual dysfunction, sleep disturbances, fatigue, and disordered eating. You will also see how gastropsychologists might work with special populations, including adolescents transitioning into adult-centered care or patients with a trauma history.

There are a few themes, however, that are *not* featured prominently. We did not cover pediatric psychogastroenterology; this could be its own special issue! Second, we did not dedicate an article to cooccurring mental health disorders, such as anxiety and depression, while present in up to 30% of individuals living with a chronic digestive disorder and a key driver of poor outcomes, these have not only been the focus of several previous articles for the past decade but their presence often distracts our gastroenterologist colleagues from recognizing the disease-interfering self-management factors that drive the majority of GI symptoms and outcomes in the other *70% of patients*. By demonstrating the range of roles and services offered by a gastropsychologist outside of traditional mental health services, we hope to underscore our contribution to value-based care and acquire buy-in for our services from our health system administrators, pharmacy benefit managers, employers, and insurance companies.

Finally, I would also encourage those of you whose interest is piqued by reading this special issue to consider joining the Rome Foundation's gastropsychology group, whose mission is to train, educate, and connect professionals from around the world interested in advancing the field of psychogastroenterology.

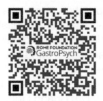

Laurie Keefer, PhD
Division of Gastroenterology
Icahn School of Medicine at Mount Sinai
17 East 102nd Street, #1134
New York, NY 10029, USA

E-mail address:
Laurie.keefer@mssm.edu

The Pervasive Impact of the Stigmatization of Gastrointestinal Diseases—A Patient's Perspective

Johannah Ruddy, MEd[a],*, Tiffany Taft, PsyD, MIS[b]

KEYWORDS

• Stigmatization • Discrimination • Stereotypes • Patient outcomes

KEY POINTS

• Stigma is a highly impactful psychological and social condition that affects the quality of life of patients with gastrointestinal (GI) illnesses.
• Stigma can be experienced in different ways by patients and lead to worsening health outcomes.
• Stigma is highly prevalent in a variety of chronic illnesses but especially in GI illnesses.
• This leads to a further decline in quality of life for patients with these conditions.

INTRODUCTION

Stigma, defined as social devaluation and discrimination, involves identifying and labeling a person with a socially undesirable trait and subjecting them to corresponding punitive behaviors. Stigma is a very common issue in health care that undermines the quality of care for patients with chronic health conditions, including patients with gastrointestinal (GI) issues. The word "stigma" or "stigmata" is thousands of years old, dating back to ancient Greece, and persists due to the need for humans to have group cohesiveness that is necessary for survival.

The origins of stigma in health care can be traced to a prevailing Western medicine paradigm of "mind-body dualism," first popularized by Rene Descartes in the seventeenth century[1] as a way to position the mind and body as separate entities to allow for surgical dissection and an increased understanding of human anatomy. This practical dichotomization of mind and body lingered and ultimately led to a belief that if symptoms were to be valid, there had to be an observable phenomenon and physical

a Campbell University, School of Pharmacy and Health Sciences, The Rome Foundation, 14460 Falls of Neuse Road #149-116, Raleigh, NC 27614, USA; b Division of Gastroenterology and Hepatology, Northwestern University Feinberg School of Medicine, 676 North Saint Clair Street, Suite 1400, Chicago, IL 60611, USA
* Corresponding author.
E-mail address: jruddy@theromefoundation.org

Gastroenterol Clin N Am 51 (2022) 681–695
https://doi.org/10.1016/j.gtc.2022.06.010
0889-8553/22/© 2022 Elsevier Inc. All rights reserved.

evidence; otherwise, symptoms were presumed to be "mind," or in modern terms, psychological. To date, any illness lacking structural evidence, including irritable bowel syndrome (IBS) and other disorders of gut–brain interaction (DGBI), are prone to stigma.[2] Stigma toward DGBIs pervades patient care, policy development, research investment, and clinician interest in treating these patients.[3] However, as we describe in later discussion, most GI illness is stigmatized.

Modern social stigma theory started in the 1960s when Erving Goffman described stigma as a "spoiled identity."[4] Early research focused on mental illnesses,[5,6] followed by HIV/AIDS,[7] and obesity[7,8] as highly stigmatized conditions. The first studies into the stigmatization of GI diseases were published in 1991 by Drossman and colleagues in patients with inflammatory bowel disease (IBD).[9] Since then, GI stigma research expanded to IBS,[10,11] gastroparesis (GP),[12] and eosinophilic gastrointestinal disorders (EGIDs).[13,14] Logically, stigmatization of people with GI disease reduces the quality of care and is associated with poor outcomes across medical, psychological, and quality of life domains.[15,16] It benefits those involved in treating these patients to understand how stigma may manifest in their patients.

In this article, we will describe the types of stigma experienced by patients living with GI illnesses, including IBS, IBD, and the impact it can have on clinical outcomes as well as on the overall quality of life of patients. We will also attempt to provide simple solutions to reduce this stigma beginning with the providers and extending to patients.

Stigma Types and Illness Traits

Stigma includes 3 highly interrelated yet unique constructs (**Fig. 1**): (1) Enacted stigma or the behaviors of others toward the stigmatized person including discrimination and social avoidance, (2) Perceived (felt) stigma, when the stigmatized person is aware enacted stigma may be occurring, and (3) Internalized stigma, seen as the most damaging for the patient, is when the stigmatized person accepts discriminatory beliefs as true and applicable to themselves. Within the internalized stigma construct is a person's resistance to stereotypes, serving as a protective factor.[17]

Jones and colleagues (1984) identified 6 key traits that make an illness more likely to be stigmatized (**Fig. 2**). All of these can be applied to GI diseases: they are generally concealable, can be highly disruptive to a person's life, and, by proxy their friends' and families' lives, are relapsing and remitting, and aesthetically unpleasing. The notion GI diseases can be controlled via diet and stress management adds to others perceiving a person's symptoms are caused by their behavior.[18]

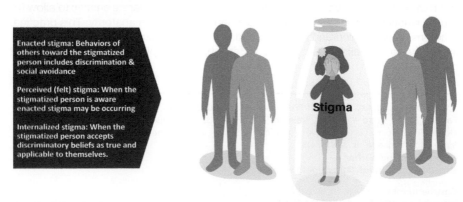

Fig. 1. Stigma types defined.

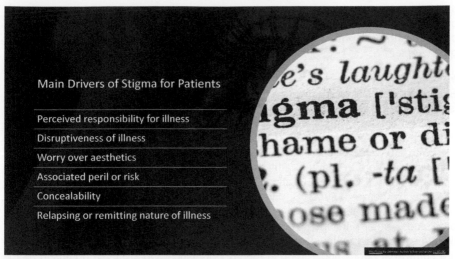

Main Drivers of Stigma for Patients

Perceived responsibility for illness

Disruptiveness of illness

Worry over aesthetics

Associated peril or risk

Concealability

Relapsing or remitting nature of illness

Fig. 2. The associated drivers of stigma in patients with chronic illness, including GI illnesses.

Most literature on GI illness focuses on perceived and internalized stigma, and how these influence health-care utilization, psychological distress (eg, depression, anxiety, self-esteem), and quality of life. Studies on enacted stigma include both the general population and medical professional cohorts.

Enacted Stigma Toward gastrointestinal Illnesses

Irritable bowel syndrome and other disorders of gut–brain interaction

Research on enacted stigma centers around the taboo nature of digestive function. In most cultures, discussing vomiting or diarrhea is generally considered off-limits. The children's book "Everybody Poops" demonstrates quite aptly how socially constructed attitudes around defecation and its association to public shame is introduced early in life. Unfortunately, although it is true everybody poops, discussing bowel movements and the passing of gas is highly embarrassing for many people, making the presence of a chronic GI condition particularly harrowing.

Enacted stigma, or the discriminatory and avoidance behaviors of others toward the stigmatized person, is prevalent in almost all functional somatic conditions, including IBS, noncardiac chest pain, chronic pelvic pain, fibromyalgia, and chronic migraine.[15] Recent studies suggest approximately 40% of patients with IBS or other "functional" disorders, now called DGBI, make up a typical gastroenterology patient cohort. Patients presenting with DGBIs can prove especially challenging because these conditions are frequently characterized by physical symptoms, sometimes quite severe but are unexplained by medical pathology. The medical ambiguity around their origin has caused a ripple effect on the public who may also view DGBIs as less valid, less in need of consistent medical care, and even psychological in origin.[19]

Recent advances in understanding clear pathophysiology for DGBIs via the brain–gut explanatory model move us closer to understanding how and why these conditions exist. However, many providers continue to adhere to the biomedical model of care despite growing support for a biopsychosocial, integrated care model in digestive disease.[20,21] In the absence of specific, identifiable pathologic condition, health-care providers may resolve themselves to the idea that there is no treatable illness present and therefore nothing can be done medically. Unfortunately, this leaves the patient without a diagnosis or treatment plan and with feelings of hopelessness, convinced something "organic" as the root cause was missed, thereby driving health care-seeking behaviors, increasing anxiety and depression, and impairment in their quality of life.[22,23]

Inflammatory bowel disease

Stigma toward IBD often occurs across interpersonal relationships but is potentially less than seen in IBS, especially from medical providers.[24,25] In a 2016 study comparing people's attitudes toward patients with IBD, IBS, or adult-onset asthma as a nonstigmatized comparator group, participants viewed those with IBS poorest. Specifically, men with IBS were most stigmatized, whereas IBD patients were significantly less stigmatized and more in line with attitudes toward adult-onset asthma.[26] However, this does not imply IBD is without stigma. A 2017 study on attitudes toward 7 diseases (IBD, genital herpes, HIV/AIDS, cancer, alcoholism, obesity, diabetes) found participants held substantial social stigma toward IBD, second only to genital herpes. In both studies, male participants held more stigmatizing attitudes toward IBD, and all participants had generally low levels of familiarity with IBD. Even today, both IBS and IBD are somewhat poorly understood in the lay population and are even confused as the same condition in medical news reporting (eg, irritable bowel disease).

Studies on disclosing IBD status to others also identify enacted stigma.[25] People living with concealable illnesses may opt to try to pass as healthy or cover the severity of the disease by downplaying symptoms. The nature of IBD treatments (eg, infusions, pills taken multiple times a day) risks accidental outing of the illness. Disclosure may be especially precarious in the workplace, with 24% of patients in one study being denied promotion due to their IBD. Alternatively, disclosing IBD status at work may relieve stress from trying to pass or cover up their disease with 77% of patients in a separate study reporting a generally helpful response from their employer.[27] Students report negative reactions from educators, with 8% of college-aged IBD patients reporting "hostility" regarding their disease.[28] These wide differences underscore the variability in response IBD patients face when opting to disclose their disease to others.

Gastroparesis

In the only study of stigma toward GP, the majority limited disclosing their illness at work for fear of repercussions. Three out of 23 interviewees (13%) reported losing a job or promotion due to the number of sick days taken.[12] More research is critically needed to understand stigmatization toward GP and those living with it.[12]

Patient Perceptions of Stigma

Across GI diseases, patients can perceive stigma from family, friends, colleagues, and medical providers. Perception of stigma is influenced by a patient's past interactions, trauma experience (medical and nonmedical), and individual rules about themselves, other people, and the world.[29] Perceiving others hold extremely negative views toward you because of an illness can be detrimental to any patient (**Fig. 3**). Chronic illness creates vulnerability, and when an illness is met with disparaging comments or dismissiveness, stigma perceptions can become internalized and part of the person's identity. Isolation occurs by intentionally avoiding interaction with others, even with family and close friends because of a belief they are seen as a burden or as not truly ill.

Outside of IBS and IBD, very little perceived stigma research exists with 2 studies on EGIDs, 2 on functional dyspepsia (FD), and 1 on GP.[12,30,31]

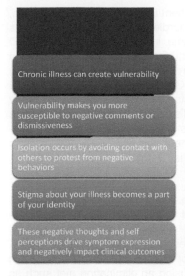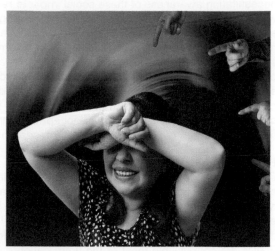

Fig. 3. Cycle of stigma impact in chronic illness.

Irritable bowel syndrome and functional dyspepsia

Similar to enacted stigma, IBS patients perceive the most stigma. In a 2009 qualitative study, 57% of 49 patients reported feeling IBS-related social stigma.[18] In this study, patients reported as feeling that their IBS was not taken seriously, that their providers implied that their symptoms are self-inflicted, and that IBS was "all in their head." In a larger survey comparing IBD and IBS patient perceptions of stigma, 27% of IBS patients reported moderate-to-high levels of stigma compared with 8% of patients with IBD.[32] Furthermore, IBS patients were significantly more likely to report stigma from health-care professionals with a large effect size (d = .90). Conversely, a greater proportion of IBD patients (44%) reported mild levels of social stigma compared with IBS (38%).

Most patients with FD (89% of 138) also perceive stigma about their illness.[30,31] Men and patients with lower educational levels were more likely to report more stigma. Interestingly, the use of antidepressants as neuromodulators to treat FD increased perceived stigma in 75% of patients; this occurred regardless of the type of antidepressant prescribed. The more stigma a person perceived, the less likely they were to adhere to neuromodulator treatment and reported more FD symptoms after 8 weeks.[2] Provider education is critical to the rationale for neuromodulators use (see later discussion for recommendations), in part to dispel the stigma attached their use for GI conditions, and for assurance, the recommendation is based on the science of dysregulation of gut–brain axis communication and not symptoms are due to a psychological condition.[23]

Inflammatory bowel disease

The perception of stigma is also prevalent in IBD. A 2016 review of 26 studies found that up to 84% of patients reported some perceived stigma.[25] Patients with IBD may feel different from others, feel shame, think that they are labeled as "difficult" or "needy" as a patient in the context of pain management, and feel a level of dismissiveness toward extraintestinal symptoms such as fatigue. Unfortunately, stigma perceptions do not tend to improve when an IBD patient achieves disease remission, necessitating awareness of these social impacts regardless of how well treatment is working. Further, the presence of perceived stigma increases worry about IBD symptoms[33] and makes IBD seem more intrusive and increases depression. Stigma may be especially salient in IBD patients with ostomy[34] and having an understanding support system can mitigate stigma and its impacts. Greater resilience, or the ability to bounce back from adversity, can reduce the effects of perceived stigma and may serve as a potential intervention point.[35] However, discussing resilience with patients requires a supportive approach to avoid additional stigma regarding a person's psychological fortitude or their ability to accept their illness and find productive ways to handle the impact of it in their life. Further research is needed.

Eosinophilic gastrointestinal diseases

One study exists on perceived stigma in EGIDs. In 209 patients (78% eosinophilic esophagitis), female patients perceived more social stigma than male patients from health-care providers and their significant others.[14] Patients with non-eosinophilic esophagitis (EoE) (EGIDs) also experienced higher levels of stigma from their health-care providers. Dietary therapy was also a factor for EGID-related stigma. Although EGIDs are concealable most of the time, patients using an elimination diet such as the 6-food elimination diet for EoE will garner questions in social situations and potential frustration among friends and family who find navigating these diets difficult (ie, high degree of peril).[13]

Gastroparesis

The only study on stigma in GP found that 100% of 23 patients interviewed reported feeling stigma related to their condition.[12] GP patients thought health-care professionals dismissed the severity of symptoms and GP's impact on daily functioning, lacked knowledge about weight gain in GP, and held racial stereotypes toward African Americans about topics such as nutrition and diet. Similar to IBS, those with GP reported feeling others believed symptoms were "all in their head" or due to a psychiatric disorder (eg, eating disorder, anxiety). Patients who reported unsolicited advice about diet or eating behaviors felt stigmatized as well, implying the person was naïve or simply not trying hard enough to get better. These findings are quite striking, considering GP has a distinct biomarker, in slow gastric emptying, so the high level of perceived stigma suggests better education about GP is needed. Additionally, recognizing stigma is prevalent in diseases that are interpreted as "controllable" by behavior or other life choices, such as HIV and obesity, and other GI illness.

Internalization and Resistance of Disease Stigma

By far, internalized stigma is associated with the poorest patient outcomes. Internalized stigma includes thoughts of alienation, social withdrawal, stereotype endorsement, and discrimination experiences. Conversely, stigma resistance is the rejection of enacted stigma and is associated with better outcomes.[36] In a study by Taft, and colleagues in 2014, patients who met Rome III criteria for IBS who reported greater internalized stigma had higher levels of anxiety and depression, more negative impacts on quality of life, a reduced sense of health competence, and an increase in health-care utilization.[16] In fact, internalized stigma contributed almost twice the variance for increases in anxiety, depression, and poorer quality of life outcomes than perceived stigma in patients with IBS. Alienation and social withdrawal tend to be more common in IBS than endorsing stereotypes about their disease.[16]

Similar trends exist in IBD, with most internalized stigma related to social withdrawal (41%) and alienation (48%). Importantly, 88% of patients reported moderate to high stigma resistance behaviors.[37] Unlike stigma perception, rates of stigma internalization decreased and stigma resistance increased with disease remission. The experience of non-White patients may differ. In a 2022 study of 90 underrepresented minority (URM) IBD patients, 27% reported high levels of internalized stigma, which is considerably higher than non-URM groups. Alienation (54%) and social withdrawal (39%) remained the most common. However, only 19% of URM patients reported stigma resistance.[38]

Patients with EGIDs also report some internalized stigma, with female patients reporting more alienation, social withdrawal, and discrimination than male patients.[13] Similar to stigma perception, using elimination diets increased internalized stigma in patients.[13] The only EGID study on this topic did not report any rates of stigma resistance.

Stigma and Treatment Adherence

Many studies on stigma in GI illness evaluate its complex relationship to treatment adherence. For example, certain medications may increase internalized stigma. In FD, patients reported minimal-to-mild internalized stigma before initiating antidepressant (ie, neuromodulator) treatment. More than half (68%) reported increases in internalized stigma after 8-weeks of treatment with 24 participants reporting moderate-to-severe internalized stigma not seen at baseline in any patients.[31] Almost all stated they did not want to tell others about their antidepressant use and 53% felt shame regarding this treatment. Over time, these proportions did decrease some but more than 80% still did not want others outside their family to know. While neuromodulators are part of the treatment guidelines for many GI conditions, these come with both perceived and internalized stigma that must be addressed during treatment planning to mitigate these outcomes.[31]

Many participants in the GP stigma study reported very little internalized stigma and more stigma resistance. Some found meaning or positive benefits from their diagnosis including being more in tune with their bodies and no longer taking things for granted in life.[12] In a study published in 2019 by Krok, and colleagues, 317 patients with GI undergoing cancer treatments were evaluated on illness perception, affective symptoms, meaning in life, and coping. The more patients with cancer perceived their illness negatively affecting their lives, the more likely they were to use such passive coping strategies such as helplessness, hopelessness, or fatalism.[39] Conversely, finding meaning was critical to reducing depression, hopelessness, and physical symptoms of distress. Thus, a patient's beliefs and goals play a critical role in their illness experience, including any stigmatization. Health-care providers can reduce the impacts of stigma by encouraging patients to focus equally on efforts to reduce the physical and psychological effects of the GI illness, and seeking meaning in their experiences which may, in turn, improve resilience and coping.[39]

Stigma's impact on patient outcomes

It should be no surprise that all stigma types are associated with poorer outcomes: symptoms are more severe, treatment adherence is reduced, health-care utilization is increased, anxiety and depression increase, self-esteem and self-efficacy decline, and HRQoL domains suffer.[2,16,26] Most of these relationships are modest and consistent across the GI disease groups. Regression models also find perceived and internalized stigma to be significant predictors of these outcomes, with internalized stigma typically more predictive of poor outcomes. When stigma heightens, a person's sense of internalized shame motivation to maintain their health can decline. Additionally, concerns about accidental disclosure of a concealed illness are associated with medication regimens not being followed.[16,37] Therefore, it is impossible to conceptualize psychosocial impacts on GI illness outcomes without considering stigma, whether clinically or in research settings.

Mitigating the Impacts of Stigma Toward Gastrointestinal Disease Through Education

Multiple studies exist to evaluate what methods work best in reducing stigmatizing beliefs and behaviors but show mixed results in their effectiveness. A lack of knowledge or familiarity with a disease will drive stigma. Unfortunately, despite efforts to create educational campaigns to increase awareness and disease state educational programming in GI and other chronic health conditions, these programs often yield less than remarkable results on their own.[40,41]

One important approach to reduce stigma in GI illness is targeting stigmatizing beliefs early in medical training.[42] Implicit bias includes subconscious attitudes or stereotypes that affect our understanding, actions, or decisions about a person or class, and can be pervasive. Multiple implicit bias studies exist for medical training as it relates to mental illness,[43] addiction,[44] and obesity[45]; none exist for GI disease. However, in a recent study by Luo and colleagues, interesting data showed that as early as GI fellowship, negative perceptions exist regarding caring for patients with DGBI, including IBS. In fact, 21.4% felt frustrated or burned out when seeing patients with DGBI and 15.9% reported that their attendings demonstrated a dismissive attitude toward patients with DGBI.[46]

Some studies find implicit bias decreases when a person is exposed to examples counter to held stereotypes.[47] Countering stereotypes associated with GI illness in medical education could normalize perceptions and reduce both implicit bias and external stigma. Further, people learn by modeling social behaviors of respected others. Recognizing and reducing stigmatizing language and behaviors used by medical school educators leverages social learning theory for stigma reduction.[41] Research is needed in GI education to gauge trainee perceptions of patients with GI illnesses and their care and generate solutions to reduce any stigmatizing beliefs.

The Roles of the Patient and Provider in Reducing Stigma

Patients with chronic GI illnesses come to appointments feeling a myriad of emotions stemming from their illness perceptions and perceived stigma, including from the health-care system and past interactions. Some patients feel stigma from the lack of a diagnosis and worry they will never find the answers they seek, and others may think past providers dismissed their symptoms and implied a psychological cause for their illness. Whatever the case, it is up to the clinician to understand and adequately address these feelings for patients to feel validated, understood, and agree to treatment.[48]

An excellent means of provider–patient communication to reduce stigma is the narrative approach to history taking which identifies key points in the patient's story useful in making a diagnosis. Patients are encouraged to tell their illness story in their own words so the events can naturally unfold. Discussion is guided by using open-ended questions to obtain additional information, and positive reinforcements such as head nodding, eye contact, and proximity encourage the patient to continue sharing. Medical and social histories are gathered at the same time and, when done well, a narrative approach to history taking does not take any longer than a typical clinical history. Added benefits include insight into the patient's emotional intelligence, stigma experiences, health perceptions, and resilience. Additionally, the narrative history can inform the physician about the patient's beliefs about behavioral health, any history of trauma, and even substance abuse. The biological, psychological, and social influences of the illness emerge to guide shared decision-making for possible diagnostic testing, a diagnosis, and treatment recommendations.[40]

Another way health-care providers can reduce stigma is by providing a clear, positive diagnosis, which allows patients to feel confident in treatment recommendations and reduce internal stigma. In a study examining the diagnosis of patients with a "functional" illness versus an "organic" illness, gastroenterologists used more qualified or uncertain language when diagnosing patients with DGBI than patients with organic diseases.[49] This can contribute to patients discarding the diagnosis and requesting additional, unwarranted investigations and drive stigma.

Health-care providers should use the Rome IV diagnostic criteria for DGBIs to provide a diagnosis after ruling out any alarm features or red flags. Validation studies comparing the Rome IV IBS criteria to Rome III fine Rome IV criteria have a positive likelihood ratio of 4.82 compared with 2.45 for Rome III, although the clinical relevance of this is uncertain.[50] A positive diagnosis of IBS, or other DGBI, can be made confidently by a health-care provider who can then clearly communicate and educate a patient about the diagnosis.

Once any GI illness diagnosis is given in a clear, positive manner, the health-care provider can further reduce illness stigma by validating patient concerns about the diagnosis and involving them in the decision-making process regarding treatment.[51] Patients will use their education about the illness and treatment rationale to educate their friends and family members, reducing both the external and perceived stigma that they previously felt.[52] For patients with low health literacy skills, providers should seek to dispel any myths or misconceptions that might exist related to an illness. Disease state education can be provided through dialog with any member of the medical care team. Handouts and other educational resources should begin by defining key terms and concepts that reiterate previously reviewed information.[23,53–55]

Language is key in reducing the stigma associated with recommendations of neuromodulators (ie, antidepressants, mood stabilizers) for DGBIs and chronic abdominal pain syndrome, including in IBD. It is critical to provide rationale via education on the pathophysiology of the brain–gut axis and the gate control theory of pain to justify the use of this class of drugs. Explaining how the brain and the gut are hardwired through the spinal cord with the brain's ability to downregulate/block, or gate, the pain signals it receives from the body, including the gut, fosters agreement to use neuromodulators while reducing feelings of stigma or shame. These concepts can also be applied to meditation, gut-directed hypnotherapy, or cognitive–behavioral therapy (CBT) as part of the treatment planning process.[2,23]

Health-care providers should acknowledge that neuromodulators are used to treat psychological disorders, with clarification they are also used to treat chronic pain and altered bowel habits when used at lower doses. Emphasizing the direct connection of the gut to the brain will help patients better understand treatments are not being recommended due to a suspected psychological illness but because of the current science pointing to the dysregulation in the communication between the gut and the brain.[23]

For brain–gut behavioral therapies, similar education when making a recommendation should provide a clear explanation of the types of behavioral therapies found to benefit patients with GI illnesses. These therapies include CBT, mindfulness-based approaches, and gut-directed hypnotherapy. Studies continue to show efficacy rates at or above pharmacologic treatments for both abdominal and pelvic pain, as well as altered bowel habits, in many patients.[56] Evidence-based behavioral therapies[57] exist to address mental health concerns, such as symptom-specific anxiety or hypervigilance to gut sensations, across all digestive disease states. They generally do not

Table 1
Ways providers can help reduce the stigma felt by patients with gastrointestinal illnesses during a clinical visit

Seek to improve patient satisfaction and engagement to reduce feelings of stigma	Patient satisfaction will help to lower stigma because it relates to their perception of the doctor's humaneness, technical competence, interest in psychosocial factors, and provision of relevant medical information. Engagement relies on nonverbal communication: good eye contact, affirmative nods, gentle tone of voice
Obtain the history through a nondirective, nonjudgmental, patient-centered interview. Consider the use of facilitated narrative history taking	This involves active listening, as well as asking questions based on the patient's thoughts, feelings, and experiences rather than using a personal or preset agenda of items. The interview can begin with: "*It's very nice to meet you, how can I help?*" This sets the stage for the patient to know you are interested and available
Determine the immediate reason for the patient's visit without preconceived ideas for their visit	The doctor can ask: "*What led you to see me at this time?*" and evaluate the patient's verbal and nonverbal responses. Consider the following possibilities: new or exacerbating factors (dietary change, concurrent medical disorder, side effects of new medication), personal or family stressors leading to worsening or development of depression, anxiety around symptoms, and impairment in daily function
Conduct a careful physical examination and cost-efficient investigation	A well-conducted physical examination has therapeutic value
Determine what the patient understands about the illness and what their concerns are	Questions to ask include: "*What do you think is causing your symptoms?*" and "*What concerns or worries do you have about your condition?*" The responses help the doctor understand the patient's inner thoughts and feelings
Elicit the patient's understanding of their symptoms and then provide a thorough explanation of the disorder that considers their views	For example, the doctor may say, "*I understand you believe you had an infection that had not been diagnosed. The infection is now gone. However, your nerves were affected by it, so that you feel as though the infection is still there, just like a 'phantom limb.'*"
When possible, provide a link between stressors and symptoms that are consistent with the patient's understanding	Many patients are unable or unwilling to associate stressors with illness but most will understand that the illness causes distress and can affect their emotional state. For example, the doctor may say: "*I understand you don't see stress as causing your pain, but you've mentioned how severe and disabling your pain is. How much do you think that is causing your emotional distress and symptoms?*"

(continued on next page)

Table 1 (continued)	
Provide explanations to help patients understand the recommendations	If the patient is reluctant to take a neuromodulator due to the stigma of the drug, believing it is for stress or psychiatric diagnosis, the doctor can say: *"Yes, we use antidepressants for depression, but medications can have more than one effect. Aspirin can treat pain and can also treat a heart attack. In this case, the medication can also turn down the pain by blocking pain pathways through the brain-gut axis, and this benefit happens with doses lower than those used for depression."*
Involve the patient in the treatment	The doctor should allow the patient to make choices and participate in care to feel less stigmatized and more empowered. For example: *"Let me suggest some treatments for you to consider. Medication 'A' has 'B' benefits and 'C' side effects. Medication 'B' has 'D' benefits and 'E' side effects. Let's discuss the pros and cons of each so you can make a decision."*
End the visit but not the care	Closing the visit should only occur after the doctor asks, *"Have I answered all your questions?"* This allows the patient to reflect and bring up any final items; if the visit was properly done, there might not be any. Patients do not want to be abandoned in their care. The best way for the doctor to reinforce their commitment is to say: *"Remember that regardless of how things go, we will continue to work on this together."*

Adapted from Drossman DA, Ruddy J. Gut Feelings: Disorders of Gut-Brain Interaction (DGBI) and the Patient-Doctor Relationship. Chapel Hill NC: DrossmanCare; 2021; with permission

have side effects but have the potential to empower patients to reduce avoidance behaviors and counterproductive thinking patterns. It is important to communicate that the behavioral treatment may address pain management needs and may also help with associated illness-related anxiety or depression, stigma, shame, and feelings of helplessness and hopelessness. Patients may initially resist seeing a therapist due to mental illness stigma, and they may think that they are not depressed or sense insinuation that their symptoms are due to a psychological condition.[40] Providing reassurance and education on the role of behavioral health treatments early in disease management can help to alleviate these fears and create buy-in for the treatment plan.[58]

The following is a table of statements and tips to help guide health-care providers in an attempt to reduce the stigma experienced by patients with gastrointestinal illnesses (**Table 1**).

SUMMARY

Stigma in GI illnesses is prevalent with a profound impact on patients. Health-care providers can play an integral role in either perpetuating or reducing this stigma, and in turn, influence clinical outcomes for patients with IBS and other GI illnesses. Being intentional in their communication about the illness, providing a clear, positive diagnosis, and education on the pathophysiology of the condition can all reduce stigma. In addition, the stigma associated with certain therapies can be reduced by providing a clear rationale for use and benefits for symptom improvement over time. This will not just reduce stigma for patients but also help in the reduction of stigma in the health-care system and society because it relates to GI illnesses.

CLINICS CARE POINTS

- Patients with gastrointestinal (GI) illness can experience stigma in a variety of ways but health-care providers can help to reduce this stigma by providing empathy and not dismissing symptoms not fully explained by (or out of proportion to) diagnostic testing.

- As championed by the American College of Gastroenterology and the Rome Foundation, patients with irritable bowel syndrome and other disorders of gut–brain interaction need a clear, confident diagnosis, after limited diagnostic testing and a physical examination. This will help legitimize the diagnosis and lead to earlier intervention, better uptake of recommended therapies and better clinical outcomes.

- Patients with GI illnesses need to be provided with clear education on their condition and the significance of the brain–gut-microbiome axis in digestive health. In addition, they need a clear rationale for the use of neuromodulators as well as behavioral health treatments. This will reduce the stigma of the proposed treatments and help improve clinical outcomes.

DISCLOSURE

T. Taft has served as a consultant for Takeda, Reckitt, and Healthline. J. Ruddy currently serves as a consultant for Mahana Therapeutics and Biomerica Inc,.

REFERENCES

1. Duncan G. Mind-body dualism and the biopsychosocial model of pain: what did Descartes really say? J Med Philos 2000;25(4):485–513.
2. Feingold JH, Drossman DA. Deconstructing stigma as a barrier to treating DGBI: Lessons for clinicians. Neurogastroenterol Motil 2021;33(2):e14080.
3. Mearin F, Sans M, Balboa A. Relevance and needs of irritable bowel syndrome (IBS): Comparison with inflammatory bowel disease (IBD). (Please, if you are not interested in IBS, read it.). Gastroenterol Hepatol 2022. https://doi.org/10.1016/j.gastrohep.2021.12.008.
4. Bates L, Stickley T. Confronting Goffman: how can mental health nurses effectively challenge stigma? A critical review of the literature. J Psychiatr Ment Health Nurs 2013;20(7):569–75.
5. Dobener LM, Fahrer J, Purtscheller D, et al. How Do Children of Parents With Mental Illness Experience Stigma? A Systematic Mixed Studies Review. Front Psychiatry 2022;13:813519.
6. O'Connor C, Brassil M, O'Sullivan S, et al. How does diagnostic labelling affect social responses to people with mental illness? A systematic review of experimental studies using vignette-based designs. J Ment Health 2022;31(1):115–30.
7. Armoon B, Fleury MJ, Bayat AH, et al. HIV related stigma associated with social support, alcohol use disorders, depression, anxiety, and suicidal ideation among

people living with HIV: a systematic review and meta-analysis. Int J Ment Health Syst 2022;16(1):17.

8. Fruh SM, Graves RJ, Hauff C, et al. Weight Bias and Stigma: Impact on Health. Nurs Clin North Am 2021;56(4):479–93.

9. Drossman DA, Leserman J, Li ZM, et al. The rating form of IBD patient concerns: a new measure of health status. Psychosom Med 1991;53(6):701–12.

10. Hearn M, Whorwell PJ, Vasant DH. Stigma and irritable bowel syndrome: a taboo subject? Lancet Gastroenterol Hepatol 2020;5(6):607–15.

11. Drossman DA, Chang L, Schneck S, et al. A focus group assessment of patient perspectives on irritable bowel syndrome and illness severity. Dig Dis Sci 2009; 54(7):1532–41.

12. Taft TH, Craven MR, Adler EP, et al. Stigma experiences of patients living with gastroparesis. Neurogastroenterol Motil 2022;34(4):e14223.

13. Guadagnoli L, Taft TH. Internalized Stigma in Patients with Eosinophilic Gastrointestinal Disorders. J Clin Psychol Med Settings 2020;27(1):1–10.

14. Guadagnoli L, Taft TH, Keefer L. Stigma perceptions in patients with eosinophilic gastrointestinal disorders. Dis Esophagus 2017;30(7):1–8.

15. Ko C, Lucassen P, van der Linden B, et al. Stigma perceived by patients with functional somatic syndromes and its effect on health outcomes - A systematic review. J Psychosom Res 2022;154:110715.

16. Taft TH, Riehl ME, Dowjotas KL, et al. Moving beyond perceptions: internalized stigma in the irritable bowel syndrome. Neurogastroenterol Motil 2014;26(7): 1026–35.

17. Ahmedani BK. Mental Health Stigma: Society, Individuals, and the Profession. J Soc Work Values Ethics 2011;8(2):41–416.

18. Jones MP, Keefer L, Bratten J, et al. Development and initial validation of a measure of perceived stigma in irritable bowel syndrome. Psychol Health Med 2009; 14(3):367–74.

19. Black CJ, Drossman DA, Talley NJ, et al. Functional gastrointestinal disorders: advances in understanding and management. Lancet 2020;396(10263): 1664–74.

20. Chey WD, Keefer L, Whelan K, et al. Behavioral and Diet Therapies in Integrated Care for Patients With Irritable Bowel Syndrome. Gastroenterology 2021;160(1): 47–62.

21. Lores T, Goess C, Mikocka-Walus A, et al. Integrated Psychological Care is Needed, Welcomed and Effective in Ambulatory Inflammatory Bowel Disease Management: Evaluation of a New Initiative. J Crohns Colitis 2019;13(7):819–27.

22. Looper KJ, Kirmayer LJ. Perceived stigma in functional somatic syndromes and comparable medical conditions. J Psychosom Res 2004;57(4):373–8.

23. Ruddy J. Review article: the patients' experience with irritable bowel syndrome and their search for education and support. Aliment Pharmacol Ther 2021;(54 Suppl 1):S44–52.

24. Fourie S, Jackson D, Aveyard H. Living with Inflammatory Bowel Disease: A review of qualitative research studies. Int J Nurs Stud 2018;87:149–56.

25. Taft TH, Keefer L. A systematic review of disease-related stigmatization in patients living with inflammatory bowel disease. Clin Exp Gastroenterol 2016;9: 49–58.

26. Taft TH, Bedell A, Naftaly J, et al. Stigmatization toward irritable bowel syndrome and inflammatory bowel disease in an online cohort. Neurogastroenterol Motil 2017;29(2). https://doi.org/10.1111/nmo.12921.

27. Mayberry MK, Probert C, Srivastava E, et al. Perceived discrimination in education and employment by people with Crohn's disease: a case control study of educational achievement and employment. Gut 1992;33(3):312–4.
28. Mayberry JF. Impact of inflammatory bowel disease on educational achievements and work prospects. J Pediatr Gastroenterol Nutr 1999;28(4):S34–6.
29. Jackson-Best F, Edwards N. Stigma and intersectionality: a systematic review of systematic reviews across HIV/AIDS, mental illness, and physical disability. BMC Public Health 2018;18(1):919.
30. Yan XJ, Qiu HY, Luo QQ, et al. Improving Clinician-Patient Communication Alleviates Stigma in Patients With Functional Dyspepsia Receiving Antidepressant Treatment. J Neurogastroenterol Motil 2022;28(1):95–103.
31. Yan XJ, Luo QQ, Qiu HY, et al. The impact of stigma on medication adherence in patients with functional dyspepsia. Neurogastroenterol Motil 2021;33(2):e13956.
32. Taft TH, Keefer L, Artz C, et al. Perceptions of illness stigma in patients with inflammatory bowel disease and irritable bowel syndrome. Qual Life Res 2011; 20(9):1391–9.
33. Roberts CM, Baudino MN, Gamwell KL, et al. Illness Stigma, Worry, Intrusiveness, and Depressive Symptoms in Youth With Inflammatory Bowel Disease. J Pediatr Gastroenterol Nutr 2021;72(3):404–9.
34. Wang Y, Li S, Gong J, et al. Perceived Stigma and Self-Efficacy of Patients With Inflammatory Bowel Disease-Related Stoma in China: A Cross-Sectional Study. Front Med (Lausanne) 2022;9:813367.
35. Luo D, Zhou M, Sun L, et al. Resilience as a Mediator of the Association Between Perceived Stigma and Quality of Life Among People With Inflammatory Bowel Disease. Front Psychiatry 2021;12:709295.
36. Yu BCL, Chio FHN, Mak WWS, et al. Internalization process of stigma of people with mental illness across cultures: A meta-analytic structural equation modeling approach. Clin Psychol Rev 2021;87:102029.
37. Taft TH, Ballou S, Keefer L. A preliminary evaluation of internalized stigma and stigma resistance in inflammatory bowel disease. J Health Psychol 2013;18(4): 451–60.
38. Veracruz N, Taft T. Stigma perceptions in non-white IBD patients and relationships with patient outcomes. Gastroenterology 2022;162(3):97–9.
39. Krok D, Telka E, Zarzycka B. Illness perception and affective symptoms in gastrointestinal cancer patients: A moderated mediation analysis of meaning in life and coping. Psychooncology 2019;28(8):1728–34.
40. Drossman DA, Chang L, Deutsch JK, et al. A Review of the Evidence and Recommendations on Communication Skills and the Patient-Provider Relationship: A Rome Foundation Working Team Report. Gastroenterology 2021;161(5): 1670–88.e7.
41. Sabin J, Guenther G, Ornelas IJ, et al. Brief online implicit bias education increases bias awareness among clinical teaching faculty. Med Educ Online 2022;27(1):2025307.
42. Drossman DA, Ruddy J. Improving Patient-Provider Relationships to Improve Health Care. Clin Gastroenterol Hepatol 2020;18(7):1417–26.
43. Sandhu HS, Arora A, Brasch J, et al. Mental Health Stigma: Explicit and Implicit Attitudes of Canadian Undergraduate Students, Medical School Students, and Psychiatrists. Can J Psychiatry 2019;64(3):209–17.
44. Cernasev A, Frederick KD, Hall EA, et al. "Don't Label Them as Addicts!" Student Pharmacists' Views on the Stigma Associated with Opioid use Disorder. Innov Pharm 2021;12(2). https://doi.org/10.24926/iip.v12i2.3388.

45. Ginsburg BM, Sheer A. Destigmatizing obesity and Overcoming Inherent Barriers to obtain improved patient Engagement. StatPearls Publishing; 2022.
46. Luo Y, Dixon RE, Shah BJ, et al. Gastroenterology Trainees' Attitudes and Knowledge towards Patients with Disorders of Gut-Brain Interaction. Neurogastroenterol Motil 2022;e14410. https://doi.org/10.1111/nmo.14410.
47. Dasgupta N, Asgari S. Seeing is believing: Exposure to counterstereotypic women leaders and its effect on the malleability of automatic gender stereotyping. J Exp Soc Psychol 2004;40(5):642–58.
48. Drossman D, Ruddy J. Gut feelings: disorders of gut brain interaction and the patient-provider relationship. Drossman Center; 2021.
49. Linedale EC, Shahzad MA, Kellie AR, et al. Referrals to a tertiary hospital: A window into clinical management issues in functional gastrointestinal disorders. JGH Open 2017;1(3):84–91.
50. Black CJ, Craig O, Gracie DJ, et al. Comparison of the Rome IV criteria with the Rome III criteria for the diagnosis of irritable bowel syndrome in secondary care. Gut 2021;70(6):1110–6.
51. Ruddy J. From Pretending to Truly Being OK: A Journey From Illness to Health With Postinfection Irritable Bowel Syndrome: The Patient's Perspective. Gastroenterology 2018;155(6):1666–9.
52. Halpert A, Dalton CB, Palsson O, et al. Irritable bowel syndrome patients' ideal expectations and recent experiences with healthcare providers: a national survey. Dig Dis Sci 2010;55(2):375–83.
53. Halpert A, Dalton CB, Palsson O, et al. Patient educational media preferences for information about irritable bowel syndrome (IBS). Dig Dis Sci 2008;53(12): 3184–90.
54. Halpert AD, Thomas AC, Hu Y, et al. A survey on patient educational needs in irritable bowel syndrome and attitudes toward participation in clinical research. J Clin Gastroenterol 2006;40(1):37–43.
55. Regula CG, Miller JJ, Mauger DT, et al. Quality of Care From a Patient's Perspective. Arch Dermatol 2007;143(12). https://doi.org/10.1001/archderm.143.12. 1592.
56. Keefer L, Ballou SK, Drossman DA, et al. A Rome Working Team Report on Brain-Gut Behavior Therapies for Disorders of Gut-Brain Interaction. Gastroenterology 2022;162(1):300–15.
57. Ruddy J, Taft T, Keszthelyi D. Gut-Brain Interactions in Patients with Inflammatory Bowel Disease and the Role of Hypnotherapy in Managing Symptoms. J Crohns Colitis 2021;15(10):1780–1.
58. Palsson OS, Whitehead WE. Psychological Treatments in Functional Gastrointestinal Disorders: A Primer for the Gastroenterologist. Clin Gastroenterol Hepatol 2013;11(3):208–16.

Stress, Resilience, and the Brain–Gut Axis

Why is Psychogastroenterology Important for all Digestive Disorders?

Sarah Ballou, PhD[a],*, Jordyn H. Feingold, MD, MSCR, MAPP[b]

KEYWORDS

- Psychogastroenterology • Psychology • Gastroenterology
- Disorders of gut–brain interaction (DGBI) • Organic disorders

KEY POINTS

- Approaches to clinical care that aim to treat the gut without attention to mind–body factors may be insufficient to adequately address the impact of stress on the brain–gut axis.
- Despite current medical practice that largely treats the mind and body as distinct and separate entities, psychogastroenterology offers a path to treat the brain and gut synergistically, accounting for biological, psychological, and social phenomena.
- Psychogastroenterology approaches can mitigate the impact of stress on the brain–gut axis by enhancing coping and resilience. These approaches may be applied across all digestive disorders, including disorders of gut–brain interaction, motility disorders, as well autoimmune and immune-mediated disorders such as Crohn's disease, ulcerative colitis (UC), and celiac disease.

INTRODUCTION

The concept of mind–body dualism—the notion that the mind and body are distinct and separate entities—served an important function in the 17th century by allowing the mechanics of the body to become the study of medicine while the workings of the mind could remain under the scope of religious study.[1] Only after the mind was liberated from the body was the field of medical science able to make important advances in dissection, and subsequently, our modern understanding of physiology, anatomy, pathology, and the "organic" basis of disease.[2] However, it has become

[a] Division of Gastroenterology, Beth Israel Deaconess Medical Center, 330 Brookline Avenue, Dana 501, Boston, MA 02215, USA; [b] Department of Psychiatry, Icahn School of Medicine at Mount Sinai, 1468 Madison Avenue, 4th floor, New York, NY 10128, USA
* Corresponding author.
E-mail address: sballou@bidmc.harvard.edu
Twitter: @Jordynfeingold (J.H.F.)

Gastroenterol Clin N Am 51 (2022) 697–709
https://doi.org/10.1016/j.gtc.2022.07.001

abundantly clear in the intervening centuries that health and disease are multidimensional experiences, extending far beyond the biology or mere mechanics of disease to include the lived experience of illness, suffering, and coping, and reciprocal relations among the physical body, the brain and mind, and the social fabric of an individual's life.[3]

Consideration of the complexities of the mind–body relationship has been particularly important in the study of chronic conditions, especially in those associated with chronic pain[4] This focus on the mind–body relationship has been most widely applied in the treatment and conceptualization of so-called "functional" conditions, including functional gastrointestinal (GI) disorders [which have been recently renamed to the less stigmatizing "disorders of gut–brain interaction" (DGBI)][5] that lack a clear organic etiology or structural basis, but nonetheless may cause debilitating physical and psychological distress.[6] However, it is important to consider the complexities of the mind–body relationship as they apply to all chronic illness, as virtually all chronic conditions interact reciprocally within a patient's psychosocial context. The idea of such a "biopsychosocial" model was coined in 1977 by internist and psychoanalyst George Engel to describe clinical care that integrates the reciprocal biological, psychological, and social aspects of life that influence an organism's health.[3] Following Engel's legacy, in recent decades, an ethos and practice of *psychogastroenterology* has approached digestive disorders from the biopsychosocial perspective, with a goal of reducing symptom burden and remediating psychosocial vulnerabilities.[7–9] Although DGBIs represent the most obvious targets for psychogastroenterology treatments, all chronic digestive disorders may be susceptible to the impact of stress on the brain–gut axis. Additionally, chronic digestive disorders may be associated with chronic pain, fatigue, psychological distress, shame, and stigma. A psychogastroenterology-informed approach may offset disease burden, disability, low quality of life, as well as health care costs for all patients with GI.[10–12]

Here, we will expand on the importance of the biopsychosocial model and the mind–body relationship as it pertains to all chronic digestive disorders, with a specific emphasis on the brain–gut axis and the role of stress and resilience in the experience of chronic digestive conditions. We will end with a brief discussion of evidence-based brain–gut behavioral therapies that are available for all patients with these conditions.

The Brain–Gut Axis

The brain–gut axis is among the most widely studied and well-understood pathways for mind–body communication. The brain–gut axis is a broad term used to describe the reciprocal, complex interactions among the central nervous system (CNS), the autonomic nervous system (ANS), the hypothalamic–pituitary–adrenal (HPA) axis, and the GI tract. Through these systems, the brain (CNS) interprets afferent signals from the gut and regulates GI functioning, a complex process that has been shown to be significantly affected by emotional states.[13] For example, an organism under psychological duress—be it from the presence of disturbing physical symptoms or from general acute or chronic life stressors—may experience a "fight-or-flight" state, mediated by the sympathetic branch of the ANS, or a "freeze" state, mediated by the dorsal vagus nerve. Both states of nervous system arousal reroute blood flow away from the GI tract, which can lead to alterations in gut sensation, motility, and immunity.[14] The pathways involved in brain–gut communication may become highly dysregulated in response to chronic stress, especially in patients with chronic digestive conditions. Indeed, dysregulation of this axis is a hallmark feature of DGBI [eg, irritable bowel syndrome (IBS), nausea and vomiting disorders, functional dyspepsia, functional dysphagia, and so forth]

Additionally, it is important to keep in mind that there is a high prevalence of overlap between organic GI disorders and DGBIs.[15] For example, aberrations in the brain–gut axis may lead to superimposed IBS-like symptoms in people with inflammatory bowel disease (IBD) (eg, Crohn's disease and UC), causing a dissociation between symptom burden and pathologically identified inflammation.[16] In fact, in one study, up to 32.5% of patients with IBD in remission met criteria for IBS,[17] a significantly higher incidence than the rate of IBS in the general population.[18] In these cases, medical management of the underlying organic disorder will not provide sufficient relief of symptoms and treatments targeting dysregulation in the brain–gut axis (eg, treatments aimed at reducing stress and improving coping and resilience) will likely be necessary.

Additionally, even among individuals with healthy brain–gut communication, alterations in one's internal and/or external environments can easily trigger GI symptoms produced by brain–gut communication (eg, "butterflies in one's stomach" in response to stress or apprehension, mediated by the sympathetic nervous system and dorsal vagus nerve). With this in mind, it is reasonable to consider the role of the brain–gut axis among patients with any chronic digestive condition, regardless of whether their symptoms are thought to be driven primarily by *disordered* brain–gut communication.

The Biopsychosocial Model in Gastrointestinal Disorders

Factors that are commonly associated with disruption or dysfunction in the brain–gut axis include many of the same constructs that would be assessed in a typical biopsychosocial evaluation of a patient with chronic illness, which can broadly be divided into environmental factors, psychosocial factors, and biological factors. Depending on the diagnosis, the biological factors will vary (eg, genetics, underlying disease process, microbiome, body habitus, anatomy, and so forth). Environmental factors known to be associated with dysfunction in the brain–gut axis include the history of GI infections/enteritis, early life experiences, and social stress/support.[6] Finally, psychological factors associated with dysfunction or dysregulation in the brain–gut axis may include psychiatric comorbidity (eg, mood disorders, anxiety disorders, trauma-related disorders, and substance-use) and maladaptive cognitive, affective, and behavioral processes (eg, health-related anxiety, neuroticism, catastrophization, somatization, internalized stigma, avoidance behaviors).[6]

As stated above, although most of the research regarding the brain–gut axis has been applied to DGBIs, all patients with chronic digestive conditions can benefit from evaluation and intervention in each of these areas, whether or not symptoms are driven primarily by dysregulation of the brain–gut axis. See **Fig. 1** for an example of how this might be applied in a gastroenterology setting in the evaluation of patients with and without DGBI. The main difference in the psychosocial evaluation of patients with and without DGBI lies in the primary treatment goal of symptom improvement with psychotherapy for patients with features of disordered brain–gut interaction[19] compared with a primary treatment goal of improved coping or quality of life among patients with organic conditions, which we elaborate on later in the article. Regardless of the treatment goal, however, psychosocial evaluation and intervention for chronic digestive disorders will focus on identifying stressors and improving resilience and healthy coping techniques in the context of stress.

Stress, Resilience, and Digestive Disorders

As in our discussion of the brain–gut axis, the role of psychological stress is often discussed exclusively in the context of DGBI. Psychological stress may result from a variety of triggers including life's daily hassles (eg, work-related strain or financial strain), chronic life stressors (eg, early life adversity such as childhood neglect or abuse,

Framing

"I'd like to talk about some factors that connect your experience as a patient to who you are as a whole person. The experience of living with a disorder such as _____ can take a toll mentally, and when we are feeling unwell mentally, it can also worsen symptoms. On the other hand, when things are going well in our lives, sometimes symptoms can be less bothersome, which can lead to feeling better overall. That is why I like to talk to all of my patients about the brain-gut axis, or the connectivity between our minds (including our thoughts, feelings, behaviors) and our digestive system (the experience of symptoms, pain, diarrhea, constipation, etc.)"

Impact

- How has this illness impacted your life on a daily basis?
  Consider: social interactions, work/school productivity, quality of life, self-esteem
- What does a good day look like?
- What does a bad day look like?

Coping

- How are you currently managing your illness? What has been difficult? What has been easier?
  Consider: medication, symptom management, school/work-related issues
- Who in your life is available to help you manage your illness? From whom do you seek support?
- What are some ways you currently manage stress (both in general and illness-related stress?

Integration

- Has your illness impacted your sense of identity? If so, how?
- Do you know others with this same illness?
- Some patients feel that they grow in unexpected ways after being diagnosed with a chronic illness. How does this apply to you?[a]
  [a]*Use clinical judgement to ascertain whether patient is ready to engage with this question*

Brain-gut factors

- What does stress feel like in your body?
- Have you noticed that stress/anxiety affects your GI symptoms?
- Have GI symptoms caused stress/anxiety?

Follow-up

"I'd like for us to keep track of some of these topics if you're interested as we continue to work together, so that we can try to intervene on some of the stressors and really optimize your strengths to better manage your symptoms and quality of life. Based on what we've discussed, there may be other treatments that I can recommend that can help, would you like to talk about these now?"

Opportunity to discuss brain-gut directed treatments

Fig. 1. Key discussion points for applying psychogastroenterology to all patients.

poverty, tumultuous family relationships), or major life events (eg, loss of a loved one, loss of employment, divorce, and so forth) What defines an event as "stressful" is that such a stimulus induces alterations in one's neuroendocrine, autonomic, or immunologic functioning. Indeed, given its vast impacts on the human body, which we elaborate on later in discussion, stress should be evaluated as part of a biopsychosocial approach to any chronic illness. However, stress is only part of the equation. The link between stressful events and the resultant psychobiological changes is mediated by *resilience:* the factors that enable patients to bounce back, or even bounce forward in the wake of significant stress and adversity. Increasingly, strengths-based, resilience-promoting approaches are seen as central to high-quality psychogastroenterology practice. Here, we will address stress and resilience separately to more fully describe their roles in the experience of chronic illness and their influence on disease outcomes and quality of life across a broad range of chronic digestive conditions.

The influence of stress on the body. The general health consequences of chronic stress have been widely researched, although the specific effects of stress are mitigated by coping and resilience and tend to vary widely among individuals. Generally speaking, stress can affect the following systems: musculoskeletal (chronic pain, tension headaches),[20,21] respiratory (shortness of breath, asthma exacerbations),[22] endocrine (increased risk of obesity, diabetes),[23,24] cardiovascular (increased risk of heart attack, hypertension, and stroke),[25,26] reproductive (changes in sexual functioning, changes in fertility, changes in menstruation),[27] and GI (see later in discussion).

The influence of stress on the digestive tract. The impact of chronic stress on the digestive tract is multifaceted. For example, chronic stress may lead to alterations in one's diet (eating less healthfully, binge eating, eating less due to poor appetite), health behaviors (physical activity, sleep, substance use), and overall self-care. Additionally, chronic stress is associated with increased visceral sensitivity to pain and discomfort,[28] and may reduce pain thresholds in patients who suffer from painful illnesses.[29] Further, chronic stress can affect colonic motility as well as gastric emptying times via activation of corticotropin-releasing factor (CRF, the primary hormonal pathway involved in the activation of the hypothalamic-pituitary axis).[30] CRF pathways mediate the inhibition of gastric emptying and, conversely, stimulation of colonic motility as part of the visceral stress response.[31] Such alterations in motility may then result in symptoms of dyspepsia, nausea, constipation, and/or diarrhea.

Finally, chronic stress may impact the composition of the microbiome, which can influence both symptom experience as well as emotions and mood.[32] These effects apply to all individuals experiencing chronic stress, but they are more prominent and bothersome among people with digestive disorders. For example, in gastroesophageal reflux disease (GERD), patients exposed to stress may experience increased esophageal sensitivity[33,34] as well as altered esophageal motility,[35] mediated by corticotropin response hormone. In IBD, higher levels of perceived stress, experiencing a major life event, and negative mood have been associated with increased odds of experiencing a subsequent flare.[36,37] And, finally, research in IBS has long supported a strong association between chronic or sustained stress and onset/exacerbation of IBS symptoms.[38]

Chronic illness is a source of stress. Beyond the complex brain–gut communication and the specific effects of stress on digestive health, having a chronic medical condition is inherently stressful and can be marked by emotional challenges, especially in the context of learning to manage one's condition, build autonomy,[39] and identify one's sense of identity.[40] Research in chronic digestive conditions suggests that there is a great deal of stigma surrounding chronic digestive disorders that operates at many levels (see Johannah Ruddy and Tiffany Taft's article, "The Pervasive Impact of the Stigmatization of Gastrointestinal Diseases- A Patient's Perspective," in this issue.). For example, patients with organic conditions, DGBI, or both may experience stigma from others as well as internalized stigma related to poor body image, frequent bathroom visits, dietary restrictions, as well as school and work absences related to symptoms, flares, and doctor's visits. Those without an organic diagnosis may experience further stigma from society and the medical establishment when they perceive a message that symptoms are "all in your head" or seen as psychosomatic and therefore, illegitimate.[12] Further, given that psychotherapy and neuromodulators are some of the mainstays of treatment for both DGBI[41] and organic conditions like as IBD,[42] patients may face stigma for taking these "anti-depressant" drugs, or engaging in behavioral therapy, which is more traditionally geared toward patients with psychiatric diagnoses. Such stigma may be a source of stress that actually exacerbates symptoms and prevents patients from accessing high-quality, evidence-based treatments.[12] Given the well-established role of stress as a mediator of symptoms in patients with digestive disorders,[43] attention to stress reduction strategies as well as efforts to enhance coping with stress warrant clinical attention and are a core feature of psychogastroenterology.

Resilience as an Early Brain–Gut Target

Resilience has recently been introduced as an important protective factor in the relationship between stress and dysregulation of the brain–gut axis.[7,10] Specifically, increased resilience in the setting of chronic and/or acute stress may mitigate the impact that stress has on the brain–gut axis. Physiologically, resilience is associated with optimal functioning of the ANS including vagal nerve functioning as well as healthy brain development.[44] For example, neurohormones associated with the brain–gut axis (including norepinephrine, CRH, and cortisol, serotonin, and dopamine) mediate transitions in autonomic arousal that may result in the experience of GI symptoms (eg, by shunting blood away from the GI tract during sympathetic activation) as well as symptom-related distress.

Work by Park and colleagues[45] has shown elevated levels of glucocorticoids in individuals with reduced resilience that differentiated healthy people from those who develop a DGBI.[46] While such biological factors are perhaps the least directly modifiable in a clinical setting, work has shown that interventions such as relaxation response meditation has been effective in IBS[47] and associated with the modified expression of inflammatory marker NF-kappaB in both IBS and IBD.[48] Helping patients with digestive disorders understand that resilience-promoting practices can ultimately modify the nervous system in positive ways to help them not only cope with illness-related stress but other forms of anxiety as well, may inspire patients to pursue evidence-based therapies.

A resilience framework considers first and foremost the patient's biological, psychological, and social strengths that help them cope with disease and more successfully adapt to symptoms, stress, stigma, and the illness experience.[10] Psychological and social interventions may also have great promise in supporting patients with both organic disorders and DGBI, both via reducing stress and by promoting distinct resilience-enhancing skills. Recent qualitative research among a cohort of adolescents with IBD found that the presence of optimism and positivity, support from within the IBD community (eg, through organizations such as the Crohn's & Colitis Foundation), social support from within existing social networks (parents, friends, siblings, and so forth), and support from a mental health professional were all protective in helping teenagers and young adults transition in their identity from pediatric to adult patients.[49] Social support has further been shown to be associated with reduced disease activity in patients with UC and improved physical and mental health-related quality of life in patients with both UC and Crohn's disease.[50] In DGBI-like IBS, social support has been associated with reduced global symptom severity and pain scores.[51] In particular, a positive, trusting, and effective patient–physician relationship is one of the most significant predictors of long-term prognosis, even irrespective of pharmacologic treatments used to treat the disorder.[52,53]

Explicitly screening for resilience and/or other character strengths has become increasingly adopted by academic IBD centers and other clinical settings to connect vulnerable patients with psychological interventions to bolster resilience *before* negative outcomes ensue.[10] One such practice at the Mount Sinai IBD Center in NYC has shown that mind–body approaches that screen for and target resilience are associated with reductions in health care utilization (71% reduction in emergency department visits and 94% reduction in unplanned hospitalizations), a 49% reduction in opioid use and 73% reduction in corticosteroid use compared with those not receiving mind–body care.[54]

How can psychogastroenterology be applied to patients with and without obvious symptoms of brain–gut axis dysregulation?

The most widely studied psychogastroenterology interventions, also known as brain–gut behavioral therapies (BGBT), include cognitive behavioral therapy and gut-focused hypnosis.[55,56] Other evidence-based therapies include mindfulness-based interventions, psychodynamic, Acceptance and Commitment Therapy, and interpersonal therapies.[43] Most of the research conducted has focused on the application of BGBTs in DGBIs,[55,57] although there have also been studies in other, chronic GI disorders.[58–60] Many aspects of these treatments are similar, regardless of the etiology of the underlying illness they are used to treat. As stated previously, the most important difference in the application of BGBTs for DGBIs compared with other chronic GI disorders lies in the treatment goals: the primary treatment target of BGBTs for disorders characterized by the dysregulation of the brain–gut axis is symptom reduction or relief.[19,61] Stress reduction, stigma reduction, and enhanced coping skills often also improve in tandem, but these are not the primary goals of therapy. On the other hand, the primary treatment target of BGBTs for "organic" conditions include stress, coping, building resilience, and disease self-management,[62] with secondary goals of possible symptom reduction. See **Fig. 2** for similarities and differences in treatment targets of these therapies.

Beyond specific psychogastroenterology interventions, there are several therapeutic approaches that can be initiated in a clinic visit with a treating physician (vs with a specialized mental health provider). Broadly, these will all fall under the approach of prioritizing and creating a strong patient–provider relationship, the importance of which cannot be underestimated. Establishing a strong and trusting patient–provider relationship requires time, effective communication, empathy, active listening, and validation of the patient's experiences and concerns.[63] Engaging patients as active and valued participants in their own care can increase satisfaction

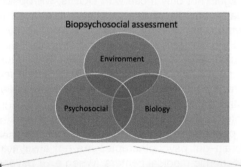

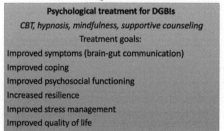

Fig. 2. Similarities and differences in psychogastroenterology treatment targets for DGBI and other GI conditions.

and improve clinical outcomes.[64,65] Importantly, effective communication is not limited to the physician's choice of words, but also includes nonverbal communication such as making eye contact, sitting facing the patient (vs facing a computer), and nodding one's head (or otherwise indicating that you are listening).[65,66]

As primary care and gastroenterology clinicians balance increasing clinical demands on their time and attention, centering this approach in more traditional treatment paradigms may have great utility in improving patient's symptoms and quality of life, and help patients feel partnered with and seen by their clinicians. Doing so will require that clinicians treating digestive disorders become adept at (1) screening for and identifying which patients will have the greatest benefit from brain–gut behavior therapies, (2) amassing an arsenal of high-quality resources, including digital resources, to provide to patients to learn more about the brain–gut axis (3) investing in training opportunities to learn to prescribe and titrate neuromodulators (at least 1 or 2 go-to medications) and hold supportive conversations with patients about the brain–gut axis, and (4) establishing referral pathways to local clinicians who can administer additional therapies, which may be beyond the scope of the gastroenterologist's role and expertise.

SUMMARY AND FUTURE DIRECTIONS

Stress, resilience, and dysregulation of the brain–gut axis should be considered for all patients with chronic digestive conditions, not only those with diagnosed DGBI.[56] Psychogastroenterology, which is a field specially dedicated to the study of psychosocial factors affecting digestive disorders, can be applied by a range of clinicians and to patients with a variety of GI symptoms and diagnoses. Physicians who embody a biopsychosocial approach and who are committed to developing a strong patient–provider relationship are considered to be operating within the field of psychogastroenterology and their approach to patient care is vital to introducing the importance of psychosocial and brain–gut factors in the experience of chronic digestive conditions. Many patients, again not only those with DGBIs, will benefit from referral to a specialized mental health provider who can assist with stress management, coping with a diagnosis or symptoms, building resilience, and/or specific gut-focused psychotherapies (such as CBT or gut-directed hypnotherapy). These should be introduced early in treatment and to all patients, so as to reduce the potential for stigmatization if a referral is made. Such topics (as those introduced in **Fig. 1**) should be revisited and followed up on in all future visits to reinforce patient–physician alignment and build a positive patient–physician relationship.

Ideally, all gastroenterologists would have at least one local GI psychologist to whom they can refer patients with chronic digestive disorders. Unfortunately, clinicians specialized in brain–gut psychotherapies are not always available, and most are located in large academic medical centers. When a GI psychologist is not available, referral to therapists in the community can be an acceptable alternative, especially when goals are to improve stress, coping, and quality of life. Fortunately, the field of psychogastroenterology continues to grow, with an increasing number of health psychologists seeking training in GI-specific interventions, as well as a recent increase in the number of available digital treatment options.

To fully take advantage of the benefits of psychogastroenterology interventions, we need to prioritize destigmatization among both providers and patients with the goal to incorporate evidence-based psychological approaches into clinical care. Investing in models of integrated care, with mental health providers available as part of a multidisciplinary care team in gastroenterology clinics, can address this stigma and improve access to care.

FURTHER READING

Keefer L, Palsson OS, Pandolfino JE. Best Practice Update: Incorporating Psychogastroenterology Into Management of Digestive Disorders. *Gastroenterology*. 2018;154(5):1249-1257. doi:10.1053/j.gastro.2018.01.045.

CLINICS CARE POINTS

- Stress, resilience, and dysregulation of the brain-gut axis should be considered for all patients with chronic digestive conditions, not only those with diagnosed DGBI.

- A specialized mental health provider can assist with stress management, coping with a diagnosis or symptoms, building resilience, and/or specific gut-focused psychotherapies (such as CBT or gut-directed hypnotherapy).

- The role of Brain Gut Behavioral Therapy should be introduced early in treatment and to all patients, so as to reduce the potential for stigmatization if a referral is made.

DISCLOSURE

The authors have nothing to disclose.

REFERENCES

1. Mehta N. Mind-body Dualism: A critique from a Health Perspective. Mens Sana Monogr 2011;9(1):202–9.
2. Drossman DA. Functional Gastrointestinal Disorders: History, Pathophysiology, Clinical Features, and Rome IV. Gastroenterology 2016;150(6):1262–79.e2.
3. Engel GL. The need for a new medical model: a challenge for biomedicine. Science 1977;196(4286):129–36.
4. Duncan G. Mind-body dualism and the biopsychosocial model of pain: what did Descartes really say? J Med Philos 2000;25(4):485–513.
5. Schmulson MJ, Drossman DA. What Is New in Rome IV. J Neurogastroenterol Motil 2017;23(2):151–63.
6. Van Oudenhove L, Levy RL, Crowell MD, et al. Biopsychosocial Aspects of Functional Gastrointestinal Disorders: How Central and Environmental Processes Contribute to the Development and Expression of Functional Gastrointestinal Disorders. Gastroenterology 2016;150(6):1355–67.e2.
7. Feingold J, Murray HB, Keefer L. Recent Advances in Cognitive Behavioral Therapy For Digestive Disorders and the Role of Applied Positive Psychology Across the Spectrum of GI Care. J Clin Gastroenterol 2019;53(7):477–85.
8. Kinsinger SW, Ballou S, Keefer L. Snapshot of an integrated psychosocial gastroenterology service. World J Gastroenterol 2015;21(6):1893–9.
9. Riehl ME, Kinsinger S, Kahrilas PJ, et al. Role of a health psychologist in the management of functional esophageal complaints. Dis Esophagus 2015;28(5):428–36.
10. Keefer L. Behavioural medicine and gastrointestinal disorders: the promise of positive psychology. Nat Rev Gastroenterol Hepatol 2018;15(6):378–86.
11. Taft TH, Keefer L, Artz C, et al. Perceptions of illness stigma in patients with inflammatory bowel disease and irritable bowel syndrome. Qual Life Res 2011;20(9):1391–9.

12. Feingold JH, Drossman DA. Deconstructing stigma as a barrier to treating DGBI: Lessons for clinicians. Neurogastroenterology Motil 2021;33(2):e14080.
13. Mayer EA, Tillisch K. The brain-gut axis in abdominal pain syndromes. Annu Rev Med 2011;62:381–96.
14. Porges SW. The Polyvagal theory: Neurophysiological Foundations of emotions, Attachment, communication, and self-Regulation. W.W. Norton & Company; 2011.
15. Aziz I, Simrén M. The overlap between irritable bowel syndrome and organic gastrointestinal diseases. Lancet Gastroenterol Hepatol 2021;6(2):139–48.
16. Halpin SJ, Ford AC. Prevalence of symptoms meeting criteria for irritable bowel syndrome in inflammatory bowel disease: systematic review and meta-analysis. Am J Gastroenterol 2012;107(10):1474–82.
17. Fairbrass KM, Costantino SJ, Gracie DJ, et al. Prevalence of irritable bowel syndrome-type symptoms in patients with inflammatory bowel disease in remission: a systematic review and meta-analysis. Lancet Gastroenterol Hepatol 2020;5(12):1053–62.
18. Sperber AD, Bangdiwala SI, Drossman DA, et al. Worldwide Prevalence and Burden of Functional Gastrointestinal Disorders, Results of Rome Foundation Global Study. Gastroenterology 2020. https://doi.org/10.1053/j.gastro.2020.04.014.
19. Lackner JM, Jaccard J, Krasner SS, et al. How does cognitive behavior therapy for irritable bowel syndrome work? A mediational analysis of a randomized clinical trial. Gastroenterology 2007;133(2):433–44.
20. McFarlane AC. Stress-related musculoskeletal pain. Best Pract Res Clin Rheumatol 2007;21(3):549–65.
21. Viero FT, Rodrigues P, Trevisan G. Cognitive or daily stress association with headache and pain induction in migraine and tension-type headache patients: a systematic review. Expert Rev Neurother 2022. https://doi.org/10.1080/14737175.2022.2041414.
22. Chen E, Miller GE. Stress and inflammation in exacerbations of asthma. Brain Behav Immun 2007;21(8):993–9.
23. Pouwer F, Kupper N, Adriaanse MC. Does emotional stress cause type 2 diabetes mellitus? A review from the European Depression in Diabetes (EDID) Research Consortium. Discov Med 2010;9(45):112–8.
24. Scott KA, Melhorn SJ, Sakai RR. Effects of Chronic Social Stress on Obesity. Curr Obes Rep 2012;1(1):16–25.
25. Batty GD, Russ TC, Stamatakis E, et al. Psychological distress and risk of peripheral vascular disease, abdominal aortic aneurysm, and heart failure: pooling of sixteen cohort studies. Atherosclerosis 2014;236(2):385–8.
26. Nabi H, Kivimäki M, Batty GD, et al. Increased risk of coronary heart disease among individuals reporting adverse impact of stress on their health: the Whitehall II prospective cohort study. Eur Heart J 2013;34(34):2697–705.
27. Nakamura K, Sheps S, Arck PC. Stress and reproductive failure: past notions, present insights and future directions. J Assist Reprod Genet 2008;25(2–3):47–62.
28. Meerveld BGV, Johnson AC. Mechanisms of Stress-induced Visceral Pain. J Neurogastroenterol Motil 2018;24(1):7–18.
29. Reinhardt T, Kleindienst N, Treede RD, et al. Individual Modulation of Pain Sensitivity under Stress. Pain Med 2013;14(5):676–85.
30. Taché Y, Mönnikes H, Bonaz B, et al. Role of CRF in stress-related alterations of gastric and colonic motor function. Ann N Y Acad Sci 1993;697:233–43.

31. Stengel A, Taché Y. Neuroendocrine Control of the Gut During Stress: Corticotropin-Releasing Factor Signaling Pathways in the Spotlight. Annu Rev Physiol 2009;71:219–39.
32. Lyte M, Vulchanova L, Brown DR. Stress at the intestinal surface: catecholamines and mucosa-bacteria interactions. Cell Tissue Res 2011;343(1):23–32.
33. Fass R, Naliboff BD, Fass SS, et al. The effect of auditory stress on perception of intraesophageal acid in patients with gastroesophageal reflux disease. Gastroenterology 2008;134(3):696–705.
34. Yamasaki T, Tomita T, Takimoto M, et al. Intravenous Corticotropin-releasing Hormone Administration Increases Esophageal Electrical Sensitivity in Healthy Individuals. J Neurogastroenterol Motil 2017;23(4):526–32.
35. Broers C, Melchior C, Van Oudenhove L, et al. The effect of intravenous corticotropin-releasing hormone administration on esophageal sensitivity and motility in health. Am J Physiol Gastrointest Liver Physiol 2017;312(5):G526–34.
36. Bernstein CN, Singh S, Graff LA, et al. A Prospective Population-Based Study of Triggers of Symptomatic Flares in IBD. Official J Am Coll Gastroenterol ACG. 2010;105(9):1994–2002.
37. Bernstein CN. The Brain-Gut Axis and Stress in Inflammatory Bowel Disease. Gastroenterol Clin North Am 2017;46(4):839–46.
38. Chang L. The role of stress on physiologic responses and clinical symptoms in irritable bowel syndrome. Gastroenterology 2011;140(3):761–5.
39. Ng JYY, Ntoumanis N, Thøgersen-Ntoumani C, et al. Self-Determination Theory Applied to Health Contexts: A Meta-Analysis. Perspect Psychol Sci 2012;7(4): 325–40.
40. Charmaz K. The Body, Identity, and Self: Adapting To Impairment. Sociological Q 1995;36(4):657–80.
41. Drossman DA, Tack J, Ford AC, et al. Neuromodulators for Functional Gastrointestinal Disorders (Disorders of Gut–Brain Interaction): A Rome Foundation Working Team Report. Gastroenterology 2018;154(4):1140–71.e1.
42. Mikocka-Walus A, Ford AC, Drossman DA. Antidepressants in inflammatory bowel disease. Nat Rev Gastroenterol Hepatol 2020;17(3):184–92.
43. Keefer L, Ballou SK, Drossman DA, et al. A Rome Working Team Report on Brain-Gut Behavior Therapies for Disorders of Gut-Brain Interaction. Gastroenterology 2021. https://doi.org/10.1053/j.gastro.2021.09.015.
44. Russo SJ, Murrough JW, Han MH, et al. Neurobiology of resilience. Nat Neurosci 2012;15(11):1475–84.
45. Park SH, Naliboff BD, Shih W, et al. Resilience is decreased in irritable bowel syndrome and associated with symptoms and cortisol response. Neurogastroenterol Motil 2018;30(1). https://doi.org/10.1111/nmo.13155.
46. Parker CH, Naliboff BD, Shih W, et al. The Role of Resilience in Irritable Bowel Syndrome, Other Chronic Gastrointestinal Conditions, and the General Population. Clin Gastroenterol Hepatol 2021;19(12):2541–50.e1.
47. Keefer L, Blanchard EB. The effects of relaxation response meditation on the symptoms of irritable bowel syndrome: results of a controlled treatment study. Behav Res Ther 2001;39(7):801–11.
48. Kuo B, Bhasin M, Jacquart J, et al. Genomic and clinical effects associated with a relaxation response mind-body intervention in patients with irritable bowel syndrome and inflammatory bowel disease. PLoS One 2015;10(4):e0123861.
49. Feingold JH, Kaye-Kauderer H, Mendiolaza M, et al. Empowered transitions: Understanding the experience of transitioning from pediatric to adult care among

adolescents with inflammatory bowel disease and their parents using photovoice. J Psychosomatic Res 2021;143:110400.

50. Slonim-Nevo V, Sarid O, Friger M, et al. Effect of Social Support on Psychological Distress and Disease Activity in Inflammatory Bowel Disease Patients. Inflamm Bowel Dis 2018;24(7):1389–400.

51. Lackner JM, Brasel AM, Quigley BM, et al. The ties that bind: perceived social support, stress, and IBS in severely affected patients: Support, stress, and IBS. Neurogastroenterology Motil 2010;22(8):893–900.

52. Owens DM, Nelson DK, Talley NJ. The irritable bowel syndrome: long-term prognosis and the physician-patient interaction. Ann Intern Med 1995;122(2):107–12.

53. Jayaraman T, Wong RK, Drossman DA, et al. Communication breakdown between physicians and IBS sufferers: what is the conundrum and how to overcome it? J R Coll Physicians Edinb 2017;47(2):138–41.

54. Keefer L, Gorbenko K, Siganporia T, et al. Resilience-based Integrated IBD Care Is Associated With Reductions in Health Care Use and Opioids. Clin Gastroenterol Hepatol 2021. https://doi.org/10.1016/j.cgh.2021.11.013. S1542356521012258.

55. Ford A, Lacy B, Harris L, et al. Effect of Antidepressants and Psychological Therapies in Irritable Bowel Syndrome: An Updated Systematic Review and Meta-Analysis. Am J Gastroenterol 2019;114(1):21–39.

56. Keefer L, Palsson OS, Pandolfino JE. Best Practice Update: Incorporating Psychogastroenterology Into Management of Digestive Disorders. Gastroenterology 2018;154(5):1249–57.

57. Rodrigues DM, Motomura DI, Tripp DA, et al. Are psychological interventions effective in treating functional dyspepsia? A systematic review and meta-analysis. J Gastroenterol Hepatol 2021;36(8):2047–57.

58. Timmer A, Preiss JC, Motschall E, et al. Psychological interventions for treatment of inflammatory bowel disease. Cochrane Database Syst Rev 2011;(2): CD006913.

59. Keefer L, Doerfler B, Artz C. Optimizing management of Crohn's disease within a project management framework: results of a pilot study. Inflamm Bowel Dis 2012; 18(2):254–60.

60. Riehl ME, Pandolfino JE, Palsson OS, et al. Feasibility and acceptability of esophageal-directed hypnotherapy for functional heartburn. Dis Esophagus 2016;29(5):490–6.

61. Windgassen S, Moss-Morris R, Goldsmith K, et al. Key mechanisms of cognitive behavioural therapy in irritable bowel syndrome: The importance of gastrointestinal related cognitions, behaviours and general anxiety. J Psychosomatic Res 2019;118:73–82.

62. Bernabeu P, van-der Hofstadt C, Rodríguez-Marín J, et al. Effectiveness of a Multicomponent Group Psychological Intervention Program in Patients with Inflammatory Bowel Disease: A Randomized Trial. Int J Environ Res Public Health 2021;18(10):5439.

63. Drossman DA, Ruddy J. Improving Patient-Provider Relationships to Improve Health Care. Clin Gastroenterol Hepatol 2020;18(7):1417–26.

64. Weiland A, Van de Kraats RE, Blankenstein AH, et al. Encounters between medical specialists and patients with medically unexplained physical symptoms; influences of communication on patient outcomes and use of health care: a literature overview. Perspect Med Educ 2012;1(4):192–206.

65. Drossman DA. 2012 David Sun Lecture: Helping Your Patient by Helping Yourself—How to Improve the Patient–Physician Relationship by Optimizing Communication Skills. Official J Am Coll Gastroenterol ACG 2013;108(4):521–8.
66. Beck RS, Daughtridge R, Sloane PD. Physician-patient communication in the primary care office: a systematic review. J Am Board Fam Pract 2002;15(1): 25–38.

Practical Approaches to Working with a Gastrointestinal Psychologist

Sarah W. Kinsinger, PhD

KEYWORDS

- Psychogastroenterology • Brain–gut axis • Cognitive-behavioral therapy
- Gut-directed hypnotherapy • GI psychology

KEY POINTS

- Assessing GI-specific psychological factors and quality of life is an essential first step for evaluating whether a patient is a candidate for referral to a GI Psychologist.
- Patients with good psychological insight, openness to learning about the brain–gut axis, and willingness to commit to behavioral treatment are ideal candidates for GI Psychology referral.
- Referrals for GI Psychology services should include a discussion of the brain–gut axis as the primary rationale for a referral.
- GI clinicians who do not have access to a GI Psychologist within their institution can provide access to brain–gut behavior therapies by proactively reaching out to a community mental health provider to build a referral pathway.

INTRODUCTION

There has been a rapid increase in the acceptance and utilization of psychological treatments (now referred to as brain–gut behavior therapies; BGBT) for gastrointestinal (GI) disorders over the past decade. Although the scientific basis for these approaches has existed since the 1940s, their application in clinical settings has grown exponentially in recent years. In fact, the American College of Gastroenterology now recommends Brain–Gut Psychotherapies in their clinical guidelines for treating irritable bowel syndrome (IBS) and there is growing interest from both physicians and patients to use an integrated approach to care that includes psychological treatment.[1] As stated by Chey and colleagues, integrated care, "is becoming the rule not the exception for IBS."[2] Similarly, a multidisciplinary model of care for patients with inflammatory bowel disease (IBD) that incorporates psychological treatment is being

Division of Gastroenterology and Nutrition, Loyola University Medical Center, 2160 South First Avenue, Building 54, Room 167, Maywood, IL 60153, USA
E-mail address: Sarah.Kinsinger@lumc.edu

Gastroenterol Clin N Am 51 (2022) 711–721
https://doi.org/10.1016/j.gtc.2022.07.002
0889-8553/22/© 2022 Elsevier Inc. All rights reserved.

adopted by a growing number of health care systems and has been shown not only to improve patient outcomes but also reduce health care utilization.[3]

Unfortunately, the vast majority of gastroenterologists have not been trained in settings that include psychological services and may not be familiar with brain–gut behavior therapies and the role of a GI psychologist. This lack of exposure to GI Psychology does not have to be a barrier to adopting an integrated care approach. GI clinicians can learn to successfully incorporate brain–gut behavior therapies into their clinical management approach and typically find it to be a highly rewarding collaboration that improves clinical care. The goal of this article is to provide guidance on practical considerations that can facilitate the successful integration of BGBT into a GI practice, including proper assessment of psychosocial factors impacting symptom presentation, identifying patients most likely to benefit from a psychological approach, effective communication strategies when making a referral, and identifying mental health professionals equipped to work with patients with GI.

ASSESSMENT

Successful integration of BGBT starts with routinely assessing psychological factors that may be contributing to a patient's GI condition to determine which patients are most likely to benefit from a referral to a psychologist. The biopsychosocial model can be used as the foundation for this assessment. This model takes into account the complex interaction of multiple factors that influence the onset and maintenance of symptoms in chronic digestive disorders.[4] Using this framework allows clinicians to validate the complex nature of the patient's condition, including the role of genetic predisposition, environmental factors, as well as true biological factors that may be playing a role (eg, infection, low-grade inflammation, abnormalities of the microbiome). This model also highlights the role of specific cognitive, emotional, and behavioral factors and their influence on gut symptoms via the brain–gut axis. For example, it is well documented that experiencing early life adversity is a risk factor for developing a disorder of gut–brain interaction (DGBI) and the presence of GI-specific maladaptive cognitions contributes to more severe GI symptoms and health care seeking behaviors.[5–7] The biopsychosocial model also applies to structural diseases such as IBD whereby psychological factors (eg, depression, anxiety, impaired coping) have been shown to influence the course of the illness and contribute to more severe disease outcomes.[8,9] The clinical information gained through a biopsychosocial assessment will inform treatment recommendations as well as strengthen the patient–provider relationship which will improve the likelihood that the patient will be receptive to a referral to a psychologist.

Given the time constraints on outpatient clinic visits, it may not be realistic to conduct a thorough psychosocial history during an initial appointment; however, a few open-ended questions related to the quality of life and the role of stress can set the stage for introducing the biopsychosocial model and highlight certain issues you may want to follow-up on at a later visit. Additionally, this assessment process does not have to add substantial time if you focus on the key psychological processes that are known to contribute to brain–gut dysregulation in GI disorders.

The use of patient-centered communication skills when discussing these sensitive topics is important as this will encourage patients to open up and will strengthen their rapport. These patient-centered techniques include the use of open-ended questions, active listening, offering empathy, and validating the patient's feelings.[10] One of the many benefits of this communication style is that it can actually save clinician time by capturing key clinical information and lead you toward a more effective treatment

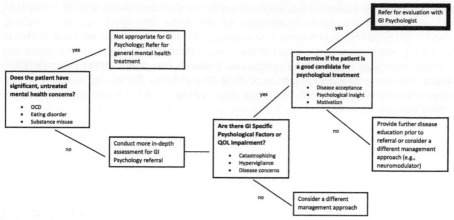

Fig. 1. Assessment process to determine if a patient is an appropriate candidate for referral to a GI psychologist.

strategy. Furthermore, patients will be appreciative of your interest in their illness experience and these conversations can create a natural segue to discuss a referral to a GI psychologist.[a] The psychosocial assessment can be introduced by informing the patient that you are using a biopsychosocial framework to understand their condition and asking permission to ask about psychosocial and behavioral factors (eg, *"Is it okay if I ask a few questions about other areas of your life so that I can understand you better and how these symptoms are impacting your life?"*). The following specific domains should be included in your assessment process and can help to determine which patients will be well-suited for a BGBT approach. **Fig. 1** summarizes these key domains and the process for determining a patient's appropriateness for GI Psychology referral.

Gastrointestinal-Specific Psychological Factors

An important goal of the assessment process is to identify the presence and severity of *GI-specific* psychological factors and disease-specific quality of life. Research supports the role of specific cognitive, emotional, and behavioral meditators associated with brain–gut dysregulation and as predictors of GI symptom severity. These factors are modifiable through behavioral interventions and are therefore key indicators of whether or not a patient may be a good candidate for a referral for BGBT. Common psychological factors include visceral anxiety and hypervigilance (anticipatory worry and preoccupation with GI symptoms), catastrophic thinking (tendency to dwell on the awfulness of the GI symptoms and underestimate that one is able to cope), and maladaptive coping (tendency to use problem-focused coping irrespective of the type of stressor).[11–13] For example, a patient with functional heartburn may express fears of developing esophageal cancer despite having a normal medical work-up. These are referred to as *GI-specific* psychological factors and can occur independent of psychopathology. It is not uncommon for patients to deny symptoms of a mental health disorder (eg, major depressive disorder, generalized anxiety disorder), yet

---

[a] Additional information and training resources related to effective communication skills can be found at https://theromefoundation.org/programs-projects/rome-foundation-communication-program/educational-resources-on-communication-skills/.

endorse these GI-specific psychological patterns. Clinician awareness of these factors can inform the conceptualization of the case and guide decision-making regarding a psychological referral. For example, it is not uncommon for these patterns to develop secondary to the onset of the GI condition due to the often embarrassing and unpredictable nature of the symptoms. Patients can often relate to experiencing stress and worry as a consequence of their GI condition. Explaining to patients that these patterns likely developed as a reaction to their symptoms and are now perpetuating the condition via brain–gut dysregulation can be a helpful framework to gain buy-in for a BGBT approach. Finally, patients with chronic digestive conditions often experience impairments in quality of life. For example, patients with IBD, celiac disease, or chronic pancreatitis may struggle with disease-specific concerns (eg, pain, fatigue, body image disturbance, fear of flare-ups) that negatively impact their quality of life. Patients who endorse these types of concerns and/or significant life disruption as a result of their condition often benefit from working with a psychologist to improve coping and optimize functioning with a chronic illness. See **Box 1** for a list of sample questions for assessing GI-specific anxiety, quality of life, and early life adversity.

Psychological Comorbidity

In addition to identifying GI-specific psychological factors, the assessment process should consider the presence of mental health disorders that are unrelated to the patient's GI condition. Often times this can be determined through chart review or when taking a clinical history. The presence of severe psychopathology such as obsessive–compulsive disorder, major depressive disorder, an eating disorder, substance use disorder, psychotic disorder, or active posttraumatic stress disorder would preclude the patient from working with a GI psychologist on BGBT. Patients with severe untreated mental health conditions typically do not respond well to GI-specific therapy and should be referred for appropriate mental health services as a top priority. In some cases, the patients can be re-evaluated for BGBT after the primary mental health concerns have been treated (it may be necessary to speak with the treating mental health provider to confirm this). Keep in mind, that is not uncommon for patients with chronic digestive disorders to have comorbid mild to moderate mental health comorbidities, such generalized anxiety disorder or panic disorder, and as long as the condition is stable and the patient is receiving appropriate treatment by an outside mental health professional (ie, medication management or therapy), they may still be a candidate for BGBT and the GI psychologist can coordinate care with their outside provider.

Box 1
Key assessment topics and examples of open-ended questions

GI Specific Anxiety and Hypervigilance
Are your GI symptoms a source of stress for you?
How much of your day is spent thinking about or worrying about your symptoms?
How often are you avoiding situations due to concerns about your symptoms (eg, travel, socializing)?

Role of Stress and Quality of Life
What worries or concerns do you have about your GI symptoms?
To what extent do you think that stress is contributing to your condition?
How has your life been impacted by your GI condition?

Early Life Adversity
How would you describe your home environment as a child?
Have you experienced abuse or sexual assault in your life?

Additional Considerations

There are additional factors to consider when determining who might be a good candidate for working with a GI psychologist. The first is disease acceptance. Patients who do not fully accept their diagnosis, particularly when diagnosed with a DGBI, are not likely to buy-in to the rationale for psychological intervention. Typically patients who are not accepting of their diagnosis are requesting additional work-up and believe there are physiologic abnormalities to explain their symptoms that will eventually be discovered with further testing. In some cases, patients with poor disease acceptance may be willing to go along with a referral to a psychologist, saying "I'm willing to try anything," but these patients typically do not respond well as they are not fully engaged in treatment and are simply wanting to "check the box" of having seen a psychologist based on your recommendation. In these cases, it is more beneficial to focus your time on further education about their diagnosis, providing reassurance, and building a strong patient–provider relationship before referring the patient for psychological services.

It is also important to consider the patient's level of psychological insight. Patients who have a good awareness of their emotions and the impact of stress on their body typically respond well to BGBT. Some degree of skepticism around their diagnosis and the role of the brain–gut axis is to be expected, but the patient needs to be open to learning about these concepts.

Finally, the patient's level of motivation is important to consider when referring for BGBT. These treatments require a commitment to attend multiple treatment sessions with a psychologist over the course of several months as well as implementing homework assignments outside of the appointments. Consider whether the patient seems to have sufficient time and motivation to fully engage in this type of treatment before making a referral. See **Table 1** for an overview of who is an appropriate candidate for BGBT.

HOW TO MAKE A SUCCESSFUL REFERRAL

Providers may be hesitant to recommend psychological treatment for a GI condition due to concerns that it will be an awkward conversation or poorly received by the patient. Indeed, patients may be surprised by the recommendation given that most individuals have never heard of a GI psychologist. However, when the rationale for the

Table 1 Appropriate and inappropriate candidates for BGBT	
Appropriate Referrals for BGBT	**Inappropriate Referrals for BGBT**
Patients who present with *symptom-related anxiety* and/or maladaptive coping related to their GI condition	Patients with *severe or untreated* mental health conditions unrelated to their GI condition (eg, major depressive disorder, obsessive–compulsive disorder)
Patients who report significant *quality of life impairment* related to their GI condition	Active *substance misuse*
Patients who are *open to the role of stress* impacting the brain–gut axis	Untreated eating disorder or risk for malnutrition (*BMI <17*)
Patients with a preference for a *nonpharmacological* approach	Patients who are *not accepting* of their GI diagnosis and are seeking additional testing
Patients who are *motivated* and willing to commit to a course of treatment and practice behavioral skills outside of sessions	Patients who *lack insight* into the role of stress and emotions impacting GI symptoms

referral is explained using patient-friendly language and the timing of the referral is appropriate, patients are often quite receptive. Keep in mind, BGBT approaches are incredibly safe and have high satisfaction rates among patients. In fact, a recent study of patients undergoing gut-directed hypnotherapy found that even the subset of patients that did not experience symptom relief had very positive impressions of the treatment and still found it worthwhile.[14] Therefore, there is much to be gained from recommending this approach and very little risk. The following 4 steps can serve as a helpful guide for making a successful and confident referral to a GI Psychologist:

1. Discuss the role of the brain–gut axis as the primary rationale for the referral. It is helpful to introduce this concept early in the treatment process, even if you don't make the referral recommendation at that time. If the concept of the brain–gut connection is already familiar to the patient, then the recommendation for a mind-based treatment will not come as a surprise. Use patient-friendly language and metaphors whenever possible when discussing the brain–gut axis and the impact of stress on the gut. See **Box 2** as well as Keefer and colleagues, for examples of patient-friendly brain–gut explanations.[15]

2. Explain the scientific support for BGBT for GI conditions. For example, when recommending treatment of IBS, highlight that BGBT approaches have been studied for >30 years and have been evaluated in numerous clinical trials which consistently show that 60% to 70% of patients have significant improvement in GI symptoms following a course of treatment. Similarly, cognitive-behavioral therapy has been shown to improve quality of life and enhance coping skills and resilience in patients with IBD.[3,16]

3. Emphasize that these are GI-specific psychological interventions that differ from traditional psychotherapy. These are short-term, skills-based treatments that are provided by health psychologists who have specialized training in working with medical populations. As the referring physician, you don't need to recommend a

---

Box 2
Patient-friendly language to explain the brain–gut axis

The gut has its own nervous system with more than 100 million nerve endings (it has been nicknamed our second brain!) and this nervous system is highly interconnected with our brain through nerves and chemical signals. This complex, bidirectional communication network between the 2 organ systems is referred to as the brain–gut axis. The interconnectedness of these two systems explains why we can experience stress or emotions in our gut, such as feeling butterflies in our stomach.

In some cases, this communication between the brain and the gut can go awry due to some type of disruption, such as infection, chronic stress, or in response to surgery. As a result, the brain starts to perceive sensations from the gut too strongly, as if the brain is on high alert for discomfort (you can think of this like a volume knob on a stereo being turned up). This may cause you to experience normal sensations, like feelings of fullness or the presence of acid in the esophagus, as highly uncomfortable. The brain also starts to send inappropriate signals back down to your digestive system causing the nerves and muscles to work in an uncoordinated manner. It is this disrupted communication that causes the uncomfortable symptoms you are experiencing.

Brain–gut behavior therapies use psychological and behavioral techniques to help restore normal communication patterns between the brain and gut. For example, a treatment like gut-directed hypnotherapy can help your mind learn to more effectively filter out and "turn down the volume" on those uncomfortable sensations in your gut and also helps to regulate your physiologic stress response so that your gut is not as reactive to stress.

specific type of treatment, this will be determined by the psychologist at the time of intake, but you can provide examples of the common brain–gut behavior therapies (eg, cognitive-behavioral therapy, gut-directed hypnotherapy).
4. Express commitment to stay engaged in the patient's care. Communicate to the patient that you view the psychologist as a member of the patient's treatment team and you are willing to communicate with the psychologist as needed to coordinate care. You may also request to receive feedback from the psychologist on the patients' progress and inform the patient that you are happy to see them back in the clinic as needed.

Patients may have a variety of responses to this referral recommendation. If the patient remains hesitant or skeptical about participating in BGBT treatment after you have made the recommendation, you can encourage the patient to at least meet with the psychologist for an initial consultation and this appointment can be an opportunity for the psychologist to provide further psychoeducation and to increase buy-in for the approach. See **Box 3** for a list of common questions that patients may have about a GI Psychology referral and suggested responses.

Communication Method

The referral recommendation is best delivered in-person during a clinic appointment. This will allow sufficient time to explain the rationale for the referral, and provide the patient with an opportunity to ask questions and to address any areas of concern. It may be helpful to supplement this referral recommendation with a program brochure developed by the psychologist, handouts on GI psychology treatments (see IFFGD. org and crohnscolitisfoundation.org/mental-health for patient education materials), or use a smart phrase built into the electronic medical record to provide further information on the referral process and treatment approach. An electronic referral should not be used as the primary method for communicating the referral, but rather as a way to reinforce the information that has already been provided and to set expectations for what to expect during the consultation visit with the psychologist.

Timing of the Referral

Appropriate timing of the referral to a psychologist for BGBT is important. Ideally, the referral should be introduced early in the treatment process; however, not before the patient's medical work-up is complete and you have communicated their diagnosis. If the referral is made prematurely and the patient is still awaiting a colonoscopy or CT scan, they may be confused as to the reason they are seeing a GI Psychologist and are less likely to buy-in to the diagnosis of a brain–gut disorder and reason for psychological treatment. On the other hand, if the referral is made long after diagnosis and only after the patient has failed multiple treatments, the patient may view this as a last resort or perceive that you are "dumping" them on the psychologist. In these cases, patients are less likely to follow through or fully engage with treatment.

Once the patient is engaged in a course of behavioral therapy, it is helpful to hold off on ordering additional tests or starting the patient on a new medication unless the patient develops new symptoms or alarm features. The psychologist and patient are better able to gauge treatment gains without introducing these additional variables. If a patient with a DGBI condition reaches out mid-way through treatment due to a flare-up of their symptoms, it would be appropriate to provide reassurance and redirect the patient to continue with the course of behavioral treatment. This will communicate to the patient that you have confidence in the psychological treatment approach and expect the patient to improve.

Box 3
Common questions related to a GI psychology referral and suggested responses

Common question:
  Does this mean that you think my symptoms are all in my head? I've been told that before!

Suggested response:
  Absolutely not! You have a medical condition that is influenced by disrupted communication between the brain and the gut's nervous system. Because the brain is part of the control system of the gut, I think it would be helpful to use mind-based treatments to help restore normal communication between the two organ systems and to help reduce stress since that can aggravate symptoms. This is a complex condition and we will work together to find the best combination of treatments to help you manage this.

Common question:
  Do you think that stress is causing all of my symptoms?

Suggested response:
  Stress can certainly contribute to this condition, but we don't think of it as the sole cause. We know from research that this is a stress-sensitive disorder and chronic stress, even early in life, can contribute to brain–gut dysregulation. The stress response can directly influence muscle contractions in your gut and also influence how your brain perceives sensations in your gut, like gas or stool moving through your intestines. We also know from research that some patients with chronic digestive conditions have abnormalities in their physiologic stress response, so you may experience more significant disruption in gut symptoms in response to everyday stressors, meaning you are a "gut responder."

Common question:
  I already see a therapist, why do I also need to see a GI psychologist?

Suggested response:
  A GI Psychologist provides short-term skills-based psychological treatments that are specifically designed to treat your GI symptoms and help you cope with this chronic health condition. This differs from general mental health care. In many cases, you can continue working with your therapist while participating in brain–gut behavior therapy.

Common question:
  I'm not sure I have the time to invest in this right now.

Suggested response:
  This treatment does require a commitment, but it is not long-term psychotherapy. This is considered short-term, skills-based treatment aimed at helping you learn skills to better manage your symptoms. You will likely need to commit to treatment for 3 to 4 months. The good news is, most patients that improve with this approach continue to experience benefits long after the treatment is completed, so you can think of this as a short-term investment that will provide long-term benefits.

How to Create a Referral Pathway

There are various models for integrating GI psychology services into a GI practice. The ideal scenario for truly integrated and collaborative care is to hire a full-time GI Psychologist to provide care on-site within a practice. This improves access for patients, allows for interdisciplinary discussions around care, and is beneficial for patients with more complex and severe presentations. Over the past several years, many academic medical centers have created GI Psychology positions to fill this need. However, this may not be realistic for all institutions or practice settings. Hiring a GI Psychologist requires buy-in from hospital administrators and a commitment from the division to provide the financial and logistical support needed for this type of program to be successful.

As an alternative, gastroenterologists can partner with health psychologists working in other departments within their institution to create a referral pathway. There may be psychologists housed within psychiatry or other medical departments (eg, primary care, pain clinic) that would be well equipped to treat patients with GI and willing to develop a care pathway with GI. You can consider arranging a co-located clinic 1 day per week as a way to create greater collaboration and move toward an integrated care approach.

Finally, GI psychology services can be integrated by developing a referral pathway with private practice therapists in the community. There are several therapist directories that can be used to identify private practice therapists in your area. The Rome Foundation Psychogastroenterology section has a searchable directory of mental health professionals that treat patients with GI conditions. There are also a number of general therapist directories that allow you to search by region, area of specialization, and even insurance panels (**Table 2** for a list of recommendations). Therapists with experience treating chronic illness or chronic pain and with training in cognitive-behavioral therapy are typically well suited to work with patients with GI conditions. Consider setting up a call or in-person meeting to discuss your interest in collaborating and to learn more about the therapist's specific training and areas of specialization. You will also want to understand the therapist's fee structure, waitlist for new patients, and their preferred method of communication. If the therapist is new to the field of psychogastroenterology, you can consider providing financial support for them to obtain continuing education through the Rome Foundation (https://theromefoundation.org/rome-gi-psych-committee).

Telemedicine has broadened access to mental health care and may be a mechanism to connect your patients to a GI psychologist located further away or even out of state. However, be aware of licensing limitations when making these referrals (ie, the therapist must be licensed in the states in which the patient is located). Some psychologists are licensed in multiple states or are authorized to practice under PSYPACT, meaning their license in their home state allows them to practice telepsychology in other states that have adopted PSYPACT legislation (https://psypact.site-ym.com/page/psypactmap).

Finally, be mindful of patient complexity and be judicious with referrals when developing a new referral pathway with private practice clinicians. Start by referring patients with more straightforward presentations and who are motivated to work with a psychologist. As your relationship with the therapist builds, you can request consultation on more complex cases and will learn the clinician's level of comfort with certain issues (eg, eating disorders, posttraumatic stress disorder). If you are unsure whether a particular patient would be a good candidate, it is always best to reach out and request a consultation before making the referral.

Table 2 Therapist directories for locating a mental health professional	
Therapist Directories	**Website**
Rome Foundation GastroPsych	www.RomeGIPsych.org
Psychology Today Therapist Finder	www.psychologytoday.com/us/therapists
American Psychological Association	locator.apa.org
Association for Behavioral and Cognitive Therapies	www.findcbt.org
Directory of GI Hypnosis Providers	www.ibshypnosis.com

SUMMARY

BGBT approaches are backed by more than 30 years of clinical research and provide demonstrated benefits for treating a wide range of digestive conditions. Ideally, these treatments are provided in an integrated care setting whereby GI clinicians work collaboratively with a GI psychologist to provide care. Successful collaboration can be achieved through appropriate patient assessment, delivering the referral for BGBT with confidence using patient-friendly language, and good communication with the treating mental health provider. Effective use of these strategies will result in better care for patients and a highly rewarding experience for both the GI clinician and psychologist.

CLINICS CARE POINTS

- Use open-ended questions and patient-centered communication techniques when assessing the role of psychological factors and discussing sensitive topics
- Introduce the concept of the brain–gut axis and the role of stress early in the care pathway
- Recommend brain–gut behavior therapy as an evidence-based treatment once the patient has been conclusively diagnosed
- To identify a mental health provider in the community to work with, search for providers who specialize in chronic illness or chronic pain and have training in cognitive-behavioral therapy and/or hypnotherapy.
- When in doubt regarding a patient's appropriateness for GI Psychology services, reach out and ask for consultation from the psychologist before making the referral

DISCLOSURE

Dr S. Kinsinger serves on Advisory Boards for Mahana Therapeutics and Allay Health and has received speaker fees from The Rome Foundation.

REFERENCES

1. Lacy BE, Pimentel M, Brenner DM, et al. ACG clinical guideline: management of irritable bowel syndrome. Am J Gastroenterol 2021;116(1):17–44.
2. Chey WD, Keefer L, Whelan K, et al. Behavioral and diet therapies in integrated care for patients with irritable bowel syndrome. Gastroenterology 2021;160(1):47–62.
3. Keefer L, Gorbenko K, Siganporia T, et al. Resilience-based integrated IBD care is associated with reductions in health care use and opioids. Clin Gastroenterol Hepatol 2021;S1542-3565(21):01225–8.
4. Van Oudenhove L, Crowell MD, Drossman DA, et al. Biopsychosocial aspects of functional gastrointestinal disorders. Gastroenterology 2016;S0016-5085(16):00218–23.
5. Ringel Y, Drossman DA, Leserman JL, et al. Effect of abuse history on pain reports and brain responses to aversive visceral stimulation: An FMRI study. Gastroenterology 2008;134(2):396–404.
6. Drossman DA. Abuse, trauma, and GI illness: Is there a link? Am J Gastroenterol 2011;106(1):14–25.
7. Jerndal P, Ringstrom G, Agerforz P, et al. Gastrointestinal-specific anxiety: an important factor for severity of GI symptoms and quality of life in IBS. Neurogastroenterol Motil 2010;22(6):646-e179.

8. Gaines LS, Slaughter JC, Horst SN, et al. Association between affective-cognitive symptoms of depression and exacerbation of crohn's disease. Am J Gastroenterol 2016;111(6):864–70.

9. Mikocka-Walus A, Pittet V, Rossel JB, et al, Swiss IBD Cohort Study Group. Symptoms of depression and anxiety are independently associated with clinical recurrence of inflammatory bowel disease. Clin Gastroenterol Hepatol 2016;14(6): 829–35.e1.

10. Drossman DA, Ruddy J. Improving patient-provider relationships to improve health care. Clin Gastroenterol Hepatol 2020;18(7):1417–26.

11. Cheng C, Yang FC, Jun S, et al. Flexible coping psychotherapy for functional dyspeptic patients: A randomized, controlled trial. Psychosom Med 2007; 69(1):81–8.

12. Labus JS, Mayer EA, Chang L, et al. The central role of gastrointestinal-specific anxiety in irritable bowel syndrome: Further validation of the visceral sensitivity index. Psychosom Med 2007;69(1):89–98.

13. Lackner JM, Quigley BM. Pain catastrophizing mediates the relationship between worry and pain suffering in patients with irritable bowel syndrome. Behav Res Ther 2005;43(7):943–57.

14. Donnet AS, Hasan SS, Whorwell PJ. Hypnotherapy for irritable bowel syndrome: Patient expectations and perceptions. Therap Adv Gastroenterol 2022;15. 17562848221074208.

15. Keefer L, Palsson OS, Pandolfino JE. Best practice update: Incorporating psychogastroenterology into management of digestive disorders. Gastroenterology 2018;154(5):1249–57.

16. Li C, Hou Z, Liu Y, et al. Cognitive-behavioural therapy in patients with inflammatory bowel diseases: A systematic review and meta-analysis. Int J Nurs Pract 2019;25(1):e12699.

Future of Brain–Gut Behavior Therapies: Mediators and Moderators

Helen Burton Murray, PhD[a,b,c,]*, Brjánn Ljótsson, PhD[d]

KEYWORDS

- Cognitive-behavioral therapy • Exposure therapy • Disorders of gut–brain interaction
- Functional gastrointestinal disorders • Irritable bowel syndrome

KEY POINTS

- Brain–gut behavior therapies for disorders of gut–brain interaction have included therapies with different theorized targets.
- There is a large knowledge gap regarding the processes through which brain–gut behavior therapies achieve change in disorders of gut–brain interaction.
- Consistent evidence suggests that gastrointestinal-specific cognitive, affective, and behavioral processes are the primary targets of brain–gut behavior therapies, leading to clinical improvements.
- Future research is needed to evaluate other target mechanisms and moderators, including understanding of which treatment techniques are most potent and why and for whom they are most beneficial.

INTRODUCTION

Brain–gut behavior therapies are efficacious treatments for disorders of gut–brain interaction (DGBI; also known as functional gastrointestinal [GI] disorders).[1] There is a large body of evidence supporting the efficacy of brain–gut behavior therapies for irritable bowel syndrome (IBS)[2,3] and emerging evidence for other DGBI (eg, supragastric belching,[4] functional dyspepsia).[5,6] Often used in combination with other approaches (eg, neuromodulation),[7] brain–gut behavior therapies are increasingly

Funding: This article was supported by the National Institute of Diabetes and Digestive and Kidney Diseases, K23 DK131334 (H.B. Murray).
[a] Division of Gastroenterology, Massachusetts General Hospital, 55 Fruit Street, Boston, MA 02114, USA; [b] Harvard Medical School, 25 Shattuck St, Boston, MA 02115, USA; [c] Department of Psychiatry, Massachusetts General Hospital, Boston, MA, USA; [d] Department of Clinical Neuroscience, Division of Psychology, Karolinska Institutet, Nobels väg 9, Solna, Stockholm 171 65, Sweden
* Corresponding author. Massachusetts General Hospital, Division of Gastroenterology, 55 Fruit Street, Boston, MA 02114
E-mail address: hbmurray@mgh.harvard.edu

viewed as no longer having to be reserved for the refractory patient. In fact, as Chey and colleagues pointed out, "integrated care is becoming the rule not the exception for IBS."[8] We suspect that many other DGBI will follow suit, with integrated care already in place in specialty medical centers. However, brain–gut behavior therapies are not uniform and instead include a variety of techniques.

Recently, a summary of and recommendations for different brain–gut behavior therapies was published by the Rome Working Team Report on Brain–Gut Behavior Therapies for DGBI.[9] The focus of the working team report was to provide a consensus on what brain–gut behavior therapies are and their mechanistic framework/targets as well as recommendations for their inclusion in DGBI care. Brain–gut behavior therapies have included approaches with varying purported targets. Building on the Rome report, our conceptual review focuses on target engagement—how (ie, mechanisms) and for whom (ie, moderators) brain–gut behavior therapies work (as hypothesized and/or supported by evidence). Of note, we share our opinions and the overarching premise of the perspective we share in this review is that the active ingredients (ie, techniques) of brain–gut behavior therapies involve *DGBI-specific targets* and aim to reduce *central symptoms* of the DGBI treated (eg, reduced abdominal pain, reduced regurgitations). We describe in detail the hypothesized targets, the interventions that are proposed to intervene on/be appropriate for those targets, available evidence for the role of proposed targets, and conclude with future research directions.

OVERVIEW OF BRAIN–GUT BEHAVIOR THERAPY TARGETS

Although brain–gut behavior therapies include approaches that can apply across the GI disorder spectrum, not one protocol is the same as the other. Brain–gut behavior therapy protocols can be classified as cognitive behavioral therapy (CBT), gut-directed clinical hypnosis (or hypnotherapy), mindfulness-based stress reduction, and emotional processing and interpersonal therapies (**Table 1**). All brain–gut behavior therapies include education about DGBI and how the therapy theoretically can improve DGBI outcomes. However, outside of education, even when two protocols share the same class name, the treatments, especially CBT, can include different techniques and emphasize

Table 1 Overview of general classes of brain–gut behavior therapies and typical components			
Cognitive Behavioral Therapies[a]	**Gut-Directed Clinical Hypnosis**	**Mindfulness-Based Stress Reduction**	**Emotional Processing and Interpersonal Therapies**[b]
• Habit-reversal training • Cognitive techniques • Exposure techniques • Relaxation training • Other general health behavior skills (eg, eating at regular intervals, physical activity)	• Relaxation training • Clinical hypnosis	• Relaxation training • Mindfulness training	• Emotional processing techniques • Interpersonal effectiveness skills

[a] Cognitive-behavioral therapy protocols vary in inclusion and emphasis of techniques; some protocols include or primarily focus on only one technique, whereas others are multicomponent protocols. Some multicomponent protocols have also been called "self-management."
[b] We created this class based on similar components that exist between Emotional Awareness and Expression Training and Psychodynamic Interpersonal Therapy protocols that have been created for disorders of gut–brain interaction.

different techniques over others. Moreover, there are different strands of stated targets hypothesized to be mechanisms of action between and within the brain–gut behavior therapy classes. Thus, separating brain–gut behavior therapies into distinct types, each one with their own set of components and purported mechanisms of action, is a challenging task. In this review, we instead focus on delineating the proposed targets of different brain–gut behavior therapies and describe which techniques are used to target them (ie, mechanisms of action) or are most appropriate for whom (ie, target moderators). The core purported targets are:

- Conditioned physiologic alterations
- GI-specific anxiety and avoidance behavior
- Trait anxiety
- Visceral hypersensitivity
- General stress exacerbation
- Emotional processing difficulties
- General interpersonal difficulties

For each target, we summarize which techniques are hypothesized to act on to improve central (DGBI) symptoms. Because CBT interventions are quite dissimilar, we chose to separate therapies within the CBT class into specific behavioral techniques (eg, habit reversal training, exposure techniques) and cognitive techniques, whereas the other classes have been retained as separate techniques. The eight brain–gut behavior therapy techniques we delineate are

- Habit-reversal training
- Cognitive techniques
- Exposure techniques
- Relaxation training
- Clinical hypnosis
- Mindfulness training
- Emotional processing techniques
- Interpersonal effectiveness

The above components have been included in brain–gut behavior therapy protocols with varying levels of emphasis. For example, some CBT protocols for DGBI mostly focus on one technique (eg, habit-reversal training for rumination syndrome[10]; exposure techniques for functional abdominal pain),[5] whereas others are multicomponent interventions (eg, a package of relaxation training targeting general stress, cognitive techniques targeting general anxiety/cognitive inflexibility, and exposure techniques targeting GI-specific anxiety).[11] This inevitably makes the separation of CBT into different techniques somewhat arbitrary and artificial. Nevertheless, we believe that it is valuable to highlight that the specific techniques within one multicomponent CBT protocol are often used for different purported targets.

A Note on Target Moderators

If there are several different interventions that lead to improvements in central symptoms, the natural question is: are all interventions equally effective for all patients or are specific interventions more effective for specific patients? We are not aware of any study that has been adequately designed and powered to compare two or more brain–gut behavior therapies to each other to identify which *type* of brain–gut behavior therapy is best for whom and which techniques produce the best clinical improvements. Furthermore, studies that have attempted to identify which patients benefit more from a specific intervention, based on baseline characteristics such as age, sex, and psychiatric comorbidity, have generally not produced meaningful predictors of treatment effects.[12] An alternative method is to investigate if patients who present with characteristics that a specific intervention is purported to target improve more from the intervention than those without the characteristic; for example, investigating if patients who report high general stress benefit more from relaxation techniques than those with lower stress. If several such treatment target ← → treatment effectiveness relationships can be established, this information can act as a guide for clinicians and patients who are selecting between different treatment options in the absence of directly comparative studies. Thus, in this review, we report if baseline severity of targets has been related to treatment effect.

RATIONALE AND EVIDENCE FOR TARGET ENGAGEMENT

For each target and corresponding techniques, we summarize empirical support or against the notion that the effects of techniques on central symptoms are either (a) actually mediated through change in the proposed targets (ie, target mechanisms of action) or (b) more effective for specific patients over others (ie, target moderators). Thus, we only report findings from studies that investigated connections between the target (as either a mechanism or a moderator) and DGBI symptom outcomes. For example, we do not include studies that evaluated change in the target across treatment without connecting it to changes in DGBI outcomes. We weave together the techniques (**Table 2**) with which techniques are likely most appropriate for whom, based on the target that they are hypothesized to act on. We also note any target evidence for techniques that do not hypothesize those targets as mechanisms or moderators. We synthesize our conceptual model in **Fig. 1**.

Conditioned Physiologic Alterations

Description of the target
A subset of DGBI are conceptualized to have physiologic conditioned processes that the body developed over time, such as with regurgitations, supragastric belching, and upright reflux.[4,10,13] Other less-studied conditioned processes in DGBI may include dysregulation in rectal signaling and appetite signaling. Habit-reversal training is hypothesized to recondition these physiologic responses.

Habit-reversal training
Habit-reversal training is specific to the type of conditioned process. For regurgitation/belching/reflux, diaphragmatic breathing is intended as a direct competing response to abdominal wall contraction (ie, the abdomen cannot contract and relax at the same time).[4,10,13,14] For rectal hyposensitivity, pediatric constipation protocols involve structured toilet-sitting with a schedule for the approximate time of day and the length of sitting time even if the individual does not produce a bowel movement. For appetite dysregulation, creating a regular schedule for eating (and increasing food volume intake when appropriate) has been proposed to recondition appetite signaling.[15]

Evidence for target
To our knowledge, no studies to date have investigated mediators or moderators of treatments that have included conditioned physiologic targets.

Gastrointestinal -Specific Anxiety and Avoidance Behavior

Description of the target
A conditioned process is also hypothesized in other DGBI, but a conditioning of cognitive (ie, thoughts), affective, and behavioral fear responding to GI symptoms. A GI-specific

Table 2
Future directions for brain–gut behavior therapies for disorders of gut–brain interaction

	What Is Known	Knowledge Gap
Which techniques are necessary	• All types of brain–gut behavior therapies (except habit-reversal training) have shown some degree of utility for irritable bowel syndrome (IBS) • Habit-reversal training is the primary brain–gut behavior therapy technique studied for functional regurgitation, belching, and upright reflux symptoms	• There is some promise for other conditions (eg, functional dyspepsia), but which techniques are needed for one DGBI over another are unknown • Protocols have had varying emphasis on different techniques, for example, the relative efficacy and optimal dosing of cognitive vs exposure vs relaxation training techniques in multicomponent treatments is unknown
How treatment works	• Decreases in GI-specific anxiety and avoidance behaviors have mediated treatment outcomes in treatments with exposure techniques and treatments focused on mindfulness training, and have been associated with symptom improvements after hypnosis for IBS • Decreases in trait anxiety are not consistent, with some research showing that decreases in trait anxiety are not associated with improvements but other research showing that cognitive flexibility (a specific aspect of trait anxiety) is associated with improvements • Preliminary evidence that changes in biomarker targets are associated with significant IBS symptom improvements in hypnosis and a multicomponent CBT but are also associated with improvements in other targets (eg, GI-specific anxiety; general stress exacerbation)	• More research is needed on target engagement, particularly for specific brain–gut behavior therapy techniques • GI-specific anxiety may be a key mechanism across brain–gut behavior therapies but needs to be studied in relation to techniques across the brain–gut behavior therapy spectrum • Data on the timing of mechanistic changes are lacking (eg, proximal vs distal mechanisms) • Biomarker targets have been limited to pilot studies and require further research with formal mediator and moderator analyses

(continued on next page)

Table 2
(continued)

	What Is Known	Knowledge Gap
Which treatment is for whom	• Individuals with IBS who have high GI-specific avoidance behaviors may benefit most from exposure techniques	• Moderation findings for other DGBI outside of IBS are unknown • More research is needed on socio-cultural-demographic factors related to better treatment outcomes • Differential outcomes when brain–gut behavior therapy is combined with a neuromodulator are unknown
What is optimal treatment delivery	• Brain–gut behavior therapies have been successful in various formats (unguided or guided self-management, individual or group formats with psychology provider or allied health professional provider)	• Moderator findings for delivery modalities are unknown • Stepped care delivery models have yet to be evaluated • Inferiority of non-psychology providers delivering treatment has not been studied

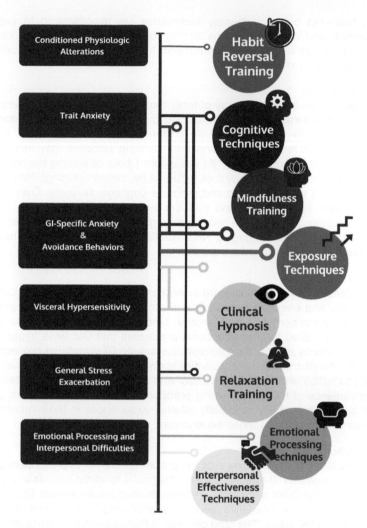

Fig. 1. Conceptual model of why and for whom brain–gut behavior therapies best work based on hypothesized targets. *Note.* Based on clinical expertise, theoretic mechanistic targets, and limited research. Thicker lines represent greater evidence supporting target engagement for a technique (from studies that at minimum correlated change in the target with change in the DGBI symptom outcome).

anxiety and avoidance model has been specifically proposed for IBS[16,17] and has more recently been applied to other DGBI including functional abdominal pain and functional dyspepsia/idiopathic gastroparesis.[5,18] In this model, aversive experiences with GI symptoms over time become associated with certain stimuli (eg, situations, foods), resulting in fear of those stimuli.[19] Patients then attempt to avoid negative predicted outcomes around their GI symptoms—they may do this by a complete avoidance of stimuli predicted to be associated with the outcomes and/or through safety/control behaviors aimed to lessen the likelihood of the predicted outcomes. It is hypothesized that the conditioned fear responding is associated with psychophysiological arousal that induces altered motility which in turn contributes to DGBI maintenance.[19]

Various brain–gut behavior therapy techniques are hypothesized to target GI-specific anxiety and avoidance, some aiming to target via primarily cognitive processes (eg, cognitive techniques, mindfulness training) versus primarily behavioral processes (eg, exposure techniques).

Cognitive techniques

Cognitive techniques involve an array of tools that aim to increase awareness of (unhelpful) thinking patterns that have developed over time around GI symptoms. Patients learn to identify unhelpful thinking patterns around GI symptoms (either in anticipation of or in response to). Unhelpful thinking patterns may include initial thoughts around GI symptoms (eg, "If I eat within 1 hour of leaving the house, I will have a diarrhea accident") or a spiral of thoughts (ie, catastrophizing). Patients learn tools to counteract these thoughts and promote cognitive flexibility. Over time with these techniques, patients may find that the frequency of experiencing unhelpful thoughts decreases, they can use "coping thoughts" (go-to thoughts to help in-the-moment), and/or they start engaging with situations/foods/activities they had previously avoided or had been cautious around.

Mindfulness training

With mindfulness training, patients learn to increase the awareness of physical sensations, thoughts, and emotions around GI symptoms and to view these experiences nonjudgmentally and perhaps with curiosity. Through these processes, mindfulness training is hypothesized to alter attentional processes that decrease hypervigilance around GI sensations and increase acceptance around GI symptoms processes. Patients practice mindfulness through activities such as guided breathing or imagery; patients learn to notice when thoughts wander and to nonjudgmentally re-attend to the sensory experience of the activity being practiced. With these techniques, patients learn to increase their ability to identify internal experiences in-the-moment and to *choose* how they respond to those experiences.

Exposure techniques

With exposure techniques, reducing avoidance/control behavior to prevent symptoms is hypothesized to maintain GI-specific anxiety. The goal is to retrain associations between situations/foods and DGBI symptoms. Patients systematically expose themselves to stimuli predicted to have a negative outcome as well as to GI sensations and remove avoidance/control behaviors. The core concept is that patients learn through repeated exposure that the likelihood of the feared outcome is much lower than predicted and/or that the outcome is not as bad as predicted. Over time, these new learning experiences are hypothesized to decrease cognitive and affective fear responding.

Evidence for target

Studies of exposure techniques for IBS and pediatric pain-related functional GI disorders show that reduction in GI-specific anxiety and avoidance behaviors mediated[17,20–23] and preceded reductions in GI symptom severity[17,22,23] and the exposure techniques were particularly effective for IBS patients who showed a high baseline avoidance behavior.[24] GI-specific anxiety has also mediated improvement in GI symptoms following mindfulness training for IBS[25] and a multicomponent protocol with an emphasis on exposure techniques.[26]

Other multicomponent CBT interventions for IBS to some extent address GI-specific anxiety and/or avoidance behavior. However, they also address other putative targets, and mediation studies reveal a somewhat different pattern than studies of exposure technique studies. One study showed that following the multicomponent intervention, reductions in IBS severity were significantly mediated by reductions in unhelpful GI-related cognitions and GI-specific control behaviors, but not avoidance behaviors.[27] Another study showed GI-specific anxiety did not significantly mediate GI symptom improvements in CBT with emphasis on cognitive techniques compared with education control.[28] Interestingly, a correlation analysis indicated that decreases in GI-specific anxiety were correlated with symptom improvement following gut-directed hypnosis, which does not explicitly target GI-specific anxiety.[29] Studies on the dosing of exposure techniques to adequately engage the targets of GI-specific anxiety and avoidance behaviors have not yet been conducted.

Trait Anxiety

Description of the target
Individuals with IBS have been shown to have increased trait anxiety, such as general tendencies to worry and overestimation of negative consequence.[30,31] Facets of trait anxiety vary, some of which include cognitive inflexibility, neuroticism, and anxiety sensitivity, and measures of general anxiety typically are associated with trait anxiety.

Cognitive techniques
Cognitive techniques for trait anxiety and GI-specific anxiety are similar in nature. However, for trait anxiety, the aim is to target trait-based thinking tendencies and decrease overall tendencies to worry rather than just in relation to GI symptoms.

Mindfulness training
Mindfulness training for trait anxiety and GI-specific anxiety are also similar in nature. However, the aim is to overall increase present moment awareness of physical sensations, thoughts, and emotions and to choose how to respond to them not necessarily just in relation to GI symptoms.

Evidence for target engagement
One sub-study of a controlled evaluation of CBT with emphasis on cognitive techniques showed that reductions in trait anxiety (specifically cognitive inflexibility) was significantly associated with reductions in IBS symptoms severity and quality of life.[30] Interestingly, the same controlled study showed that individuals with lower levels of trait anxiety were more likely to benefit from CBT compared with the control condition and there were no significant differences between groups in IBS outcomes for those with higher levels of trait anxiety.[32] This finding contradicts the notion that patients who are "higher" on the target should benefit more from an intervention aimed at that target but is consistent with other moderation findings that show that general psychological distress does not differentiate who will respond best to cognitive techniques for IBS.[33] Interestingly, emerging research suggests that any changes in trait anxiety are distal to more proximal changes in GI-specific targets. For example, one multicomponent CBT showed reductions in symptom-specific unhelpful thinking patterns reduced before generalized anxiety.[27] To our knowledge, there have been no mediation or moderation studies evaluating trait anxiety with mindfulness training.

Visceral Hypersensitivity

Description of the target
Visceral hypersensitivity has been conceptualized as disturbance in perception of visceral sensations—that is, patients with visceral hypersensitivity report heightened GI sensations in response to physiologic stimulation than those without. For example, as compared with healthy subjects, individuals with IBS[34] and functional dyspepsia[35] report heightened pain/discomfort to gastric and rectal distension, respectively. However, as

visceral hypersensitivity has been identified based on self-report pain scales, it is not clear how much heightened sensitization is because of heightened visceral signaling versus heightened hypervigilance to signaling or a combination of both.

Clinical hypnosis
Hypnosis involves learning a series of techniques to induce a heightened state of focus and awareness, with scripted (personalized when possible) suggestions verbalized while in the altered awareness state. The purported active ingredient of hypnosis is suggestion—although the patient is in an altered state of arousal, specific suggestions are made by the provider (or via recording) related to improved control over and functioning of GI processes. Over time, hypnosis is hypothesized to decrease sensitivity to visceral sensations, that is "turn down the dial" on GI sensations.

Evidence for target engagement
There are limited albeit mixed findings for the effects of hypnosis on visceral sensitivity. Pretreatment to posttreatment changes in sensitivity to rectal distension was not significantly correlated with symptom changes in a pilot randomized trial of hypnosis for children with functional abdominal pain or IBS.[36,37] However, another pilot open trial of hypnosis for adults with IBS showed that only among those with the highest pretreatment rectal sensitivity, reductions in rectal sensitivity after treatment had a trend correlation with symptom improvement, suggesting heightened visceral sensitivity may be a moderator of treatment outcomes.[38]

General Stress Exacerbation

Description of the target
Heightened physiologic arousal and negative emotions related to extra-intestinal stressors (eg, work stress, family difficulties) are hypothesized to increase autonomic arousal, which then in-turn is hypothesized to contribute to gut–brain dysregulation (through multiple processes including visceral sensitivity and altered motility).

Relaxation training
Relaxation training involves a variety of techniques such as relaxed breathing (with or without diaphragm engagement), progressive muscle relaxation, autogenic training, and guided imagery, with or without mindfulness practice. Relaxation training has often been incorporated into multicomponent CBT protocols.[39] Instructions for relaxation training among protocols vary—with some suggesting in vivo utilization when experiencing GI symptoms, some suggesting regular practice (eg, daily), and others suggesting both. Relaxation training is hypothesized to downregulate autonomic arousal contribution to the stress response.

Cognitive techniques
Cognitive techniques for general stress exacerbation mainly aim to teach skills to increase ability to cope with general stressors and have been incorporated into multicomponent CBT protocols.[31]

Mindfulness training
Mindfulness training may be paired with relaxation training, and some mindfulness training protocols hypothesize general stress exacerbation as a target.[40]

Evidence for target
To our knowledge, no study has evaluated general stress exacerbation as a target mechanism of action or moderator in relaxation training, protocols with cognitive techniques, or mindfulness training interventions.

Emotional Processing and Interpersonal Difficulties

Description of the target

Low awareness of emotions, difficulty processing or expressing emotions, and general interpersonal styles have been hypothesized as factors contributing to IBS maintenance.[41] These hypothesized mechanisms are rooted in evidence of related etiologic processes that may have contributed to the onset of GI symptoms, including early life stress and traumatic experiences.[42]

Emotional processing techniques

Emotional processing techniques involve discussing the connections between previous traumatic/stressful experiences and GI symptoms and learning to identify, approach, and experience emotions. Patients may complete exercises that involve expressing thoughts and feelings related to past traumatic/stressful experiences, such as through writing example letters they might send to past people in their lives.[41]

Interpersonal effectiveness techniques

Interpersonal effectiveness techniques include learning new ways to effectively communicate emotions to others. Psychodynamic interpersonal therapy, in particular, is hypothesized to improve interpersonal functioning via the building of a collaborative relationship with the treating clinician.[43] As a result of improving interpersonal functioning, more GI-specific cognitive and emotional targets are believed to improve. Therapy typically focuses on past interpersonal (or other) difficulties, how they relate to the patient's current interactional style, and how the patient's current interactional style interacts with their current functioning including symptoms.

Evidence for target engagement

In a study of psychodynamic interpersonal therapy, improvements in abdominal pain were better accounted by decrease in general psychological distress than change in interpersonal difficulties.[43] To our knowledge, there are no other studies that have investigated this target as a potential mechanism of action or moderator.

Other Targets

Nonspecific targets

Brain–gut therapies for DGBI may also target other processes that contribute to DGBI maintenance or are not specific to one treatment or another. For example, expectancies around what treatment will involve, agreement with the provider about treatment focus, and improvements in beliefs in ability to cope with IBS (ie, self-efficacy) have significantly mediated outcomes in a randomized trial of CBT with an emphasis on cognitive techniques for IBS.[28]

Biomarker targets

Research on biomarker targets of brain–gut behavior therapies is nascent and further research is needed to understand both target mechanisms and moderators. Heart rate variability normalization (ie, via increased vagal tone and decreased sympathetic power) significantly correlated with improvements in IBS symptoms, as well as general stress exacerbation and trait anxiety, in a pilot randomized trial of a multicomponent CBT.[44] Decreases in neural response (via functional magnetic resonance imaging) during high-intensity rectal distension significantly correlated with both reductions in GI-specific anxiety (in anterior insula) and IBS symptoms severity (in hippocampus) in a pilot randomized trial of gut-directed hypnosis.[45] Of note, it is unknown whether the neural response to rectal distension may be a marker of decreased emotional/cognitive (eg, GI-specific anxiety) and/or physiologic (eg, visceral hypersensitivity) response.[45] Recently, one randomized trial of a CBT that emphasized cognitive techniques showed that brain–gut–microbiome biomarkers may moderate CBT effects, with pretreatment microbiome profiles differentiating those who responded versus did not respond to CBT.[46]

DISCUSSION

The purpose of this review was to summarize the evidence for the proposed targets of brain–gut behavior therapies that aim to reduce central symptoms of DGBI. We delineated seven therapeutic targets with examples of behavioral techniques that purportedly influence the targets in attempt to reduce DGBI symptom severity. Our overall conclusion is that there is a large knowledge gap regarding the processes through which brain–gut behavior therapies achieve change in DGBI. In **Table 2**, we provide our summary of what gaps exist which require future study, described in further detail below.

GI-specific anxiety and avoidance (in trials for IBS and pediatric functional abdominal pain disorder) has the strongest mechanistic support. GI-specific anxiety most consistently was identified as a target mechanism and moderator in CBT protocols emphasizing exposure techniques. However, there is some evidence that GI-specific anxiety is a target of mindfulness training and, perhaps surprisingly, hypnosis for IBS. Our results echo the findings in a previous meta-analysis of mediation analyses of brain–gut therapies for IBS, which found that change in GI-specific anxiety and avoidance behaviors was key mechanism of treatment effect, whereas change in trait anxiety was not.[27] However, the meta-analysis did not separate interventions based on their purported target or investigate other DGBI than IBS and more research is needed to evaluate *how* it is best targeted (eg, which techniques best target it, when change is seen).

It seems that multicomponent CBT protocols that "mix" different techniques (and therefore have multiple targets) have mixed evidence for target engagement overall. CBT protocols that include multiple components show mixed findings for GI-specific anxiety as a target, possibly because of insufficient dosing or dosing timing of techniques that target GI-specific anxiety. Multicomponent CBT protocols also do not seem to work primarily through reduced trait anxiety.[27] Instead, trait anxiety has been shown as a target mechanism in one CBT protocol that emphasizes cognitive techniques and explicitly is purported to target cognitive inflexibility.[30] Taken together, CBT protocols may best target the proposed mechanisms when particular techniques are emphasized, but this has yet to be empirically investigated.

There is mixed or a lack of evidence for other targets. There is some evidence (albeit from a pilot open trial) that visceral hypersensitivity in IBS is a target of hypnosis for those high in rectal hypersensitivity. However, other than that, to our knowledge, conditioned physiologic alterations, general stress exacerbation, or emotional processing and interpersonal difficulties do not have evidence supporting them as key targets of brain–gut behavior therapies in DGBI (that is not to say that interventions with these targets are ineffective, see below). Of note, there are possible key targets that have not yet been a key focus of protocols to date. For example, some patients over time developed a lack of interest in eating with low appetite leading to inadequate caloric intake, which could contribute to dysmotility.[15] Some patients may also have sleep disturbances (eg, insomnia) that could contribute to gut–brain dysregulation maintenance warranting specific behavioral strategies such as sleep hygiene[47] and sleep restriction.[48] Finally, other techniques are emerging that aim to increase targets largely unexplored in brain–gut behavior therapies such as acceptance of thoughts and feelings around GI symptoms or strategies to increase the regulation of emotional states.[49]

Major limitations to current target mechanism and moderator evidence for brain–gut behavior therapies relate to adequate investigation of target engagement. First, mediation analyses require that measures used accurately measure the purported target (ie, construct validity) to produce unbiased results.[50] The mixed findings regarding trait anxiety, for example, may potentially be explained by a lack of a clearly defined target and valid measurements (eg, some studies have used measures of "generalized" anxiety and not specifically trait anxiety). Second, some investigations of treatment mechanisms have been flawed, for example, by not including repeated measurements of the mediators throughout the treatment period.[51] Repeated measures allow for investigation of *when* a mechanism changes, potentially in relation to specific treatment techniques. Third, there are no adequately powered studies that have compared different brain–gut therapies with the same or different targets, thus we cannot draw conclusions regarding which target is the most important to intervene on or which intervention is most suitable for that target. To identify which techniques are most effective and for whom (and for when), increasingly used trial designs include designs from the mutliphase optimization MOST and the sequential multiple assignment randomized trial (SMART) frameworks.

We want to underline that the lack of mechanistic support for a specific brain–gut behavior therapy technique does not mean that the intervention is ineffective. On the contrary, there is no evidence that the interventions for which mechanistic data exist are more effective than interventions that lack such data. Nevertheless, stating a purported target for an intervention and conducting studies that measure change in the both the target and the outcome to conduct mediation analysis to test the hypothesized mechanism of action is a crucial part of the development of effective psychological treatments.[52] In fact, a mediation analysis found that brain–gut behavior therapies for IBS that have stated purported target are more effective than the ones who do not.[53] Moreover, it seems unlikely that all purported targets that we delineate are equally important to intervene on to achieve symptom reduction in DGBI. Although conditioned physiologic alterations have been proposed to be central for a specific subset of the DGBI (eg, rumination syndrome, supragastric belching), we show that at least six targets for interventions have been proposed for IBS and to some extent other pain-related DGBI. This is in stark contrast to the anxiety disorders where there now exist "gold-standard" psychological treatments that intervene on specific targets that are well-founded in empirical research.[51] Patients with DGBI would likely benefit from a similar development in brain–gut behavior therapies.

Thus, we believe that the research field of brain–gut behavior therapies should (1) conduct more rigorous trials that can confirm or reject the purported targets of a specific intervention, (2) compare different intervention techniques to each other (e.g., in a MOST framework design), and (3) conduct moderation analyses that can identify which interventions work best for whom.

CLINICS CARE POINTS

- Although the efficacy for brain–gut behavior therapies is strong for irritable bowel syndrome and growing for other disorders, the protocols studied have often included multiple techniques (eg, relaxation training + cognitive techniques) with varying emphasis.
- Brain–gut behavior therapy techniques have different purported mechanistic targets and may be more appropriate for certain patient presentations.

- Consistent evidence to date (largely from irritable bowel syndrome research) suggests gastrointestinal-specific anxiety is a key target, and there is mixed or lacking evidence for other targets.
- Future investigations should be designed to best test potential mechanisms of action and moderators of outcome.

DISCLOSURE

H. Burton Murray receives royalties from Oxford University Press her forthcoming book on rumination syndrome. B. Ljótsson licenses a cognitive-behavioral treatment manual for irritable bowel syndrome to Pear Therapeutics Inc.

REFERENCES

1. Drossman D, Chang L, Chey WD, et al, editors. ROME IV: functional gastrointestinal disorders – disorders of gut-brain interaction. 4th edition. Raleigh (NC): Rome Foundation; 2016.
2. Laird KT, Tanner-Smith EE, Russell AC, et al. Short-term and long-term efficacy of psychological therapies for irritable bowel syndrome: a systematic review and meta-analysis. Clin Gastroenterol Hepatol 2016;14:937–47. e4.
3. Black CJ, Thakur ER, Houghton LA, et al. Efficacy of psychological therapies for irritable bowel syndrome: systematic review and network meta-analysis. Gut 2020;69(8):1441–51.
4. Glasinovic E, Wynter E, Arguero J, et al. Treatment of supragastric belching with cognitive behavioral therapy improves quality of life and reduces acid gastro-esophageal reflux. Am J Gastroenterol 2018;113:539–47.
5. Bonnert M, Olén O, Lalouni M, et al. Internet-delivered exposure-based cognitive-behavioral therapy for adolescents with functional abdominal pain or functional dyspepsia: a feasibility study. Behav Ther 2019;50:177–88.
6. Kinsinger SW, Joyce C, Venu M, et al. Pilot Study of a Self-Administered Hypnosis Intervention for Functional Dyspepsia. Dig Dis Sci 2021. https://doi.org/10.1007/s10620-021-07183-z.
7. Drossman DA, Tack J, Ford AC, et al. Neuromodulators for Functional GI Disorders (Disorders of Gut-Brain Interaction): A Rome Foundation Working Team Report. Gastroenterology 2018;154:1140–71.
8. Chey WD, Keefer L, Whelan K, et al. Behavioral and Diet Therapies in Integrated Care for Patients With Irritable Bowel Syndrome. Gastroenterology 2021;160: 47–62.
9. Keefer L, Ballou SK, Drossman DA, et al. A Rome Working Team Report on Brain-Gut Behavior Therapies for Disorders of Gut-Brain Interaction. Gastroenterology 2022;162:300–15.
10. Burton Murray H, Zhang F, Call CC, et al. Comprehensive Cognitive-Behavioral Interventions Augment Diaphragmatic Breathing for Rumination Syndrome: A Proof-of-Concept Trial. Dig Dis Sci 2021;66:3461–9.
11. Everitt H, Landau S, Little P, et al. Assessing Cognitive behavioural Therapy in Irritable Bowel (ACTIB): protocol for a randomised controlled trial of clinical-effectiveness and cost-effectiveness of therapist delivered cognitive behavioural therapy and web-based self-management in irritable bowel syndrome in adults. BMJ Open 2015;5:e008622.

12. Ljótsson B, Andersson E, Lindfors P, et al. Prediction of symptomatic improvement after exposure-based treatment for irritable bowel syndrome. BMC Gastroenterol 2013;13:160.

13. Barba E, Accarino A, Soldevilla A, et al. Randomized, placebo-controlled trial of biofeedback for the treatment of rumination. Am J Gastroenterol 2016;111:1007.

14. Halland M, Bharucha AE, Crowell MD, et al. Effects of Diaphragmatic Breathing on the Pathophysiology and Treatment of Upright Gastroesophageal Reflux: A Randomized Controlled Trial. Am J Gastroenterol 2021;116:86–94.

15. Weeks I., Becker K.R., Ljótsson B., et al., Brief Cognitive Behavioral Treatment is a Promising Approach for Avoidant/Restrictive Food Intake Disorder in the Context of Disorders of Gut-Brain Interaction. Poster presented at the American Gastroenterological Association annual conference Digestive Disease Week, San Diego, CA; 2022 May.

16. Craske MG, Wolitzky-Taylor KB, Labus J, et al. A cognitive-behavioral treatment for irritable bowel syndrome using interoceptive exposure to visceral sensations. Behav Res Ther 2011;49:413–21.

17. Ljótsson B, Hesser H, Andersson E, et al. Mechanisms of change in an exposure-based treatment for irritable bowel syndrome. J Consult Clin Psychol 2013;81:1113.

18. Abber S, Edwards RR, Napadow V, et al. Brief cognitive-behavioral treatment for gastroparesis: a proof-of-concept open trial. San Diego (CA): Digestive Disease Week; 2022.

19. Mayer EA, Craske M, Naliboff BD. Depression, anxiety, and the gastrointestinal system. J Clin Psychiatry 2001;62(Suppl 8):28–36 [discussion: 7].

20. Lalouni M, Hesser H, Bonnert M, et al. Breaking the vicious circle of fear and avoidance in children with abdominal pain: A mediation analysis. J Psychosom Res 2021;140:110287.

21. Wolitzky-Taylor K, Craske MG, Labus JS, et al. Visceral sensitivity as a mediator of outcome in the treatment of irritable bowel syndrome. Behav Res Ther 2012;50:647–50.

22. Hesser H, Hedman-Lagerlöf E, Andersson E, et al. How does exposure therapy work? A comparison between generic and gastrointestinal anxiety-specific mediators in a dismantling study of exposure therapy for irritable bowel syndrome. J Consult Clin Psychol 2018;86:254–67.

23. Bonnert M, Olén O, Bjureberg J, et al. The role of avoidance behavior in the treatment of adolescents with irritable bowel syndrome: A mediation analysis. Behav Res Ther 2018;105:27–35.

24. Hesser H, Hedman-Lagerlöf E, Lindfors P, et al. Behavioral avoidance moderates the effect of exposure therapy for irritable bowel syndrome: A secondary analysis of results from a randomized component trial. Behav Res Ther 2021;141:103862.

25. Garland EL, Gaylord SA, Palsson O, et al. Therapeutic mechanisms of a mindfulness-based treatment for IBS: effects on visceral sensitivity, catastrophizing, and affective processing of pain sensations. J Behav Med 2012;35:591–602.

26. Mohsenabadi H, Zanjani Z, Shabani MJ, et al. A randomized clinical trial of the Unified Protocol for Transdiagnostic treatment of emotional and gastrointestinal symptoms in patients with irritable bowel syndrome: evaluating efficacy and mechanism of change. J Psychosom Res 2018;113:8–15.

27. Windgassen S, Moss-Morris R, Goldsmith K, et al. Key mechanisms of cognitive behavioural therapy in irritable bowel syndrome: The importance of gastrointestinal related cognitions, behaviours and general anxiety. J Psychosom Res 2019;118:73–82.

28. Lackner JM, Jaccard J. Specific and common mediators of gastrointestinal symptom improvement in patients undergoing education/support vs. cognitive behavioral therapy for irritable bowel syndrome. J Consult Clin Psychol 2021; 89:435–53.

29. Gonsalkorale WM, Toner BB, Whorwell PJ. Cognitive change in patients undergoing hypnotherapy for irritable bowel syndrome. J Psychosom Res 2004;56:271–8.

30. Lackner JM, Gudleski GD, Radziwon CD, et al. Cognitive flexibility improves in cognitive behavior therapy for irritable bowel syndrome but not nonspecific education/support. Behav Res Ther 2022;104033.

31. Blanchard EB, Schwarz SP, Suls JM, et al. Two controlled evaluations of multicomponent psychological treatment of irritable bowel syndrome. Behav Res Ther 1992;30:175–89.

32. Lackner JM, Jaccard J. Factors Associated With Efficacy of Cognitive Behavior Therapy vs Education for Patients With Irritable Bowel Syndrome. Clin Gastroenterol Hepatol 2019;17:1500–8.e3.

33. Lackner JM, Jaccard J, Krasner SS, et al. How does cognitive behavior therapy for irritable bowel syndrome work? A mediational analysis of a randomized clinical trial. Gastroenterology 2007;133:433–44.

34. Mertz H, Naliboff B, Munakata J, et al. Altered rectal perception is a biological marker of patients with irritable bowel syndrome. Gastroenterology 1995;109: 40–52.

35. Tack J, Caenepeel P, Fischler B, et al. Symptoms associated with hypersensitivity to gastric distention in functional dyspepsia. Gastroenterology 2001;121:526–35.

36. Palsson OS, Turner MJ, Johnson DA, et al. Hypnosis treatment for severe irritable bowel syndrome: investigation of mechanism and effects on symptoms. Dig Dis Sci 2002;47:2605–14.

37. Vlieger AM, van den Berg MM, Menko-Frankenhuis C, et al. No change in rectal sensitivity after gut-directed hypnotherapy in children with functional abdominal pain or irritable bowel syndrome. Am J Gastroenterol 2010;105:213–8.

38. Lea R, Houghton LA, Calvert EL, et al. Gut-focused hypnotherapy normalizes disordered rectal sensitivity in patients with irritable bowel syndrome. Aliment Pharmacol Ther 2003;17:635–42.

39. Heitkemper MM, Jarrett ME, Levy RL, et al. Self-management for women with irritable bowel syndrome. Clin Gastroenterol Hepatol 2004;2:585–96.

40. Zernicke KA, Campbell TS, Blustein PK, et al. Mindfulness-based stress reduction for the treatment of irritable bowel syndrome symptoms: a randomized wait-list controlled trial. Int J Behav Med 2013;20:385–96.

41. Thakur ER, Holmes HJ, Lockhart NA, et al. Emotional awareness and expression training improves irritable bowel syndrome: A randomized controlled trial. Neurogastroenterol Motil 2017;29.

42. Guthrie E, Creed F, Dawson D, et al. A controlled trial of psychological treatment for the irritable bowel syndrome. Gastroenterology 1991;100:450–7.

43. Hyphantis T, Guthrie E, Tomenson B, et al. Psychodynamic interpersonal therapy and improvement in interpersonal difficulties in people with severe irritable bowel syndrome. Pain 2009;145:196–203.

44. Jang A, Hwang S-K, Padhye NS, et al. Effects of cognitive behavior therapy on heart rate variability in young females with constipation-predominant irritable bowel syndrome: a parallel-group trial. J Neurogastroenterol Motil 2017;23:435.

45. Lowén MB, Mayer EA, Sjöberg M, et al. Effect of hypnotherapy and educational intervention on brain response to visceral stimulus in the irritable bowel syndrome. Aliment Pharmacol Ther 2013;37:1184–97.

46. Jacobs JP, Gupta A, Bhatt RR, et al. Cognitive behavioral therapy for irritable bowel syndrome induces bidirectional alterations in the brain-gut-microbiome axis associated with gastrointestinal symptom improvement. Microbiome 2021; 9:236.

47. Jarrett ME, Cain KC, Burr RL, et al. Comprehensive self-management for irritable bowel syndrome: randomized trial of in-person vs. combined in-person and telephone sessions. Am J Gastroenterol 2009;104:3004–14.

48. Ballou S, Katon J, Rangan V, et al. Brief Behavioral Therapy for Insomnia in Patients with Irritable Bowel Syndrome: A Pilot Study. Dig Dis Sci 2020;65:3260–70.

49. Sebastián Sánchez B, Gil Roales-Nieto J, Ferreira NB, et al. New psychological therapies for irritable bowel syndrome: mindfulness, acceptance and commitment therapy (ACT). Rev Esp Enferm Dig 2017;109:648–57.

50. Baron RM, Kenny DA. The moderator-mediator variable distinction in social psychological research: Conceptual, strategic, and statistical considerations. J Pers Soc Psychol 1986;51:1173–82.

51. Ljótsson B. What are the mechanisms of psychological treatments for irritable bowel syndrome? J Psychosom Res 2019;118:9–11.

52. Kazdin AE. Mediators and mechanisms of change in psychotherapy research. Annu Rev Clin Psychol 2007;3:1–27.

53. Henrich JF, Knittle K, De Gucht V, et al. Identifying effective techniques within psychological treatments for irritable bowel syndrome: a meta-analysis. J Psychosom Res 2015;78:205–22.

Behavioral Digital Therapeutics in Gastrointestinal Conditions
Where Are We Now and Where Should We Go?

Ruby Greywoode, MD, MS[a], Eva Szigethy, MD, PhD[b],*

KEYWORDS

• Digital therapeutics • Behavioral therapy • Psychogastroenterology

KEY POINTS

• Mental health disorders are a great burden in various gastrointestinal disorders of brain–gut interaction.
• As digital technology transforms health care, digital therapeutics (technology-based therapeutic interventions aimed at the prevention, management, or treatment of a medical condition) have the potential to meet a critical need.
• Behavioral digital therapeutics offers an innovative approach to provide integrated mental health care to enhance (but not replace) clinical care with the potential to improve access, care efficiency, and supplement other modalities to enhance outcomes.

INTRODUCTION

Mental health disorders are increasingly recognized as part of the burden of functional gastrointestinal (GI) disorders (eg, irritable bowel syndrome, IBS) and GI diseases (eg, inflammatory bowel disease, IBD). Brain–gut interactions between the autonomic and central nervous system link stress and mood disorders to intestinal processes, such as visceral sensation, permeability, motility, and inflammation.[1,2] Many individuals with IBS experience heightened visceral abdominal pain that leads to poor quality of life and physical functioning.[3–5] Anxiety and depression are highly prevalent in IBD and left untreated lead to increased resource utilization and poor health outcomes.[6–8] As a result, there is growing interest in addressing comprehensive, integrated care among individuals with GI conditions. Behavioral interventions are recognized as an important element in addressing the psychological aspect of care. However, there are barriers to widespread availability and utilization. A national

[a] Division of Gastroenterology, Einstein-Montefiore Medical Center, 111 East 210th St, Bronx, NY 10467, USA; [b] University of Pittsburgh, 3708 Fifth Avenue, Pittsburgh, PA 15213, USA
* Corresponding author.
E-mail address: Szigethye@upmc.edu

Gastroenterol Clin N Am 51 (2022) 741–752
https://doi.org/10.1016/j.gtc.2022.07.011
0889-8553/22/© 2022 Elsevier Inc. All rights reserved.

shortage of mental health providers, cost limitations, and lack of immediate care options prevent many individuals from accessing behavioral therapy.[9] The COVID pandemic led to further demand for mental health services, and there has been a concurrent shift toward the delivery of health care via digital technology. Leveraging digital technology for mental health care may overcome some of the existing barriers to accessing behavioral health interventions through increased availability of services on a larger scale and outside of usual geographic limitations. In settings where behavioral clinicians exist, digital therapeutics can enhance the efficiency of current clinical workflows and augment or supplement other behavioral modalities.

The accelerated adoption of digital technology has transformed health care delivery and GI disease management through a broad array of tools, such as the electronic medical record used for remote disease monitoring and predictive analytics,[10] telemedicine video platforms, artificial intelligence in endoscopy for adenoma detection,[11] and smartphone applications for remote patient monitoring.[12] Digital health technology is currently not only computer-based but includes mobile devices like smartphones and tablets as well as wearable biosensors (**Fig. 1**).

A subset of digital health technology referred to as digital therapeutics is defined by the Digital Therapeutic Alliance as the delivery of evidence-based therapeutic interventions to prevent, manage, or treat a medical condition. Amidst the rapid proliferation of various forms of digital health technology, a distinguishing feature of digital therapeutics is their basis on clinical testing and focus on therapeutic outcomes. Digital therapeutics for a variety of conditions have been developed. In the context of this issue on psychogastroenterology, this article will focus on the current landscape of behavioral digital therapeutics that address the effects of brain–gut interactions in GI conditions.

EVIDENCE BASE FOR BEHAVIORAL DIGITAL THERAPEUTICS IN GASTROENTEROLOGY

Most behavioral digital therapeutics in GI with empirical support are for either the diagnosis or treatment of GI symptoms and associated mood disorders (**Table 1**). The first step in addressing mental health disorders is of course identification of symptoms and diagnosis. Computerized Adaptive Testing of Mental Health (CAT-MH) is a novel method based on multidimensional item response theory that can accurately and

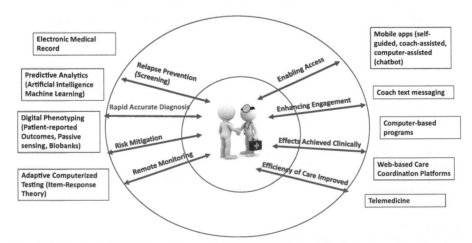

Fig. 1. Behavioral digital therapies as vehicle to improve GI care delivery.

Table 1
Selected studies of behavioral digital therapeutics for gastrointestinal conditions

Author (Year)	Condition	Study Design	Sample Size	Description of Technology	Selected Outcomes	Limitations
Karpin (2021)	IBD	Cross-sectional survey	$N = 134$	• Computerized Adaptive Testing Mental Health technology (CAT-MH) based on multidimensional item response theory; screening for major depression, generalized anxiety disorder, and suicidality	• Median survey administration time was 3.5 minutes • Screen positive patients with previously undiagnosed depression 55.9% (19/34) and anxiety in 55.5% (10/18) • Active disease significantly associated with depression and anxiety	Single center

Bonnert (2017)	IBS	Randomized control trial (Internet CBT vs. wait list control)	$N = 101$ (47 vs. 54)	• Internet-based CBT: 10 weekly online modules aimed at stepwise provocation of abdominal symptoms using short texts, examples, audio files, videos, and homework exercises
				• Therapist support: asynchronous feedback, answering questions, sending reminders
					• Internet CBT vs. control at 10 weeks:
					  ○ Global GI symptom improvement $d^a = 0.45$ (0.12–0.77)
					  ○ Quality of life improvement $d^a = 0.40$ (0.13–0.70)
					  ○ Improvements sustained at 6 months
						Waitlist control group

(continued on next page)

Table 1
(continued)

Author (Year)	Condition	Study Design	Sample Size	Description of Technology	Selected Outcomes	Limitations
Ljótsson (2010)	IBS	Randomized control trial (Internet CBT vs. wait list control)	$N = 85$ (42 vs. 43)	• Internet-delivered CBT: 10 week online program with exposure and mindfulness exercises divided into five modules • Therapist support: asynchronous corrective feedback and coaching to complete modules	• Internet CBT vs. control at 10 weeks: ○ Reduction in daily GI symptoms of pain, diarrhea, bloating, nausea, flatulence, primary symptoms ($p < 0.05$) ○ Large effect size in change in severity of weekly GI symptoms between groups, $d^a = 1.21$ (0.73–1.66) ○ Quality of life improvement: $d^a = 0.93$ (0.47–1.36)	Waitlist control group
Owusu (2021)	IBS	Randomized control trial (Internet CBT vs. TAU)	$N = 36$ (25 vs. 11)	• Internet-delivered CBT: 12 week online program of eight modules; interactive pathways tailored to participant responses • Therapist support: None. Participants received biweekly reminder emails to access program	• Internet CBT baseline vs. 3 months: ○ IBS symptom severity significantly decreased from 296.3 to 232.6 ($p < 0.0001$) • Control baseline vs. 3 months: ○ IBS symptom severity remained unchanged or slightly worsened (270.7 vs. 293.7)	Small sample size

Everitt (2019)	IBS	Parallel group, randomized trial (telephone CBT vs. web-based CBT vs. TAU)	N = 558 (186 vs. 185 vs. 187)	Web-based CBT: 8 online sessions with interactive components (eg, developing a personal model, symptom diary, goal sheets, thought records, homework) Therapist support: 30 min phone calls at weeks 1,3,5 and months 4,8	Web-based CBT vs. TAU at 12 months: ○ Decrease in severity and duration of abdominal pain (p = 0.002) ○ Improvement in work and social functioning (p = 0.001)	Participants and therapists not blinded
Szigethy (2021)	FGID	Open label, non-randomized implementation trial	N = 176	Digital CBT app for mobile devices using iOS or Android operating systems. App content consisted of brief skill-building techniques (relaxation, behavioral activation, distress tolerance, cognitive reframing, mindfulness meditation), which are customizable to patient	Patients enrolled in digital CBT app: ○ Reduction in anxiety and depression at 4 months of follow-up (mean change in anxiety: 2.71 ± 5.68, 95%CI 1.28–4.01; mean change in depression: 2.85 ± 4.58, 95%CI 1.49–4.21) ○ 50% reduction in emergency room use over subsequent 6 months compared with unenrolled patients (p < 0.012)	No control group

Abbreviations: CBT, cognitive behavioral therapy; FGID, functional gastrointestinal disorders; IBD, inflammatory bowel disease; IBS, irritable bowel syndrome; TAU, treatment as usual.

[a] Cohen's *d* (95% confidence interval).

efficiently diagnose mental health disorders.[13] Although a formal psychological diagnosis relies on structured clinical interviews that involve time with a trained clinician, mental health instruments are available for less time-intensive large-scale screening of mood disorders. To measure a particular psychological trait, traditional mental health instruments are administered and scored as individual assessments with a fixed number of questions (eg, Hospital Anxiety and Depression Scale, HADS; 9 item-Patient Health Questionnaire, PHQ-9). Computerized adaptive testing, on the other hand, uses each of an individual's responses to determine the severity of a measured trait (eg, depression) and the selection of subsequent questions from an item bank that can contain hundreds of questions. In this way, an individual receives a subset of questions within minutes that are optimized to assess his or her severity of symptoms.

In a novel trial of CAT-MH in IBD, 134 consecutive patients seen at a tertiary IBD center completed adaptive testing questions screening for depression, major depressive disorder, anxiety, and suicidality.[14] The median completion time was only 3.5 minutes. Depression (positive screening for the major depressive disorder) was identified in 34 patients of whom 19 (55.9%) were previously undiagnosed. Anxiety (positive screening for generalized anxiety disorder) was identified in 18 patients of whom 10 (55.5%) were previously undiagnosed. Patients with clinically active disease, compared with those in clinical remission, had significantly higher rates of depression and anxiety: 43% vs. 18% ($p = 0.003$) and 23% vs. 10% ($p = 0.045$), respectively. Although this is a single-center study with relatively modest sample size, it shows the potential efficiency and utility of CAT-MH in screening for mental health disorders among patients with IBD. Additional studies using CAT-MH in GI disorders may lead to a more widespread and efficient diagnosis of mental health disorders as the first step in behavioral digital therapy.

With respect to behavioral digital therapeutics for the treatment of GI and psychological symptoms, several trials have shown the efficacy of Internet-delivered cognitive behavioral therapy (CBT) in GI conditions (see **Table 1**). In a trial among 101 adolescents with IBS randomized to Internet-based CBT aimed at the stepwise provocation of abdominal symptoms compared with waitlist control, there was high adherence (89%) with the majority of intervention participants completing more than half of the modules.[15] The 10-week online program consisted of text as well as audio-video presentations of exposure-based exercises aimed at reducing symptom-fear and avoidance. Accompanying modules for parents focused on encouraging their adolescents to engage in treatment. The Internet-based CBT program was supported by clinical psychologists who provided asynchronous feedback, homework assignment planning, and responses to participant questions. Participants also received text messages and phone call reminders to complete the program. After 10 weeks, there was a significantly greater reduction in the primary outcome of global GI symptoms on the Gastrointestinal Symptoms Rating Scale for IBS (GSRS-IBS) among participants in the Internet-based CBT program compared with controls, Cohen's $d = 0.45$ (95% confidence interval, CI 0.12–0.77). Improvements in secondary outcomes, such as reduction in pain intensity, pain frequency, and quality of life were also observed in the Internet-based CBT group.

A similar trial was conducted among 85 adults with IBS who were randomized to either a 10-week program of Internet-based CBT with asynchronous therapist support or waitlist control.[16] Participants in the Internet-based CBT group compared with controls experienced a significant reduction in the primary outcome of daily GI symptoms of pain, diarrhea, bloating, nausea, flatulence, and primary symptoms ($p < 0.05$). There was also a large effect size between groups with respect to GI symptom severity measured on the GSRS-IBS (Cohen's $d = 1.21$, 95% CI 0.73–1.66). Large and moderate size treatment effects were also observed in secondary outcomes of quality of life and visceral sensitivity, Cohen's $d = 0.93$, (95% CI 0.47–1.36), $d = 0.64$ (95% CI 0.20–1.07), respectively. Adherence to the program was high with 74% of Internet-based CBT participants completing at least five online sessions.

Of note, both of the above trials were designed with waitlist controls who received the Internet-based CBT program on completion of post-study assessment. One limitation of waitlist design is the inability to control participant attention and expectation of improvement. Both trials also incorporated some degree of therapist support. Minimal contact therapist support is considered an important component of ensuring participant engagement in behavioral digital therapeutics, although there is also evidence backing behavioral digital therapeutics without any therapist support.[17]

A small pilot feasibility study sought to test a self-guided (no therapist support) digital therapeutics program among 36 adults with IBS. Participants were randomized to either 12 weeks of Internet-based CBT or treatment as usual (TAU), which involved no psychotherapy. Participants received biweekly email reminders to access the Internet-based CBT program. Those in the Internet-based CBT group experienced a significant reduction with respect to the primary outcome of symptom severity on the IBS symptom severity scale (IBS-SSS) at 12 weeks compared with their baseline scores (232.6 vs. 296.3, $p < 0.0001$). IBS symptom severity remained unchanged or slightly worse in the control group (270.7 vs. 293.7). At 3 months, there was a medium treatment effect on IBS symptom severity between the Internet-based CBT and control group, Cohen's $d = 0.54$.

One of the largest trials of behavioral digital therapeutics in GI disorders was a multisite parallel-group study in which 558 adults with IBS were randomized to either telephone-delivered CBT, web-based CBT, or TAU for 12 months.[18] The web-based CBT consisted of 8 online sessions with educational components as well as instruction in behavioral and cognitive techniques to improve bowel habits and healthy eating patterns, manage stress, and reduce negative thinking and symptom focusing. The web-based CBT program was supported by a 30-min therapist phone call to participants at five different time points throughout the trial. Co-primary outcomes were severity and duration of abdominal pain and work and social adjustment at 12 months. Abdominal pain was reduced by a clinically important and statistically significant difference in the web-based CBT group compared with the TAU group ($p = 0.002$). Work and social adjustment was similarly reduced by a clinically relevant and statistically significant degree between web-based CBT and TAU ($p = 0.001$). Of note, participants in the telephone-delivered CBT group also experienced significant reductions in the co-primary outcomes compared with TAU. Adherence was also high in both CBT groups with 84.4% of participants in the telephone-delivered CBT completing at least four phone calls and 69.2% of participants in the web-based CBT group completing four web sessions. Results from this trial led to the development of a mobile device app available to IBS patients by prescription, and developers have obtained FDA clearance as a class II medical device.

With the ubiquity of mobile devices, the development of behavioral digital therapeutics specifically for a mobile device application (app) is emerging as an alternative to online programs formatted for use on a computer. One example of this is a coached digital CBT app developed and tested in a large, integrated health system for adults with functional GI disorders (FGIDs), which included conditions ranging from gastroparesis and cyclic vomiting syndrome to IBS and pelvic floor dysfunction.[19] Patients with other GI conditions, such as IBD or chronic pancreatitis who had comorbid functional pain were also included. During routine clinical encounters at a dedicated behavioral neuro-gastroenterology clinic, patients who showed symptoms of anxiety and/or depression were prescribed the app, which could be accessed on iOS and Android platforms. The app was designed based on CBT principles and delivered with a brief (5–10 min) skill-building techniques, such as relaxation, behavioral activation, distress tolerance, cognitive reframing, mindfulness, and meditation.

Of the 364 patients who were prescribed the app, 176 (48.4%) downloaded it and enrolled in the study. Patients selected either the "Anxiety Track" ($n = 126$) or the "Depression Track" ($n = 50$). Each track contained dozens of techniques that could be personalized based on interaction with health coaches who were bachelor-level graduates trained in motivational interviewing and CBT and supervised by a licensed mental health provider. Coaches communicated asynchronously (to reinforce CBT principles and navigate app techniques) with any patient who engaged via app messaging. Adherence with app usage was modest, with 100 patients (56.8%) completing 3 or more techniques, and 86 (48.9%) messaging their coach at least once.

Compared with baseline, patients using the app experienced a clinically meaningful and statistically significant reduction in anxiety, as measured by the Generalized Anxiety Disorder-7 (GAD-7), and depression, as measured by the Personal Health Questionnaire Depression Scale (PHQ-8), at up to 4 months of follow-up (mean change for GAD-7 was 2.71 ± 5.68, 95% CI 1.28–4.01; mean change for PHQ-8 was 2.85 ± 4.58, 95% CI 1.49–4.21). Additionally, as compared with patients prescribed the app who did not enroll in the study, enrolled patients had fewer emergency room visits over the subsequent 6 months (odds ratio 0.503, $p < 0.012$). Results from this study suggest the feasibility of integrating behavioral digital therapeutics into GI practice. As an open-label feasibility study, there were no uniform diagnostic criteria for assessing anxiety or depression to determine study inclusion, and patients had a range of mood disorder severity. Determining the efficacy of mobile CBT apps and the level of mood disorder severity appropriate for use of the intervention will require future randomized controlled studies. In addition, the use of mobile CBT apps to enhance, rather than replace, mental health therapy is an important area for future research. Preliminary results from a small ($n = 12$) feasibility study of IBD patients with a comorbid DSM-V anxiety disorder using a coached mobile CBT app in conjunction with face-to-face therapy suggested a dose-response reduction in levels of anxiety and a concurrent reduced need for face-to-face therapy sessions.[20]

Although most behavioral digital therapeutics are based on principles from CBT, other forms of brain–gut psychotherapy exist.[21,22] Gut-directed hypnotherapy (GDH) is a type of medical hypnosis that uses metaphors and delivers posthypnotic suggestions specific to the GI tract. GDH has been successfully applied to a variety of GI disorders including IBS, functional dyspepsia, and IBD.[23–26] However, GDH requires specialized training, and there are limited clinicians who offer this form of therapy. A recent randomized trial (NCT04133519) evaluated the efficacy of a GDH mobile app among a group of adults with IBS ($n = 362$). Participants were randomized to 12 weeks of a mobile app featuring either GDH or muscle relaxation in seven 30-minute sessions with audio-video recordings that participants completed over the course of the study period. Study findings suggest significant improvement in the primary outcome of abdominal pain intensity in the 4 weeks following the study period (weeks 13–16). Based on these results, development is underway to create the program into a prescription GDH mobile app. The app has also been granted FDA clearance as a class II medical device.

CHALLENGES IN ADOPTION OF BEHAVIORAL DIGITAL THERAPEUTICS

Behavioral digital therapeutics are poised to address barriers to mental health care for individuals with various GI disorders. However, there are still knowledge gaps in developing evidence-based therapeutics as well as challenges in their implementation into routine clinical practice. An international forum composed of leaders and stakeholders from health care organizations, payors, policy makers, and patients recently convened to discuss challenges and opportunities for digital mental health treatments and issue consensus recommendations.[27] Many of the issues raised during that forum are relevant to the current landscape of behavioral digital therapeutics in GI disorders and are summarized below.

As digital behavioral therapeutics in GI disorders reviewed in this article show, there is variability in the degree of clinician involvement. Challenges to integrating digital behavioral therapeutics into routine care will vary depending on the intensity of clinical or health coach interaction (eg, text messaging, telephone calls, concomitant face-to-face therapy) and any additional workflow required. Determining the type of behavioral digital therapeutic appropriate for different levels of mood disorder severity could allow for a stepwise approach in the level of clinician support based on patient severity of symptoms. Behavioral digital therapeutics should be viewed as enhancing, and not replacing, clinical care. Health care professionals working with patients with GI disorders should be comfortable discussing brain–gut interactions, be aware of available products on the market, and explain the rationale for directing a patient to behavioral digital therapeutics.[21,28] Interoperability of behavioral digital therapeutics across data-sharing platforms (eg, electronic medical record) would also be necessary to streamline uptake and implementation.

Reimbursement is a distinct challenge for behavioral digital therapeutics. Insurance coverage is inconsistent across different health care organizations and payors. Although regulations around telemedicine were relaxed in the wake of the coronavirus disease-2019 pandemic, billing and device codes for behavioral digital therapeutics are lacking. To unlock the potential of behavioral digital therapeutics to meet the large-scale mental health care needs of individuals with GI disorders, removing cost as a barrier to implementation is essential. Equitable distribution would also eliminate barriers based on primary language, disability, mobile device access, and reliable Internet connectivity.

Currently, there are limited regulatory processes for the development of behavioral digital therapeutics that ensure appropriate and evidence-based content is provided.[29] Acknowledging that software is becoming integral to health care and in an attempt to improve regulation of Software as Medical Device, the FDA has supported recommendations from international device regulators in attempts to promote safe innovation.[30] Non-regulatory organizations, such as the American Psychiatric Association (APA) have also issued guidance to help patients and clinicians comprehensively evaluate a mobile app before using it. The APA "App Advisor" offers a step-wise series of questions about app accessibility and background, privacy and safety, clinical foundation, usability, and therapeutic goal aimed at allowing users to make more informed decisions about which apps to engage.[31]

FUTURE DIRECTIONS

On the horizon are technology applications that better use of clinical biobanks to diagnose or risk stratify patients as well as synchronous text-based conversational agents (ie, "chatbot"). Biobank examples include a digital therapeutics platform, which analyses genetic, gut microbiome, lifestyle, and demographic data of individuals with FGIDs to predict symptom severity and personalize a management plan.[32] Synchronous text-based conversational agents designed based on natural language processing with artificial intelligence have been designed to deliver CBT in brief, daily conversations in a non-GI population with preliminary support for use in augmenting mental health treatment.[33,34] As with current behavioral digital therapeutics, essential next steps for these emerging modalities are solutions for scalability[35] and improving care flow and integration across institutions and nationally.[27]

SUMMARY

Behavioral digital therapeutics can offer a range of beneficial options for patients with GI disorders, particularly in the setting of a shortage of mental health providers. Their use may be applied to a range of indications, including screening, diagnosis, risk mitigation, and remote monitoring. In addition to enabling access to care, behavioral digital therapeutics can enhance patient engagement via therapist, health coach, or computer-assisted interactions and achieve important clinical effects. Opportunities exist to interface behavioral digital therapeutics with existing technologies, such as the electronic medical record, as well as through novel methods, such as mobile applications and artificial intelligence. Improved interoperability of technology platforms with behavioral digital therapeutics and integration into clinical care will be important to the efficiency of care and to ensure that the desired clinical outcomes are optimally achieved.

CLINICS CARE POINTS

- Behavioral digital therapeutics in gastroenterology include evidence-based interventions that leverage technology to screen and manage mental health disorders among individuals with gastrointestinal conditions.
- Internet-based cognitive behavioral therapy is an emerging behavioral digital therapeutic that can be delivered effectively to enhance face-to-face therapy as well as with minimal therapist support.
- Internet-based cognitive behavioral therapy is an emerging behavioral digital therapeutic that can be delivered effectively with minimal therapist support as well as to enhance face-to-face therapy.
- Integrating behavioral digital therapeutics into gastroenterology practice is feasible, and opportunities exist to improve scalability.

FUNDING

E. Szigethy has funding of Patient-Centered Outcomes Research Institute (PCORI) HSR Project Number HSRP20193255. R. Greywoode has no funding.

DISCLOSURE

The Authors have nothing to disclose.

REFERENCES

1. Jones MP, Dilley JB, Drossman D, et al. Brain–gut connections in functional GI disorders: anatomic and physiologic relationships. Neurogastroenterol Motil 2006;18:91–103.
2. Bonaz BL, Bernstein CN. Brain–gut interactions in inflammatory bowel disease. Gastroenterology 2013;144:36–49.

3. Creed F, Ratcliffe J, Fernandez L, et al. Health-related quality of life and health care costs in severe, refractory irritable bowel syndrome. Ann Intern Med 2001; 134:860–8.
4. Monnikes H. Quality of life in patients with irritable bowel syndrome. J Clin Gastroenterol 2011;45(Suppl):S98–101.
5. Frandemark A, Tornblom H, Jakobsson S, et al. Work productivity and activity impairment in irritable bowel syndrome (IBS): a multifaceted problem. Am J Gastroenterol 2018;113:1540–9.
6. Barberio B, Zamani M, Black CJ, et al. Prevalence of symptoms of anxiety and depression in patients with inflammatory bowel disease: a systematic review and meta-analysis. Lancet Gastroenterol Hepatol 2021;6:359–70.
7. Szigethy EM, Allen JI, Reiss M, et al. White paper AGA: the impact of mental and psychosocial factors on the care of patients with inflammatory bowel disease. Clin Gastroenterol Hepatol 2017;15:986–97.
8. Nguyen NH, Khera R, Ohno-Machado L, et al. Annual Burden and Costs of Hospitalization for High-Need, High-Cost Patients With Chronic Gastrointestinal and Liver Diseases. Clin Gastroenterol Hepatol 2018;16:1284–92.e30.
9. 2022 access to care survey results: prepared for the national council for mental wellbeing by the harris poll. Available at: https://www.thenationalcouncil.org/wp-content/uploads/2022/06/2022-Access-To-Care-Report.pdf. Accessed July 13, 2022.
10. Kosinski L, Brill JV, Sorensen M, et al. Project sonar: reduction in cost of care in an attributed cohort of patients with Crohn's disease. Gastroenterology 2016;150(4): S173.
11. Wang PA-OX, Berzin TA-O, Glissen Brown JA-O, et al. Real-time automatic detection system increases colonoscopic polyp and adenoma detection rates: a prospective randomised controlled study. Gut 2019;68:1813–9.
12. Atreja A, Khan S, Szigethy E, et al. Improved quality of care for IBD patients using HealthPROMISE app: a randomized, control trial. Am J Gastroenterol 2018; 113:S1.
13. Gibbons RD, Weiss DJ, Frank E, et al. Computerized adaptive diagnosis and testing of mental health disorders. Annu Rev Clin Psychol 2016;12:83–104.
14. Karpin J, Rodriguez TG, Traboulsi C, et al. Assessment of comorbid depression and anxiety in inflammatory bowel disease using adaptive testing technology. Crohns Colitis 2021;360:3.
15. Bonnert M, Olen O, Lalouni M, et al. Internet-delivered cognitive behavior therapy for adolescents with irritable bowel syndrome: a randomized controlled trial. Am J Gastroenterol 2017;112:152–62.
16. Ljotsson B, Falk L, Vesterlund AW, et al. Internet-delivered exposure and mindfulness based therapy for irritable bowel syndrome—a randomized controlled trial. Behav Res Ther 2010;48:531–9.
17. Karyotaki E, Riper H, Twisk J, et al. Efficacy of self-guided internet-based cognitive behavioral therapy in the treatment of depressive symptoms: a meta-analysis of individual participant data. JAMA Psychiatry 2017;74:351–9.
18. Everitt HA, Landau S, O'Reilly G, et al. Assessing telephone-delivered cognitive-behavioural therapy (CBT) and web-delivered CBT versus treatment as usual in irritable bowel syndrome (ACTIB): a multicentre randomised trial. Gut 2019;68: 1613–23.
19. Szigethy E, Tansel A, Pavlick AN, et al. A coached digital cognitive behavioral intervention reduces anxiety and depression in adults with functional gastrointestinal disorders. Clin Transl Gastroenterol 2021;12:e00436.

20. Szigethy E, Oser M, Regueiro MD, et al. Feasibility of mobile CBT for generalized anxiety among IBD patients in medical home. Gastroenterology 2017;152:S844.
21. Keefer L, Palsson OS, Pandolfino JE. Best practice update: incorporating psychogastroenterology into management of digestive disorders. Gastroenterology 2018;154:1249–57.
22. Ford AC, Lacy BE, Harris LA, et al. Effect of antidepressants and psychological therapies in irritable bowel syndrome: an updated systematic review and meta-analysis. Am J Gastroenterol 2019;114:21–39.
23. Keefer L, Taft TH, Kiebles JL, et al. Gut-directed hypnotherapy significantly augments clinical remission in quiescent ulcerative colitis. Aliment Pharmacol Ther 2013;38:761–71.
24. Calvert EL, Houghton LA, Cooper P, et al. Long-term improvement in functional dyspepsia using hypnotherapy. Gastroenterology 2002;123:1778–85.
25. Flik CE, Laan W, Zuithoff NPA, et al. Efficacy of individual and group hypnotherapy in irritable bowel syndrome (IMAGINE): a multicentre randomised controlled trial. Lancet Gastroenterol Hepatol 2019;4:20–31.
26. Palsson OS. Hypnosis treatment of gastrointestinal disorders: a comprehensive review of the empirical evidence. Am J Clin Hypn 2015;58:134–58.
27. Mohr DC, Azocar F, Bertagnolli A, et al. Banbury forum consensus statement on the path forward for digital mental health treatment. Psychiatr Serv 2021;72: 677–83.
28. Riehl ME. Limited access to integral care: digital therapeutics show promise of scalable solutions to behavioral interventions. Clin Transl Gastroenterol 2022; 13:e00444.
29. Carlo AD, Hosseini Ghomi R, Renn BN, et al. By the numbers: ratings and utilization of behavioral health mobile applications. NPJ Digit Med 2019;2:54.
30. International Medical Device Regulators Forum Software as a Medical Device (SaMD) Working Group. (2014). *Software as a Medical Device: Possible Framework for Risk Categorization and Corresponding Considerations*. International Medical Device Regulators Forum. Available at: https://www.imdrf.org/sites/default/files/docs/imdrf/final/technical/imdrf-tech-140918-samd-framework-risk-categorization-141013.pdf.
31. The app evaluation model: american psychiatric association. Available at: https://www.psychiatry.org/psychiatrists/practice/mental-health-apps/the-app-evaluation-model.
32. Kumbhare SV, Francis-Lyon PA, Kachru D, et al. Digital Therapeutics Care Utilizing Genetic and Gut Microbiome Signals for the Management of Functional Gastrointestinal Disorders: Results From a Preliminary Retrospective Study. Front Microbiol 2022;13:826916.
33. Hoermann S, McCabe KL, Milne DN, et al. Application of synchronous text-based dialogue systems in mental health interventions: systematic review. J Med Internet Res 2017;19:e267.
34. Fitzpatrick KK, Darcy A, Vierhile M. Delivering cognitive behavior therapy to young adults with symptoms of depression and anxiety using a fully automated conversational agent (Woebot): a randomized controlled trial. JMIR Ment Health 2017;4:e19.
35. Prodan A, Deimel L, Ahlqvist J, et al. Success factors for scaling up the adoption of digital therapeutics towards the realization of P5 medicine. Front Med (Lausanne) 2022;9:854665.

Psychological Considerations for Food Intolerances

Celiac Sprue, Eosinophilic Esophagitis, and Non-Celiac Gluten Sensitivity

Shayna Coburn, PhD[a], Monique Germone, PhD[b],
Josie McGarva, BS[c], Tiffany Taft, PsyD, MIS[c],*

KEYWORDS

- Food intolerance • Celiac disease • Eosinophilic esophagitis • Mental health
- Disordered eating

KEY POINTS

- Digestive illness involving food intolerances bring unique challenges to clinical management due to their impacts on psychological and social functioning and reliance on elimination diets as primary treatment strategies.
- Both pediatric and adult patients with celiac disease, non-celiac gluten sensitivity, and eosinophilic esophagitis report increased anxiety-related and hypervigilance-related eating, social ramifications including stigma and isolation, and reduced quality of life directly related to food intolerances and dietary management.
- In some patients, hypervigilance regarding food and eating may become severe and lead to disordered eating behaviors including avoidant/restrictive food intake disorder and food phobia.
- Integrated approaches using properly trained registered dietitians and clinical psychologists should be a mainstay for patients requiring long-term elimination diet treatment to mitigate some of these negative impacts.

[a] Children's National Hospital 111 Michigan Avenue NW, Center for Translational Research, 6th Flr Main, Washington, DC 20010, USA; [b] Departments of Psychiatry and Pediatrics, University of Colorado Anschutz Medical Campus, Digestive Health Institute, Children's Hospital Colorado, 13123 E. 16th Ave., B130, Aurora, CO 80045, USA; [c] Division of Gastroenterology and Hepatology, Northwestern University Feinberg School of Medicine, 676 North Saint Clair Street Suite 1400, Chicago, IL 60611, USA
* Corresponding author.
E-mail address: ttaft@northwestern.edu

Gastroenterol Clin N Am 51 (2022) 753–764
https://doi.org/10.1016/j.gtc.2022.07.003
0889-8553/22/© 2022 Elsevier Inc. All rights reserved.

INTRODUCTION

Food intolerances are a common discussion point in managing chronic digestive diseases. Most patients think certain foods can trigger their disease symptoms, which a diagnostic workup may or may not confirm. At the center of some disease management approaches are exclusionary diets, whether gluten for celiac disease (CeD), the six-food elimination diet (SFED) for eosinophilic esophagitis (EoE), or the low-fermentable oligosaccharides, disaccharides, monosaccharides and polyols (FODMAP) diet for irritable bowel syndrome. Academically, food elimination often yields excellent clinical results in the resolution of symptoms across diagnoses. However, the clinical implementation of dietary treatment is much more complicated. Moreover, real-world management of food intolerance lacks the controlled research setting and is often missing multidisciplinary supports, such as dietitians, usually present in a dietary study.

The psychological and social impacts of eliminating foods, especially those common in the Western diet, are becoming more apparent in pediatric and adult cohorts. Constructs such as food-related quality of life (FRQoL), which includes anxieties around navigating eating outside the home, finding acceptable foods to eat, and the impact on interpersonal relationships and disordered eating are garnering more attention in gastroenterology (GI) practice. A delicate balance of patient expectations and beliefs about the role of food in their disease/symptoms, translating research knowledge to the examination room, dietary treatment planning, and long-term management of secondary effects (eg, poorer FRQoL and Health-Related Quality of Life (HRQoL), mental health issues, disordered eating) is needed. Herein, we focus on GI conditions in which dietary exclusion is central to their management: CeD, non-celiac gluten sensitivity (NCGS), and EoE.

Diseases Characterized by Food Intolerance(s)

Celiac Disease

CeD is an autoimmune condition in which ingestion of gliadin protein in food causes intestinal damage and systemic inflammation.[1] Approximately 1 in 133 individuals has CeD.[2] It has a genetic component, and first-degree relatives are encouraged to be screened due to the increased risk for CeD.[3] Symptoms are heterogeneous and not necessarily diagnostic. Until recent years, it was previously thought that the primary CeD symptoms were poor growth, malabsorption, and gastrointestinal symptoms such as diarrhea, constipation, gas, bloating, and nausea/vomiting.[4,5]

However, with the increased awareness, population-based screening research, and diagnostic technology, it is now increasingly recognized that individuals diagnosed with CeD have extraintestinal manifestations in addition to classic gastrointestinal symptoms. These can include joint pain, headaches and other neurologic symptoms, and emotional and behavioral symptoms.[6] In addition, there is an elevated risk for mental health disorders among individuals with CeD across the lifespan, including anxiety and depressive disorders as well as attention-deficit/hyperactivity disorder (ADHD).[7–10]

The only current treatment for CeD is a strict gluten-free diet (GFD).[1] The GFD includes eliminating wheat, barley, and rye but also requires taking care to avoid cross-contact of even trace amounts of gluten. Thus, individuals with CeD must ask questions and check packaged products regarding the food preparation or manufacturing processes. There are also concerns about oats, which may have potential cross-contact with wheat in the growing and grinding stages,[11] and is the food most often contaminated with wheat.[12,13] The GFD becomes complicated by labeling laws in the United States, which omit some sources of gluten. For instance, labeling of major allergens includes wheat, but not necessarily barley or rye. In 2013, the Food and Drug Administration (FDA) established guidelines for voluntary labeling food as "gluten-free."[14] However, labeling food as gluten-free is not required and therefore not consistent. Some naturally gluten-free products do not necessarily include the label on the package (eg, some brands of tortilla chips). Nonfood products may also contain gluten and are not regulated by the FDA or other governing bodies. Many individuals are advised to contact manufacturers of products to verify sources of medications and cosmetic ingredients, such as vitamin E, which typically comes from wheat germ.[15]

Non-Celiac Gluten Sensitivity

NCGS is recently recognized as a condition distinct from CeD.[16] It includes a heterogeneous group of individuals who experience reactivity to gluten, even in the absence of traditional diagnostic markers of CeD. Diagnosing NCGS requires thorough knowledge in the differences and overlap of clinical presentation among gluten-related disorders and other GI disorders. Unfortunately, NCGS is not well understood, leading to distress, frustration, and stigmatization among individuals living with this condition. Recent evidence suggest NCGS may have an autoimmune basis.[16] NCGS remains an area of scientific debate leaving patients and broader society without a clear understanding of other forms of gluten sensitivity beyond CeD. NCGS also tends to have extraintestinal manifestations such as bone or joint pain, muscle cramps, and chronic fatigue, all contributing to the risk for decreased quality of life (QoL) and increased psychiatric complications.[17] Prolonged diagnosis or misdiagnosis of the correct condition and lack of clarity surrounding disease process can lead to reduced quality of life of NCGS patients.[18]

Despite a debated and unknown cause, the treatment of NCGS is also dietary, such as the GFD and the low-FODMAP diet.[16] As such, the complexities of health literacy regarding gluten in foods and other products apply to NCGS as well. At times, individuals with NCGS may be dismissed by family, friends, employers, and health-care providers. They may not be granted the same care in their food preparation or accommodations as others with a clearer diagnosis such as CeD, EoE, or food allergy. Given the uncertainty surrounding NCGS, not much is known about the impact these factors play in its management.

Eosinophilic Esophagitis

EoE is an immune-mediated non-IgE allergic reaction to exposure to certain foods, and sometimes nonfood environmental allergens.[19] The estimated incidence and prevalence rates of EoE are 5.1 cases/100,000 persons/y and 19.1 cases/100,000 persons, respectively, with a bimodal peak of incidence that includes children and adults in their 30s; it is more common in White men. In patients undergoing esophagogastroduodenoscopy (EGD), 2% to 6.5% are diagnosed with EoE,[19] and when difficulty swallowing is the reason for the EGD, EoE rates increase to 12% to 22%.

In EoE, the esophagus experiences an infiltration of eosinophils, which results in edema, longitudinal furrows, the development of esophageal rings, and narrowing or forming of strictures. Symptoms of EoE in adults include dysphagia (difficulty swallowing), chest pain, and heartburn. Patients report a sensation of food moving up and down their esophagus and of food getting stuck, necessitating regurgitation to relieve the intense discomfort. In children, symptoms tend to be nausea and vomiting, and failure to thrive. People with EoE frequently have comorbid asthma, eczema, rhinitis, or food allergies.

Treatments for EoE are limited to elimination diets and swallowed steroids. However, novel therapeutics show promise to treat EoE at the immunologic level versus present strategies.[20,21] Elimination diets for EoE include the SFED, which requires a person to remove dairy, wheat, soy, eggs, nuts/peanuts, and fish/shellfish from their diet. The SFED is an incredibly challenging diet to follow due to the regularity in which most of these food types seem in the Western diet for both pediatric[22] and adult patient populations[23] and the aforementioned challenges with accurate food labeling in the United States.

More recently, abbreviated SFED approaches are being used to reduce the burden on patients of the full SFED approach.[23,24] These include Four-Food[25] and Two-Food trials, or a step-up approach whereby foods are added should the initial elimination trials (eg, dairy, wheat) neither relieve symptoms nor improve physiology. The most common food trigger seems to be dairy, followed by wheat and soy. Most patients do not have all 6 foods as triggers for EoE, but some may, whereas others may have additional triggers (eg, sesame, other grains). Logically, EoE patients with more identified food triggers are at a greater risk for negative impacts on mental health[26] and HRQoL.[27] These can include increased anxiety related to eating,[28] reduced FRQoL, and stigmatization.[29,30]

Qualitative analysis of online discussion forums used by people with EoE found that patients were generally positive about dietary therapy while universally acknowledging how difficult it can be to follow. These results were in the context of deciding between identifying the actual triggers of their EoE versus taking corticosteroids indefinitely.[31] In terms of cost–benefit analysis, patients thought the relief of symptoms was worth the challenges of EoE elimination diets.

Hypervigilance Regarding Food, Eating, and Symptoms

With conditions requiring special diets, it is necessary to adopt vigilance surrounding everything one eats, all day, every day. Vigilance is an adaptive and protective skill to check foods before eating them, determining whether they potentially contain any ingredients that are harmful to the individual. The ideal amount of vigilance can be identified

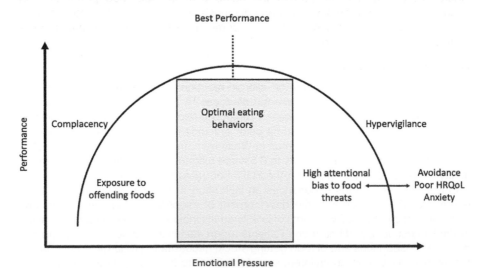

Fig. 1. Too little pressure can result in complacency and exposure to offending foods, and too much pressure can lead to poorer HRQoL and high levels of anxiety.

through Yerkes and Dodson's (1908) Inverted U Theory of Arousal,[32] in which an optimal performance is achieved through a balance between low and high "pressure." Too little pressure can result in complacency and exposure to offending foods, and too much pressure can lead to poorer HRQoL and high levels of anxiety (**Fig. 1**).

Hypervigilance occurs when pressure is too high and is characterized by a high attentional bias toward potential threats, which can precipitate or maintain a forward feedback loop in which anxiety is increased. When a person is in a hypervigilant state, the limbic system is engaged, which, on its own, does not have logical thought. Instead, the person reacts based on stimuli, or sensory information before the prefrontal cortex (PFC; ie, the thinking brain) is engaged. As a result, there may be activation of the threat response in the 1/1000th of a second it takes for that message from the limbic system to arrive at the PFC, thereby influencing the interpretation of the original stimuli and symptom experience. For example, in EoE, hypervigilance to esophageal sensations is a greater predictor of increased dysphagia symptoms and poorer HRQoL than physiologic testing.[33] Patients with a history of traumatic experiences (eg, abuse, combat, crime victim) may be at particular risk for this threat response due to the impacts trauma has on the nervous system and response to threat. Trauma may have existed before a medical diagnosis or may evolve from disease experiences.[34,35] Hypervigilance to symptoms can translate to hypervigilance regarding food and eating,[36] causing even typical sensations from eating and digestion to be amplified and difficult to ignore.[33] A person with hypervigilance may check in regularly with their body, taking pauses during meals to assess how their digestive system is responding to the ingested food. Any sign of "trouble" may be met with the person abruptly stopping eating and assumptions the food is now permanently off limits without concrete evidence that a consistent, direct link to digestive symptoms exists.

By nature, the process of identifying allergens or trigger foods and actively avoiding them requires vigilance.[28,31,36] The emphasis on consistent attention to avoiding specific foods serves as a potential foundation for those at risk for hypervigilance. Individuals are told by their health-care team that there can be short-term and long-term health risks from food exposure[37] or continued inflammation.[19] In many cases, even trace amounts of these ingredients may sicken a person. They may not experience symptoms at times but could still incur physiologic damage (eg, in asymptomatic CeD or EoE). In some cases, such as with gluten or other foods not on the major allergen list mandated under food labeling laws, individuals must be suspicious of any packaged food or food prepared outside of their home. There is often no definitive answer as to whether a product is safe unless explicitly labeled (eg, gluten-free, a voluntary label in the United States).[14] Even so, contamination is often a concern. Vigilance is not only limited to foods. Individuals are instructed to be cautious of medications, lip balms, makeup, toothpaste, and many other products, yet the quality of data informing recommendations may be insufficient.[38] In young children,[22] art supplies and other materials must be scrutinized because some of the material could be ingested (eg, Play-Doh).[39]

An aspect of vigilance in conditions with food intolerance is the concern about a potential reaction to the offending food. When there are doubts about the safety of a food ingested, individuals may use high attentional bias toward bodily functions and sensations, leading to anxiety and increased symptoms.[33,36] These doubts can confuse individuals and obscure an already murky process of recognizing potential signs of reactions, leading to functional pain and other symptoms. Furthermore, these doubts and symptoms can cause individuals to avoid foods or situations unnecessarily as a protective strategy, which eventually may reduce quality of life,[36] and/or increase symptoms of depression or other mental distress.

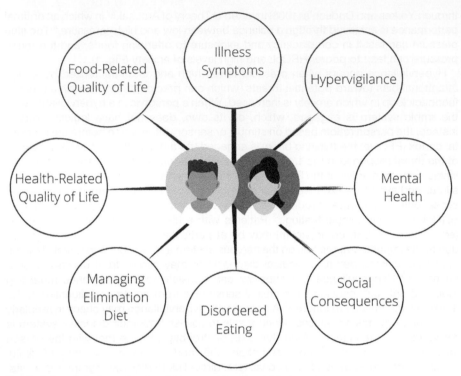

Fig. 2. Interrelated constructs when managing food intolerances.

Impact of Elimination Diets on Mental Health and Disordered Eating Behaviors

The mental health impact of food intolerance and associated dietary strategies can be pervasive and intertwined (**Fig. 2**). The initial adjustment to a chronic illness diagnosis and its dietary treatment can elicit feelings of grief and loss, which must be navigated by individuals, caregivers, and often the entire household. Changes to daily life, ranging from planning ingredients in recipes to navigating social activities, require significant adaptive coping and executive functioning skills. As mentioned, worrying about eating as a trigger of symptoms is common and can become severe, as in the case of Avoidant/Restrictive Food Intake Disorder (ARFID; Helen Burton Murray and Samantha Calabrese's article, "Identification and Management of Eating Disorders (including ARFID) in GI Patient," in this issue). People report losing enjoyment from eating, in part, due to stress related to planning activities around eating and anxiety about having symptoms in front of others or in public.[27] Embarrassment about having to advocate for dietary needs that may be heavily stigmatized, such as GFDs, which have become more popular among those without CeD, NCGS, or EoE, can lead to isolation, either self-inflicted or being intentionally or unintentionally left out of social events or work functions.[8,28,29,40]

Patients with food intolerances often must make quick decisions about whether to eat a particular food, especially in social situations or around others whom they do not know. These quick decisions can lead to regret in eating foods that make symptoms worse, with corresponding frustration about the degree of attention and focus they must pay to how food may affect their condition. Over time, a person may feel a loss of control surrounding what they can and cannot eat or feel that they do not have many options for dietary variety. In some patients, compensatory behaviors may arise, such as overly "clean" eating (ie, orthorexia), extreme emphasis on "safe" foods, or turning to dietary supplements to maintain nutritional status.

Celiac Disease

The symptoms and treatment of CeD can lay the groundwork for the development of disordered eating due to concerns about physical reactions to gluten and the nature of a strict GFD. Individuals may experience emotional distress and negative body image in response to weight gain that may occur once nutrient absorption improves, leading to anorexia nervosa or bulimia nervosa.[41] Related, but distinct from body image concerns, fears of physical symptoms and other aversive experiences in CeD[42] may lead to unnecessary additional restriction of the variety, quantity, or frequency of foods eaten, as in ARFID.[43] Alternatively, insecurities around reduced access to palatable gluten-free food options may lead to binge eating behaviors when safe or desirable foods become available.[41] Disordered eating can have a major negative impact on achieving optimal physical health and overall quality of life in CeD.[40]

Non-Celiac Gluten Sensitivity

The experiences of those with NCGS mirror those with CeD with the added burden of living with a somewhat controversial and poorly understood condition. Because of the lack of a definitive diagnosis, those with NCGS may feel even more stigmatized about the use of a GFD because "there's nothing really wrong with them." They may be more likely to be diagnosed with ARFID because their food restriction due to fear of GI symptoms may be deemed to be beyond what is "reasonable and expected" when compared with a person with a definitive disease such as CeD or EoE. The dearth of literature on NCGS and disordered eating makes it difficult to draw conclusions; however, clinicians should be aware of the added social and emotional complexities of NCGS when treating these individuals.

Eosinophilic Esophagitis

There is only a single study in pediatric patients with EoE on disordered eating, comprising 2 case studies, both of whom developed disordered eating behaviors to cope with their disease.[44] In adults, a small sample of EoE patients (N = 53) as part of a more extensive study on ARFID found that 42.9% of participants met the diagnostic cutoff using the Nine Item ARFID scale (NIAS).[45] The authors caution interpreting this finding due to limitations in the NIAS in GI populations because half the variance in NIAS score was explained by fear of GI symptoms. Worry about unpleasant symptoms, such as food impactions (which are medical emergencies), and hypervigilance to esophageal sensations act as adaptive responses to a perceived threat. The limitations in the NIAS in GI populations, combined with the use of elimination diets as a primary treatment of EoE, makes understanding disordered eating in EoE quite complicated.

Stigma and Bullying

Limited research on stigma toward GI disease finds patients with EoE and CeD do report disease-related stigmatization,[29,30,46] and dietary treatment seems to be a contributing factor. The GFD has become highly popular in recent years, although most individuals choosing the GFD have done so by choice and not due to a medical condition. The popularity of the GFD by choice has led to more misinformation and stigma in the community for those requiring the GFD for medical reasons. However, the popularity of the GFD may have led to the availability of more GF foods, especially those offered by major food manufacturers, and have facilitated the more widely available GF options at restaurants.

Bullying is unfortunately common in children with food intolerances having to follow a strict diet. Similar to stigma, bullying makes the child feel different and excluded by peers. Others lack knowledge about the child's health condition and its treatment such that children cannot necessarily go to any adult for help, adults may have judgments of parents and/or their children, and may harbor resentment in having to accommodate dietary restrictions. In a 2013 study of 251 children with food allergies and their parents, 31.5% of the children and 24.7% of the parents reported bullying or harassment specifically due to dietary restrictions, including threats with foods by classmates as a means of intimidation.[47] Similar proportions of children report bullying due to food allergy in additional studies[48,49] and children from racial minority groups may be more affected than White peers.[50] To date, no studies exist evaluating bullying specifically in children with CeD or EoE.

Psychological Interventions

Behavioral interventions adapted for chronic digestive diseases are available to reduce the psychological and social impacts of food intolerances and related treatments. These include cognitive behavioral therapy (CBT), acceptance and commitment therapy (ACT), and mindfulness-based stress reduction (MBSR).[51–54] Although research is limited in the application of these approaches to food intolerance, they are highly effective in reducing symptom-specific anxiety and hypervigilance, reducing disordered eating, and improving HRQoL across multiple GI conditions.

In CBT, patients are taught to identify counterproductive thinking about food intolerances and replace these thoughts with more adaptive responses to a chronic condition necessitating dietary changes (eg, "I will never figure out what I can and cannot eat" to "I know sometimes a food may disagree with my system but that does not mean I can never eat it again"). This thought reframing reduces catastrophizing (expecting the worst-case scenario) and introduces additional behavioral strategies to increase self-efficacy, which is often lost in catastrophic worry. Exposure therapies can also help patients who may have extreme food fears to reintroduce beyond their "safe food" list or reduce other avoidance behaviors that have become problematic.

In ACT and MBSR, which are theoretic extensions of CBT, patients are taught to focus more on the present moment versus predicting future events, engage in values-based activities, and defuse repetitive thinking or rumination about eating. In CBT, ACT, and MBSR, relaxation strategies (eg, diaphragmatic breathing, meditation) are combined with cognitive exercises to reduce autonomic nervous system arousal and corresponding hypervigilance. Clinicians working with pediatric or adult patients with food intolerances will benefit from partnering with a mental health practitioner skilled in GI behavioral therapies or, if unavailable, a practitioner with experience in chronic illness populations. The Rome Foundation Psychogastroenteorlogy Group has an online directory of GI behavioral health providers (https://romegipsych.org) for reference.

SUMMARY

Individuals with conditions requiring special diets may experience several psychosocial challenges due to the nature of their symptoms and the burden of treatment. Even with clear and effective treatments, psychological support is needed due to their inherently challenging and often stressful nature. Reactions to foods can invoke both physical and emotional distress, leading to vulnerability to developing comorbid psychological conditions (eg, anxiety, depression, and eating disorders). A special diet requires the affected individual (or caregivers) to remain constantly vigilant around food and other materials with which they make contact. In addition, significant social challenges can arise with food being a social activity in most cultures and settings. For these reasons, maintaining optimal adherence is difficult.

Psychosocial support can be an important resource to build effective coping strategies using frameworks such as CBT and ACT to address hypervigilance, anxiety, and disordered eating that may develop because of food intolerances. Psychological support also helps identify and address potential barriers and explore any ambivalence about adherence to a special diet. There has been a growing emphasis on psychological services as part of a multidisciplinary standard of care for conditions requiring special diets in recent years. Additional implementation and evaluation of these services will help advance efforts to develop and refine appropriate empirically supported interventions to optimize self-management and quality of life.

CLINICS CARE POINTS

- When managing patients with food intolerances using dietary treatment, screen for baseline anxiety especially because it relates to food and its relationship to digestive symptoms.
- Discuss the potential psychological and social impacts that may occur with patients being prescribed or using self-directed dietary approaches and monitor at each follow-up.
- If possible, establish referral relationships with qualified registered dietitians and mental health clinicians with specific training in digestive disease and food intolerances in your area as resources for patients. Introduce these early in treatment to prevent poor outcomes.
- Learn nonstigmatizing language to discuss disordered eating to demonstrate to your patients that you understand the unique challenges of long-term dietary treatment.

DISCLOSURE

T. Taft has served as a consultant for Takeda, Reckitt, and Healthline. The remaining authors have nothing to disclose.

S. Coburn's research is supported by the National Institute Of Diabetes And Digestive And Kidney Diseases of the National Institutes of Health under Award Number K23DK129826. The content is solely the responsibility of the authors and does not necessarily represent the official views of the National Institutes of Health.

REFERENCES

1. Rubio-Tapia A, Hill ID, Kelly CP, et al. ACG clinical guidelines: diagnosis and management of celiac disease. Am J Gastroenterol 2013;108:656–76, quiz 677. PMC3706994.
2. Mustalahti K, Catassi C, Reunanen A, et al. The prevalence of celiac disease in Europe: results of a centralized, international mass screening project. Ann Med 2010;42:587–95.
3. Singh P, Arora S, Lal S, et al. Risk of Celiac Disease in the First- and Second-Degree Relatives of Patients With Celiac Disease: A Systematic Review and Meta-Analysis. Am J Gastroenterol 2015;110:1539–48.
4. Uche-Anya E, Lebwohl B. Celiac disease: clinical update. Curr Opin Gastroenterol 2021;37:619–24.

5. Silvester JA, Therrien A, Kelly CP. Celiac Disease: Fallacies and Facts. Am J Gastroenterol 2021;116:1148–55. PMC8462980.
6. Durazzo M, Ferro A, Brascugli I, et al. Extra-Intestinal Manifestations of Celiac Disease: What Should We Know in 2022? J Clin Med 2022;11. PMC8746138.
7. Lebwohl B, Haggard L, Emilsson L, et al. Psychiatric Disorders in Patients With a Diagnosis of Celiac Disease During Childhood From 1973 to 2016. Clin Gastroenterol Hepatol 2021;19:2093–2101 e13.
8. Zingone F, Swift GL, Card TR, et al. Psychological morbidity of celiac disease: A review of the literature. United Eur Gastroenterol J 2015;3:136–45. PMC4406898.
9. Coburn SS, Puppa EL, Blanchard S. Psychological Comorbidities in Childhood Celiac Disease: A Systematic Review. J Pediatr Gastroenterol Nutr 2019;69: e25–33.
10. Coburn S, Rose M, Sady M, et al. Mental Health Disorders and Psychosocial Distress in Pediatric Celiac Disease. J Pediatr Gastroenterol Nutr 2020;70: 608–14.
11. Guennouni M, Admou B, El Khoudri N, et al. Gluten contamination in labelled gluten-free, naturally gluten-free and meals in food services in low-, middle- and high-income countries: a systematic review and meta-analysis. Br J Nutr 2021;1–15.
12. Pinto-Sanchez MI, Causada-Calo N, Bercik P, et al. Safety of Adding Oats to a Gluten-Free Diet for Patients With Celiac Disease: Systematic Review and Meta-analysis of Clinical and Observational Studies. Gastroenterology 2017; 153:395–409 e3.
13. Fritz RD, Chen Y. Oat safety for celiac disease patients: theoretical analysis correlates adverse symptoms in clinical studies to contaminated study oats. Nutr Res 2018;60:54–67.
14. Food, Drug Administration HHS. Food labeling: gluten-free labeling of foods. Final rule. Fed Regist 2013;78:47154–79.
15. Thompson T. The gluten-free labeling rule: what registered dietitian nutritionists need to know to help clients with gluten-related disorders. J Acad Nutr Diet 2015;115:13–6.
16. Cardenas-Torres FI, Cabrera-Chavez F, Figueroa-Salcido OG, et al. Non-Celiac Gluten Sensitivity: An Update. Medicina (Kaunas) 2021;57. PMC8224613.
17. Porcelli B, Verdino V, Bossini L, et al. Celiac and non-celiac gluten sensitivity: a review on the association with schizophrenia and mood disorders. Auto Immun Highlights 2014;5:55–61. PMC4389040.
18. Tovoli F, Granito A, Negrini G, et al. Long term effects of gluten-free diet in non-celiac wheat sensitivity. Clin Nutr 2019;38:357–63.
19. Khan S, Guo X, Liu T, et al. An Update on Eosinophilic Esophagitis: Etiological Factors, Coexisting Diseases, and Complications. Digestion 2021;102:342–56.
20. Chehade M, Aceves SS. Treatment of Eosinophilic Esophagitis: Diet or Medication? J Allergy Clin Immunol Pract 2021;9:3249–56.
21. Rokkas T, Niv Y, Malfertheiner P. A Network Meta-Analysis of Randomized Controlled Trials on the Treatment of Eosinophilic Esophagitis in Adults and Children. J Clin Gastroenterol 2021;55:400–10.
22. Hannan N, McMillan SS, Tiralongo E, et al. Treatment Burden for Pediatric Eosinophilic Esophagitis: A Cross-Sectional Survey of Carers. J Pediatr Psychol 2021; 46:100–11.
23. Lucendo AJ, Molina-Infante J. Treatment of eosinophilic esophagitis with diets. Minerva Gastroenterol Dietol 2020;66:124–35.

24. Wechsler JB, Schwartz S, Arva NC, et al. A Single Food Milk Elimination Diet Is Effective for Treatment of Eosinophilic Esophagitis in Children. Clin Gastroenterol Hepatol 2022;20(8). 1748.e11–1756.e11.

25. Molina-Infante J, Arias A, Barrio J, et al. Four-food group elimination diet for adult eosinophilic esophagitis: A prospective multicenter study. J Allergy Clin Immunol 2014;134:1093–9.e1.

26. Taft TH, Guadagnoli L, Edlynn E. Anxiety and Depression in Eosinophilic Esophagitis: A Scoping Review and Recommendations for Future Research. J Asthma Allergy 2019;12:389–99. PMC6910091.

27. Taft TH, Kern E, Keefer L, et al. Qualitative assessment of patient-reported outcomes in adults with eosinophilic esophagitis. J Clin Gastroenterol 2011;45: 769–74.

28. Wang R, Hirano I, Doerfler B, et al. Assessing Adherence and Barriers to Long-Term Elimination Diet Therapy in Adults with Eosinophilic Esophagitis. Dig Dis Sci 2018;63:1756–62. PMC6166243.

29. Guadagnoli L, Taft TH, Keefer L. Stigma perceptions in patients with eosinophilic gastrointestinal disorders. Dis Esophagus 2017;30:1–8. PMC5770239.

30. Guadagnoli L, Taft TH. Internalized Stigma in Patients with Eosinophilic Gastrointestinal Disorders. J Clin Psychol Med Settings 2020;27:1–10. PMC6688970.

31. Chang JW, Chen VL, Rubenstein JH, et al. What patients with eosinophilic esophagitis may not share with their providers: a qualitative assessment of online health communities Dis Esophagus 2021.

32. Perkins CC Jr. The relation between conditioned stimulus intensity and response strength. J Exp Psychol 1953;46:225–31.

33. Taft TH, Carlson DA, Simons M, et al. Esophageal Hypervigilance and Symptom-Specific Anxiety in Patients with Eosinophilic Esophagitis. Gastroenterology 2021; 161:1133–44. PMC8463417.

34. De Young AC, Paterson RS, Brown EA, et al. Topical Review: Medical Trauma During Early Childhood. J Pediatr Psychol 2021;46:739–46.

35. Appel PR. Post-traumatic stress in the medical setting. Am J Clin Hypn 2020;63: 112–27.

36. Wolf RL, Lebwohl B, Lee AR, et al. Hypervigilance to a Gluten-Free Diet and Decreased Quality of Life in Teenagers and Adults with Celiac Disease. Dig Dis Sci 2018;63:1438–48.

37. Mones RL. Incidence of autoimmune diseases in celiac disease: protective effect of the gluten-free diet. J Pediatr Gastroenterol Nutr 2009;48:645–6.

38. Theodoridis X, Grammatikopoulou MG, Petalidou A, et al. Dietary management of celiac disease: Revisiting the guidelines. Nutrition 2019;66:70–7.

39. Weisbrod VM, Silvester JA, Raber C, et al. A Quantitative Assessment of Gluten Cross-contact in the School Environment for Children With Celiac Disease. J Pediatr Gastroenterol Nutr 2020;70:289–94. PMC7857141.

40. Cadenhead JW, Wolf RL, Lebwohl B, et al. Diminished quality of life among adolescents with coeliac disease using maladaptive eating behaviours to manage a gluten-free diet: a cross-sectional, mixed-methods study. J Hum Nutr Diet 2019; 32:311–20. PMC6467807.

41. Satherley RM, Higgs S, Howard R. Disordered eating patterns in coeliac disease: a framework analysis. J Hum Nutr Diet 2017;30:724–36.

42. Satherley RM, Lerigo F, Higgs S, et al. An interpretative phenomenological analysis of the development and maintenance of gluten-related distress and unhelpful eating and lifestyle patterns in coeliac disease. Br J Health Psychol 2022;27: 1026–42.

43. Zysk W, Glabska D, Guzek D. Food Neophobia in Celiac Disease and Other Gluten-Free Diet Individuals. Nutrients 2019;11. PMC6722680.
44. Robson J, Laborda T, Fitzgerald S, et al. Avoidant/Restrictive Food Intake Disorder in Diet-treated Children With Eosinophilic Esophagitis. J Pediatr Gastroenterol Nutr 2019;69:57–60.
45. Fink M, Simons M, Tomasino K, et al. When Is Patient Behavior Indicative of Avoidant Restrictive Food Intake Disorder (ARFID) Vs Reasonable Response to Digestive Disease? Clin Gastroenterol Hepatol 2022;20(6):1250.
46. Olsson C, Lyon P, Hornell A, et al. Food that makes you different: the stigma experienced by adolescents with celiac disease. Qual Health Res 2009;19:976–84.
47. Shemesh E, Annunziato RA, Ambrose MA, et al. Child and parental reports of bullying in a consecutive sample of children with food allergy. Pediatrics 2013; 131:e10-7. PMC3529950.
48. Cooke F, Ramos A, Herbert L. Food Allergy-Related Bullying Among Children and Adolescents. J Pediatr Psychol 2022;47:318–26. PMC8898384.
49. Lieberman JA, Weiss C, Furlong TJ, et al. Bullying among pediatric patients with food allergy. Ann Allergy Asthma Immunol 2010;105:282–6.
50. Brown D, Negris O, Gupta R, et al. Food allergy-related bullying and associated peer dynamics among Black and White children in the FORWARD study. Ann Allergy Asthma Immunol 2021;126:255–263 e1. PMC7897313.
51. Palsson OS, Ballou S. Hypnosis and Cognitive Behavioral Therapies for the Management of Gastrointestinal Disorders. Curr Gastroenterol Rep 2020;22:31.
52. Aucoin M, Lalonde-Parsi MJ, Cooley K. Mindfulness-based therapies in the treatment of functional gastrointestinal disorders: a meta-analysis. Evid Based Complement Alternat Med 2014;2014:140724. PMC4177184.
53. Cherpak CE. Mindful Eating: A Review Of How The Stress-Digestion-Mindfulness Triad May Modulate And Improve Gastrointestinal And Digestive Function. Integr Med (Encinitas) 2019;18:48–53. PMC7219460.
54. Wynne B, McHugh L, Gao W, et al. Acceptance and Commitment Therapy Reduces Psychological Stress in Patients With Inflammatory Bowel Diseases. Gastroenterology 2019;156:935–945 e1.

Identification and Management of Eating Disorders (including ARFID) in GI Patients

Helen Burton Murray, PhD[a,b,c,*], Samantha Calabrese, CNP[a]

KEYWORDS

- Avoidant/restrictive food intake disorder • Feeding and eating disorders
- Disorders of gut–brain interaction • Functional gastrointestinal disorders
- Inflammatory bowel disorders • Celiac disease

KEY POINTS

- There is growing awareness of the intersection between eating disorders and gastrointestinal conditions, including bidirectional risk and maintenance pathways.
- The risk of avoidant/restrictive food intake disorder is of particular concern in individuals with disorders of gut–brain interaction and is differentiated from other eating disorders by a lack of body image-driven diet restriction.
- Gastroenterology providers have the ability to identify and potentially play a role in the prevention of eating disorders.
- We provide recommendations for the evaluation of eating disorder symptoms, including medical red flags, outpatient medical monitoring, and clinical history assessment.

INTRODUCTION

The intersection between gastrointestinal (GI) disorders and eating disorders has gained increasing attention in the gastroenterology field.[1–6] In particular, the emergence of a nonbody image-based eating disorder, avoidant/restrictive food intake disorder (ARFID), has become highly relevant given its comorbidity rates (13%–40%)[7–13] with disorders of gut–brain interaction (formerly known as functional GI disorders). In this conceptual review, we provide a practical guide for the gastroenterology provider for identification and management of eating disorder

[a] Division of Gastroenterology, Massachusetts General Hospital, 55 Fruit Street, Boston, MA 02114, USA; [b] Harvard Medical School, 25 Shattuck St, Boston, MA 02115, USA; [c] Department of Psychiatry, Massachusetts General Hospital, 55 Fruit Street, Boston, MA 02114, USA
* Corresponding author. Division of Gastroenterology, Massachusetts General Hospital, 55 Fruit Street, Boston, MA 02114. .
E-mail address: hbmurray@mgh.harvard.edu

Gastroenterol Clin N Am 51 (2022) 765–783
https://doi.org/10.1016/j.gtc.2022.07.004
0889-8553/22/© 2022 Elsevier Inc. All rights reserved.

gastro.theclinics.com

symptoms—we place emphasis on symptoms, as the behaviors and cognitive processes of eating disorders lie along a spectrum and may be missed if not viewed as such. In the following sections, we: (1) conceptually describe how eating disorders and GI symptoms can interact; (2) delineate ARFID from other eating disorders; and (3) provide recommendations for eating disorder assessment.

The Eating Disorder—Gastrointestinal Symptom Intersection

We classify two pathways in which eating disorders and GI disorders can be related. The first is *etiology*—how GI disorders may put some patients at risk for eating disorders and vice versa. The second is *maintenance*—how eating disorder symptoms perpetuate GI symptoms and vice versa.

Eating disorder versus gastrointestinal disorder—which comes first?

There are multiple etiologic pathways through which eating disorders may intersect with GI disorders, for which research is nascent. We summarize each potential pathway as follows:

Concurrent development

Individuals with eating disorders commonly report GI symptoms that may develop due to the eating disorder,[14] and may either resolve or persist after eating disorder resolution. For example, delayed gastric emptying has been reported in anorexia nervosa,[15] and bulimia nervosa,[16] but methods used to assess gastric emptying are now outdated. Underweight status (from studies in anorexia nervosa) has been associated with delayed colonic transit that typically normalizes with refeeding.[17–19] Among individuals with eating disorders, GI symptoms are common,[8,13,20] with some research in inpatients suggesting persistence even after eating disorder treatment resolution.[21,22] Similarly, eating disorder symptoms, such as dietary restriction, binge eating, and purging have been reported in 5%–44% of individuals with GI conditions.[14] However, whether eating disorder symptoms were the cause of the GI symptoms or vice versa from these reports is unknown.

An eating disorder may also develop in the context of a GI disorder. For example, ARFID symptoms have been reported in approximately 25% of pediatric and adult patients with disorders of gut–brain interaction (range = 13%–40%) based on studies using self-report surveys or chart review diagnosis.[7–12] While no study to date has evaluated the development of ARFID prospectively, cross-sectional data show that a history of using an exclusion diet was associated with a three-fold greater likelihood of having ARFID symptoms among pediatric and adult patients with disorders of gut–brain interaction.[23] Thus, we urge providers to use caution when prescribing dietary approaches for disorders of gut–brain interaction—a recent Rome working team report provides guidance on the psychological and nutritional considerations of diet in disorders of gut–brain interaction.[24] Recent practice guidelines for irritable bowel syndrome also suggest exclusion diets should not be prescribed for patients who already have restricted diets and provide clear guidance that exclusion diets should have predetermined durations to prevent disordered eating and/or malnutrition.[6]

ARFID can also develop in disorders with a more structural or organic etiology, such as inflammatory bowel disease—there is concern about overinflated rates of ARFID, with recent self-report survey studies indicating 14% to 53% of adults with inflammatory bowel disease screen positive for ARFID,[25,26] but these are likely lower during disease remission. Other eating disorder symptoms (eg, diet rigidity due to health concerns, laxative abuse) may also develop in the context of GI disorders. It is possible that eating disorder symptoms persist even once the GI disorder is managed, but research is lacking to support this.

Prospective risk

Risk for eating disorder development certainly applies for concurrent development (as discussed earlier). However, what may be less obvious is the potential that *past* eating disorders or GI symptoms could increase risk for one or the other. For example, the development of a new disorder of gut–brain interaction has been reported 1 year after eating disorder inpatient treatment.[22] GI symptoms (eg, abdominal pain) during childhood have also been shown to increase the risk of later eating disorder symptoms.[27] Further, prospective research has shown a heightened bidirectional risk between eating disorders and autoimmune conditions, including inflammatory bowel diseases and celiac disease.[28] It is possible neurosensory changes that occur with both GI and eating disorder symptoms may share etiologic pathways that relate to bidirectional risk, but again, research is nascent in this regard.

Bidirectional maintenance between eating and gastrointestinal disorders— Particularly Disorders of Gut–brain interaction

While eating disorders and GI symptoms may have shared factors that contribute to their respective development, what starts something is not always what keeps it going. There are multiple *maintenance* pathways through which eating disorder symptoms and GI symptoms may contribute to each other's perpetuation (**Fig. 1**). In particular, bidirectional maintenance may be most relevant for disorders of gut–brain interaction and eating disorder symptoms. For example, one cross-sectional study found that among adults with chronic constipation, GI-specific anxiety mediated the relationship between eating disorder symptoms and constipation symptom severity—suggesting that GI-specific anxiety is a possible mechanism through which eating disorder symptoms perpetuate symptoms associated with constipation.[29] In addition, avoidant/restrictive eating that leads to weight loss may maintain poor gastric accommodation and tolerance disturbances seen in functional dyspepsia.[30,31] More research is needed to understand the biologic and behavioral mechanisms at

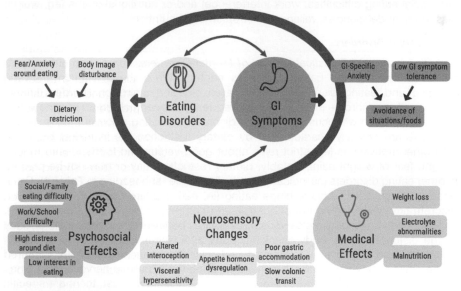

Fig. 1. Conceptual model of the eating disorder—gastrointestinal intersection.

this intersection. There are numerous candidate mechanisms that warrant further exploration to identify treatment targets; some examples are listed hereunder:

- Brain–gut dysregulation makes it difficult to tolerate eating
- Dysmotility contributes to perpetuation of eating disorder cognitions (thoughts) or behaviors
- Eating disorder behaviors contribute to GI motility and sensory disturbances (eg, through visceral hypersensitivity, appetite hormone dysregulation)
- Eating disorder cognitions (thoughts) contribute to GI hypervigilance (which in turn perpetuates brain–gut dysregulation)

WHAT ARE EATING DISORDERS?

Eating disorders include a spectrum of cognitions (ie, thought patterns) and behaviors around eating and/or body image that negatively affect nutritional status and/or quality of life. Example cognitions may be related to fear of GI symptoms around eating (eg, "If I eat X food, I will throw up") or overvaluation of body shape/weight (eg, "I will never be happy unless I lose 20 lbs"). The cognitive processes vary among eating disorders but a core behavioral manifestation is related to undereating, which includes either *attempts to* restrict or *actual* restriction of food intake. **Table 1** delineates features of the spectrum of eating disorders and separates out ARFID from other eating disorders.

Avoidant/Restrictive Food Intake Disorder

ARFID has garnered particular attention in the GI space recently. ARFID is characterized by a reduction in food volume and/or variety motivated by one or more prototypic presentation: fear of aversive consequences (eg, vomiting, abdominal pain), lack of interest in eating/low appetite (eg, forgetting to eat, high satiation), and/or sensory sensitivity (eg, to taste, smell, appearance). Avoidant/restrictive eating does lie along a spectrum, on which many GI patients may fit into. However, avoidant/restrictive eating may be considered to cross the line to ARFID when it affects quality of life (eg, social eating difficulties, work interference) and/or nutritional status (eg, weight loss, nutrient deficiencies, reliance on supplemental nutrition).[32]

Other Eating Disorders

The *Diagnostic and Statistical Manual of Mental Disorders,* fifth edition (*DSM-5*) includes a Feeding and Eating Disorders section. While the distinction between "feeding" and "eating" disorders is still debated, pica and rumination disorders (known as rumination syndrome in Rome IV) are frequently conceptualized as feeding disorders, and as such we focus on the other disorders as eating disorders. Other eating disorders are typically characterized by dietary restriction like in ARFID but often with other motivations (eg, strict rules about good versus bad foods, desire to lose weight, fear of weight gain). Notably, dietary restriction may or may not be present in other eating disorders (as indicated by the "possible" subheading in **Table 1**). Other behavioral symptoms include binge eating (ie, eating a large quantity of food in a discrete time while feeling out of control) and compensatory/purging behaviors (eg, self-induced vomiting, exercise abuse), as well as behavioral manifestations of body image disturbance (eg, body checking, body avoidance). Constellations of certain behavioral and cognitive symptoms at particular frequencies/severity are captured in the *DSM-5* as specific disorders—anorexia nervosa, bulimia nervosa, and binge eating disorders; when the criteria for these (or ARFID) are not met, there are specific examples of disorders within a catchall other specified feeding or eating disorder category (eg, atypical anorexia). In addition, ARFID symptoms can be comorbid with other eating disorder symptoms; in most cases, the ARFID diagnosis is likely only appropriate when it is the *primary* eating disorder.

EATING DISORDER ASSESSMENT

Given the bidirectional relationship between eating disorders and GI symptoms, the gastroenterology provider needs to be aware of both frank red flags and potential lower

Table 1 Characteristics of *DSM-5* eating disorders		
	Avoidant/Restrictive Food Intake Disorder	**Other Eating Disorders**
Dietary Restriction (reduced frequency, volume, or variety of food intake)	YES Motivated by (one or more) • Fear of aversive consequences (eg, choking, nausea, diarrhea) • Lack of interest in eating/low appetite • Sensitivity to sensory characteristics of food	POSSIBLE Motivated by (one or more) • Fear of weight gain • Body image disturbance • High rigidity around eating due to overconcern with "healthy" eating (known outside of the *DSM-5* as orthorexia)
Compromised Nutrition Status	YES[a] • Weight loss • Inability to gain weight/grow • Nutrient deficiencies • Dependence on supplemental nutrition	POSSIBLE • Weight loss • Inability to gain weight/grow • Nutrient deficiencies • Dependence on supplemental nutrition
Quality of Life Impairment/Distress	YES[a] • Social eating difficulties • Significant distress around eating • Family difficulties • Work difficulties • Concentration difficulties	POSSIBLE • Social eating difficulties • Significant distress around eating • Family difficulties • Work difficulties • Concentration difficulties
Overvaluation of body shape/weight	NO	POSSIBLE • Explicitly self-reported (eg, fear of weight gain, desire to lose weight) • Based on clinician's judgment that the patient is continuing to engage in persistent behavior interfering with weight gain (when indicated) • Body checking (eg, repeated mirror checking) • Body avoidance (eg, wearing loose clothing)
Binge Eating	NO	POSSIBLE A sense of loss of control (ie, feeling like one cannot stop eating) while eating a large quantity of food in a discrete period

(continued on next page)

Table 1 (continued)		
	Avoidant/Restrictive Food Intake Disorder	Other Eating Disorders
Purging Behaviors	NO	POSSIBLE Regular use of behaviors for weight/shape control that may or may not be directly related to binge eating episodes • Self-induced vomiting • Fasting • Exercise • Laxative or other medication abuse

Note. This table highlights avoidant/restrictive eating disorder (ARFID) and other eating disorders. Characteristics of other eating disorders include those of anorexia nervosa, bulimia nervosa, binge eating disorder, and other specified feeding or eating disorders. Characteristics across these diagnoses lie along spectrums of behavioral (eg, dietary restriction, binge eating, purging, problematic exercise) and cognitive (eg, fear of aversive consequences with eating, dietary rules, body image disturbance) symptoms. While some characteristics are not diagnostic of ARFID, some individuals with ARFID may have comorbid other eating disorder symptoms (eg, binge eating). Two disorders are not included, as they are beyond the scope of this review—pica and rumination disorder. YES = characteristics required for the diagnosis. POSSIBLE = characteristics present in eating disorders but presence of which vary across diagnoses. NO = not characteristic of the disorder. Examples for each characteristic are provided in bullet points.
[a] Either quality of life impairment/distress OR compromised nutrition status is required for ARFID diagnosis.

(medical) risk concerns that patients may express during their office visit. It is important to recognize that all eating disorders hold the potential for medical, physical, and psychological complications, some of which are life-threatening. An eating disorder assessment should be considered for all patients, regardless of medical/psychological comorbidities, sex, gender, race, ethnicity, sexual orientation, current height/weight, age, socioeconomic status, education, or other sociocultural factors.[33,34]

Unfortunately, the high stigma of eating disorders, both at the provider and patient level, may often pose barriers to adequate screening, detection, and intervention. In **Table 2**, we delineate examples of misconceptions about eating disorders through patient case examples. We provide clinical pearls through alternatives to consider—to increase awareness of the heterogeneity of eating disorder presentations and facilitate provider assessment of the possible relationship current (or past) eating disorder symptoms may have with presenting GI complaints.

In the following sections, we provide recommendations based on our clinical experience, guided by best practice recommendations for managing eating disorders in primary care (Lemly and colleagues[35]) and international guidelines published by the Academy for Eating Disorders.[33] We include an overview of medical assessment parameters to consider and suggestions for navigating eating disorder questions through clinical history.

Medical Assessment

While medical assessment related to eating disorder symptoms may be typically managed by primary care providers or adolescent medicine specialists, gastroenterology providers are equipped to assess for acute medical risks and other lower-risk factors that may be red flags for an eating disorder.

Table 2
Myths and misconceptions about eating disorders relevant for the gastroenterology provider

Myth	Case Example	Possible Misconceptions	Alternatives to Consider
Only anorexia nervosa is life-threatening	A 30-year-old female with IBS-D and a BMI of 33.4 kg/m² followed for 3 y, presents at follow-up with concerns about her BMI and after prompting, discloses episodes of self-induced vomiting.	• Diarrhea is a result of laxative misuse. • Self-induced vomiting is not a problem. • Patient is in obese BMI range, so weight loss could improve body image.	• Purging behaviors (eg, laxative misuse, self-induced vomiting) can lead to similar medical complications of anorexia nervosa. In this case, the patient had diarrhea but was not misusing laxatives. • Similar complications include cardiac arrhythmias, electrolyte imbalances, increased risk of hospitalization, and even death. • Purging is often not recognized if patients are never asked directly. In this case, the patient at initial consult described involuntary regurgitation, but was not asked about self-induced vomiting until 3 y later.
Eating disorders are life-long illnesses.	A 25-year-old with chronic constipation with pelvic floor dyssynergia reports having bulimia nervosa as an adolescent with laxative misuse.	• The patient's chronic constipation is due to continued underlying eating disorder. • The patient needs to see a mental health provider. • Inclination to suggest patient not take laxatives for their chronic constipation.	• Full recovery from the eating disorder is possible, which can be determined by screening for the presence of current symptoms. • Pelvic floor dysfunction may or may not have been caused by the past eating disorder. • When eating disorder symptoms are present or there is concern for risk of relapse, some laxative agents (eg, prucalopride) may pose lower risk as there is not a typical "purging" feeling with use.

(continued on next page)

Table 2
(continued)

Myth	Case Example	Possible Misconceptions	Alternatives to Consider
Only patients who have a low body mass index (BMI) or BMI percentile can have an eating disorder.	A 32-year-old female with a history of GERD presents to clinic to happily discuss a 10 lb weight loss (BMI = 28.0 kg/m²).	• Weight loss is great for GERD symptoms, so the patient should be counseled on diet and exercise. • The patient is still overweight; inclination to suggest the patient continue strategies for further weight loss.	• Even when weight loss may seem minimal or patients are not "low weight" by BMI standards, maladaptive dietary restriction may be present. In this case, the patient fasted throughout the day, only eating in the evening (with the intent of losing weight). • Identifying the motivations behind weight loss attempts is key. In this case, the patient was motivated to lose weight due to significant body image disturbance, not just for GERD symptom improvement.
Patients cannot have an eating disorder if have medically necessary diet exclusions.	A 28-year-old female diagnosed last year with celiac disease presents to clinic with a 20 lb weight loss over 3 mo (BMI = 20.3 kg/m²).	• It is normal for some patients with celiac disease to lose weight. • As long as weight stays stable, her weight is fine because her BMI is in the normal range.	• Weight loss, albeit not to an "underweight" BMI can indicate problems with food intake. In this case, the patient was concerned about her weight loss, but was fearful of eating more. • Some patients who need to follow an exclusion diet (eg, gluten-free diet) become hypervigilant around food intake, fearing disease worsening. This may lead to caloric intake reductions leading to weight loss and possibly meeting criteria for ARFID.

Misconception	Case example	Automatic assumptions	Challenge
Males do not have eating disorders.	A 31-year-old cis-gender male with significant epigastric pain, early satiation, and reduced food intake with weight loss presents to clinic.	• He must be exercising more to "get fit" for the summer, which is why he has lost weight. • As a male, he is at low risk for an eating disorder.	• Eating disorders present in individuals across sex and gender spectrums. • In some cases, particularly with ARFID, males are just as likely as females to present with an eating disorder. • Males may present with different clinical characteristics of eating disorders (eg, some with a desire for more muscle than to be smaller). As a result, males are less likely to have access to treatment due to assumptions they do not have an eating disorder.
The core pathology of eating disorders is body image disturbance.	A 70-year-old female with significant weight loss (BMI = 16.5 kg/m²) and post-prandial symptoms of nausea, high satiety, and bloating (organic causes are ruled out). She reports reduced food intake due to fear of and difficulty tolerating her GI symptoms.	• Elderly patients don't have eating disorders. • She probably has had lifelong eating disorder that emerged in adolescence.	• Patients of any age can develop an eating disorder. • Some patients may have a lack of body image disturbance driving restriction that led to weight loss (ala avoidant/restrictive food intake disorder), as in this case. • Some patients may have overconcern for health/rigidity around eating as a driver for restriction (ala "orthorexia nervosa") where they do not describe frank body image disturbance. • Dietary restriction may be exacerbating functional gastric symptoms, which in turn perpetuate drivers of restriction.

Note. BMI, body mass index; GERD, gastroesophageal reflux disease; IBS-C, IBS, constipation predominant; IBS-D, irritable bowel syndrome, diarrhea predominant. We suggest providers to consider questioning whether automatic assumptions about eating disorders and weight status that may be present due to myths and misconceptions about eating disorders. In the right column, we provide examples that challenge these misconceptions.

Box 1
Criteria for hospitalization for acute medical stabilization

≤75% median body mass index for age, sex, and height

Hypoglycemia

Electrolyte disturbance (hypokalemia, hyponatremia, hypophosphatemia, and/or metabolic acidosis or alkalosis)

Electrocardiogram abnormalities (eg, prolonged QTc >450 ms, bradycardia, other arrhythmias)

Hemodynamic instability
- Bradycardia (heart rate < 40–50 bpm)
- Hypotension (systolic blood pressure < 80/50 mm Hg)
- Hypothermia

Orthostasis: blood pressure changes >20 mm Hg or pulse >20 bpm

Acute medical complications of malnutrition (eg, syncope, seizures, cardiac failure, pancreatitis)

Comorbid psychiatric or medical condition that prohibits or limits appropriate outpatient treatment (eg, severe depression, suicidal ideation, obsessive-compulsive disorder, type 1 diabetes mellitus)

Acute Medical Stability

Medical instability that could be because of an eating disorder should serve as the bare minimum assessment. We outline medical stability benchmarks in **Box 1** based on the Academy for Eating Disorders guidelines.[33] The presence of *any* of these medical instability markers indicates that the patient most likely requires inpatient medical monitoring for stabilization and should prompt a more thorough assessment (eg, through an emergency room visit).

Outpatient Medical Assessment

In **Box 2**, we outline example questions that providers can ask patients to inform further work-up, either done by the gastroenterology provider or in collaboration with other providers (eg, primary care). Often, continued outpatient medical monitoring is provided by a primary care provider or adolescent medicine specialist. Primary care providers will likely have increased access to patient care, which is an important factor when considering close monitoring of laboratory testing, weight, and vital signs. However, a brief assessment from the gastroenterology provider allows for a check of medical stability (to inform if a patient meets an acute risk benchmark in **Box 1**) or an indication for testing that could be recommended to the patient's primary care provider. Baseline laboratories may be drawn in the GI clinic for a variety of other reasons or if medical red flags are overtly noted during a consultation visit (ie, abnormal vital signs, history of electrolyte imbalance). In the following sections, we focus on the importance of provider questions and considerations when a patient presents with a likely diagnosis of an eating disorder.

Weight status

Body mass index (BMI) is only one marker of weight status and is appropriate when considering acute risks, which include <75% median BMI for age, sex, and height (see **Box 1**). Reviewing a patient's weight trajectory is helpful to have a better understanding of a patient's weight in relation to GI symptom onset. Some patients may lose weight or have difficulty gaining or growing after GI symptom onset.

Box 2		
Medical assessment that could be related to an eating disorder		
Symptoms Assessment	Questions to Pose to Patient	Testing to Consider[a]
Palpitations/ Chest pain	Do you feel as though your heart is racing? Do you feel your heart beating fast or irregularly? Is there pain in your chest at rest or with exertion?	• Bradycardia (heart rate < 40–50 bpm) • Hypotension (systolic blood pressure < 80/50 mm Hg) • Electrocardiogram for tachycardia • Electrolyte laboratory testing
Syncope/ Near syncope	Do you feel dizzy? Lightheaded? Have you ever lost consciousness?	• Check heart rate and blood pressure • Electrocardiogram for tachycardia • Electrolyte laboratory testing
Menstrual cycle	When was your last menstrual cycle? Does this occur regularly each month?	[Collaboration with patient's primary care team or gynecologist]
Temperature intolerance	Does the heat or cold affect any of your gastrointestinal symptoms, or worsen any other physical symptoms? Do you always feel cold?	• Check for low weight • Check for hypothermia
Fatigue	Do you feel fatigued despite a full night's rest?	• Check heart rate and blood pressure • Electrolyte laboratory testing • Iron level and complete blood count (CBC)

[a]Positive responses to questions may warrant further work-up, some of which may be representative of medical instability (see **Box 1**). In most cases, the gastroenterology provider is not ordering testing; for example, testing may be recommended to the patient's primary care physician to manage.

That is, many patients are "low weight," *not* based on BMI. For adults, even if weight has stabilized after an initial loss, weight restoration may still be important—a weight suppressed state may be an indication that the patient has insufficient nutrient intake. **Table 3** includes suggested cutoffs for significant weight loss. If a patient meets criteria for ARFID or another eating disorder, their previous trajectory is used to inform a range for a weight gain goal.[35] For more information on assessing weight status, see Lemly and colleagues.[35]

Some patients may not want to know their weight or may want to self-report their weight, which can be considered, in and of itself, a red flag for current body image disturbance. While providers may feel hesitant about obtaining weight from patients who express these concerns, it is important to obtain a weight reading to monitor for unintentional body weight loss associated with GI symptoms. While it is important for patients to know their weight in eating disorder treatment, gastroenterology providers can generally consider alternative methods to obtaining weights, such as covering the weight for the patient or weighing the patient backward.[35]

Orthostatic vital signs

If a patient does report dizziness, near syncope, or syncope, orthostatic vital signs should be considered. The heart is auscultated to rule out arrhythmias, but many patients will eventually get an electrocardiogram for a variety of reasons, whether in the gastroenterology clinic for drug monitoring or, as previously discussed, deferred to the primary care provider for routine monitoring.

Laboratory abnormalities

Table 3
Eating disorder symptom-specific questions for the gastroenterology provider

Considerations	Provider Questions	Potential Red Flags
Restricted diet	Have you had issues with eating because of your GI symptoms?	"I have 5 safe foods and I can't eat anything else." "I never feel hungry." "I can only eat small amounts at a time." "I rarely eat more than 1–2 times per day." Reliance on tube feeding when not medically indicated
Dietary changes	Do you feel like you adjust your diet based on your GI symptoms?	"I have tried so many diets to eliminate trigger foods for my GI symptoms." "I have to eat really clean and healthy—I only eat raw vegetables and fruit with lean proteins." "I go all day without eating to avoid symptoms but then 'binge' at night and feel terrible." Prolonged adherence to restrictive diets (eg, the low FODMAP diet restriction phase beyond 6 wk)
Weight suppression	Have you lost weight as a result your GI symptoms?	Unintentional body weight loss of— • >5% over 1 mo • >7.5% over 3 mo • >10% over 6 mo [weight may have stabilized since initial weight loss, but many patients may be in a suppressed weight status that could be contributing to GI symptom maintenance]
Quality of life impact	How much time/effort do you feel like you spend thinking about your GI symptoms in the setting of your diet?	"Each morning I wake up, preparing my meals for the day and with each bite hoping I don't experience bloating." Patient describes spending a lot of time researching diet management strategies Patient has pursued diet sensitivity testing and has rigid beliefs about which foods are causing their symptoms

(continued on next page)

Table 3 (continued)		
Considerations	Provider Questions	Potential Red Flags
Quality of life impact	Do you feel anxious about eating or around trying new restaurants? Have other people in your life been concerned about your diet?	"I'm constantly worried about what food choices I'm making." "I often don't go out to eat with my friends unless I have been to that restaurant before and they have an option of my 'safe food.'" "I no longer eat with my family." Concern from family members Difficulty attending school/work
Laxative abuse	Do you have a history of laxative misuse?	"If I don't use an enema daily, I never feel completely empty." Unnecessary use of laxative/ reliance on laxative; if fleet enema, could lead to electrolyte abnormalities
Self-induced vomiting	Have you ever made yourself vomit for any reason?	"If I feel extremely full, I will often make myself vomit which alleviates the fullness."

Note. Example assessment questions to evaluate eating habits and screen for possible current eating disorder symptoms. All questions assume a structural cause for GI symptoms has been ruled out. When you ask a patient, "Do you have an eating disorder?", they may not understand completely what that means or may feel stigmatized. The above questions may better facilitate an open dialogue. Of note, these questions are meant to help guide screening for disordered eating, but not intended to make a diagnosis, and thus do not include comprehensive questions assessing all eating disorder symptoms (eg, binge eating, body image disturbance). Presence of any red flag may warrant referral to a behavioral health provider for further assessment.

Abnormalities for acute medical risk are shown in **Box 1**. The importance of laboratory abnormalities ties back into a patient's risk for needing acute medical stabilization and can serve as a marker of current eating disorder symptoms. Baseline laboratories often include a basic metabolic panel as well as add on magnesium and phosphorus, which are not part of the basic metabolic panel. For some GI disorders (eg, inflammatory bowel diseases), micronutrient levels may be captured routinely and could serve as additional evidence for a patient that dietary variety is insufficient (eg, when disease activity is in remission).

Enteral and parenteral nutrition

If a patient is reliant on supplemental feeding and is not able to increase oral nutrition when indicated, this may be a red flag for a potential eating disorder. If a patient has a known eating disorder, parenteral nutrition should not be used unless the patient is without a functional GI tract; supplemental enteral feeds are typically only recommended for patients who are in eating disorder treatment and who are not gaining weight as expected and receiving an inpatient specialty refeeding protocol is not an option. To prevent the development of ARFID when enteral or parenteral nutrition is medically necessary, providers are encouraged to emphasize the intended timeline for their use and educate patients that, while difficult, increasing oral nutrition as soon as possible is imperative for gastric functioning.

Clinical History

When approaching a patient's history during an office visit, it may feel easy to ask the question, "Do you have an eating disorder?" However, it is unlikely the patient will adequately respond to this question and it is more likely to result in the patient feeling uncomfortable—the patient may feel that the provider is being accusatory or presumptuous, which is detrimental to the patient–provider relationship. In the following sections, we provide practical recommendations as examples of how to use clinical history to inform assessment of eating disorder symptoms. In **Table 3**, we also delineate specific assessment considerations with example questions and corollary example patient responses that may indicate a possible eating disorder.

Basic Assessment Tools

We encourage providers to introduce eating disorder assessment questions in a sensitive and nonjudgmental manner. Patients may be afraid to discuss their history of eating disorder symptoms, thinking that their eating disorder will frame the patient–provider relationship and negatively impact their treatment. Patients may also wonder why they are being asked questions related to disordered eating in a gastroenterology clinic, which makes it imperative for providers to explain the rationale behind history taking. An example to initiate questioning is as follows:

"I next have some questions that I go through with all patients. Know that some may or may not apply to you. These questions help us better understand your GI symptoms and history of your GI symptoms so that we can come up with the best treatment plan collaboratively."

Screening tools

There are several brief screening tools that can be used to assess eating disorder symptoms, including the SCOFF Questionnaire. The SCOFF is brief and can be administered verbally by the provider or as a survey. If a patient screens positively on the SCOFF, this could warrant further questioning, as listed in **Table 3**. However, reliance on screening tools alone can be insufficient as they may have low specificity for certain eating disorder presentations (eg, excessive exercise, ARFID).

Specific Behavioral Assessment Questions

Limited diet

In **Table 3**, positive red flags related to restricted diet or dietary changes based on GI symptoms may indicate significant restrictions in food variety and/or overall caloric intake. Framing dietary changes specifically around GI symptoms can help a patient feel more comfortable expressing their difficulties with food intake. A positive red flag for a restricted diet may include a patient disclosing their "safe food" list (ie, foods perceived to not exacerbate symptoms). A positive red flag for weight suppression may also indicate limited caloric intake below energy needs, with organic causes for weight loss ruled out. Providers may also choose to get a food recall (eg, *"Can you describe a typical day of eating for you in the past month—including the times you eat and one example of food at each time?"*).

Positive red flags for a restricted diet should alert the provider to further questioning to determine the motivations for the restriction (eg, fear of GI symptoms, fear of weight gain, rigid thinking about food intake, and overall loss of interest in eating) and tie in negative consequences (either medically or in terms of quality of life). Teasing out the presence of body image concerns can be difficult, but it is helpful to think of other eating disorders as opposed to ARFID.

Quality of life impacts

The quality of life impact questions in **Table 3** may be prompted by positive red flags for limited diet or asked on their own to inform possible eating disorder symptom presence. In many cases, significant quality of life impacts around a restricted diet could technically meet criteria for ARFID, even without nutritional impairments.

Other eating disorder behaviors

The presence of other eating disorder behaviors can distinguish other eating disorders from ARFID (see **Table 1**). **Table 3** provides some specific questions for laxative misuse and self-induced vomiting. However, examples of other eating disorder behaviors may need to be described to patients—these may include excessive exercise, exercise despite inability to gain weight, eating large amounts of food with the feeling of not being able to stop (ie, binge eating), or misuse of other non-GI medications, such as diuretics.

In the gastroenterology clinic, it is particularly imperative to understand a patient's history of laxative use or misuse. Reasons for laxative misuse may include purging after a meal in an attempt to expunge calories or to decrease discomfort with abdominal bloating or distension. If a patient reports current laxative misuse, it can be helpful to educate patients that laxatives are ineffective for calorie excretion and have negative physiologic effects. If a patient with constipation reports a history of laxative misuse, ideally agents that cause a "purging" sensation (eg, stimulant laxatives) may be avoided, but this does not preclude the use of other agents.

Referral for Further Assessment and Treatment

Conveying a new (possible) diagnosis

It is not necessarily the responsibility or within the purview of the GI provider to make a diagnosis of a specific eating disorder. If any eating disorder is suspected and the patient is at acute medical risk, then inpatient medical stabilization is likely required. For medically stable patients, providers can consider referral to an eating disorder program, a behavioral health provider (eg, psychologist) specialized in eating disorders, or a GI psychologist to further assess and make a diagnosis. When behavioral health programs or providers are not an option, dietitians or primary care providers may be able to further assess and/or facilitate connections with behavioral health treatment options.

Diagnosing ARFID

As ARFID is more common in some GI populations (eg, disorders of gut–brain interaction) than other eating disorders, it is particularly relevant for gastroenterology providers to feel comfortable considering an initial diagnosis. Notably, many patients meeting criteria for ARFID express concern about being labeled with an "eating disorder." ARFID can be explained as a diagnosis that is categorized as a feeding and eating disorder—one in which patients experience difficulty with eating enough types of foods or amounts of food. The reason why the diagnosis can be important is that it can get patients to a treatment that can help them expand their diet. It may be helpful to discuss how ARFID develops in the context of the GI disorder for a subset of patients—that ARFID is not the reason for their GI symptoms, but rather a *consequence* of them. Some examples of language to facilitate patient buy-in to ARFID are as follows:

"It sounds like you are really struggling with being able to eat enough because of your GI symptoms."

"I hear from a lot of patients that GI diet limitations make it difficult to live their lives in the way they want to."

"I am concerned about the weight loss you experienced because of your GI symptoms and how little you can eat right now. Even though it will be hard, increasing how much you are eating and gaining weight is important for your GI tract. In the short term, it will feel uncomfortable, but in the longer term it is likely to help with your GI symptoms."

"In concert with the medications that you are on, there are behavioral treatments that have been shown to help patients expand their diet. Would you like to learn more about what those treatments are?"

Eating Disorder Treatment

In the sections that follow, we summarize the types of treatment options typically employed for patients with eating disorders through eating disorder treatment programs and typical outpatient management.

Eating disorder programs (higher levels of care)

Eating disorder programs that offer higher levels of care vary in what they offer—for example, some have age or sex restrictions, and some do not treat ARFID. Inpatient medical stabilization is typically required for patients who have acute medical instability (see **Box 1**) and may be facilitated either through emergency department visits or eating disorder-specific programs. Eating disorder inpatient programs are used for patients who need 24-h medical monitoring during nutrition rehabilitation. A residential level of care (where patients stay at the facility) is used for patients who need longer-term care but not necessarily 24-h medical monitoring. Day programs (where patients have several hours per day at the program) are used for patients who are either stepping down from inpatient/residential or for patients who need more intensive support (eg, intensive outpatient, partial hospitalization). There can be difficulties with the availability and patient acceptability of higher levels of care—the Academy for Eating Disorders as well as other organizations (eg, the National Eating Disorders Association) provides resources for navigating care options.

Outpatient management

The first-line treatments for all eating disorders are behavioral—the most common being cognitive-behavioral therapies (CBTs), which vary in length. For non-low weight eating disorders, 8 to 10 sessions of CBTs may be used.[36] For anorexia nervosa or low-weight ARFID, longer treatment (eg, up to 40 sessions) may be needed for weight restoration.[37,38] Family-based treatment or family supported CBTs are typically used for children and adolescents, as well as some young adults.[39,40] In particular, for patients needing to gain weight or patients who have frequent purging behavior, multidisciplinary providers are involved in the behavioral treatment. Primary care providers typically manage outpatient medical monitoring (eg, weight, laboratories) and dietitians provide diet recommendations in concert with CBT to increase caloric intake and expand dietary variety. Psychiatric medications may also be indicated for some patients.[35] From a GI perspective, avoidance of misuse of laxatives, including plans to taper laxative misuse and medication selection to target sensory and motility disturbance (eg, with neuromodulators), can be an important contribution to the patient's multidisciplinary team.

SUMMARY

Eating disorders are heterogeneous conditions that affect individuals of any weight status. There is growing awareness of the intersection between eating disorders and GI conditions—both in terms of risk for one or the other as well as shared maintenance mechanisms. ARFID may be of particular relevance to preventing the development of disorders of gut–brain interaction, but we recommend that gastroenterology providers screen for all eating disorders among their patients. At a bare minimum, markers of medical instability that could be related to an eating disorder should be evaluated (see **Box 1**).

CLINICS CARE POINTS

- Overlap between eating disorders and gastrointestinal conditions is common—patients presenting to gastroenterologists may have a history of eating disorder symptoms, concurrent eating disorder symptoms, or be at risk for developing an eating disorder.

- We recommend that current eating disorder symptoms be assessed in all patients presenting to gastroenterology, as eating disorder symptoms could contribute to gastrointestinal symptom maintenance.

- Of particular concern is the prevention of negative psychosocial and medical consequences resulting from restrictive dietary interventions (i.e., symptoms of avoidant/restrictive food intake disorder).

DISCLOSURE

H. Burton Murray receives royalties from the Oxford University Press for her forthcoming book on rumination syndrome.

FUNDING

This work was supported by the National Institute of Diabetes and Digestive and Kidney Diseases, K23 DK131334 (H. Burton Murray).

REFERENCES

1. Harer KN, Eswaran SL. Irritable bowel syndrome: food as a friend or foe? Gastroenterol Clin 2021;50:183–99.
2. Chey WD. Elimination diets for irritable bowel syndrome: approaching the end of the beginning. Am J Gastroenterol 2019;114:201–3.
3. Scarlata K, Catsos P, Smith J. From a dietitian's perspective, diets for irritable bowel syndrome are not one size fits all. Clin Gastroenterol Hepatol 2020;18:543–5.
4. McGowan A, Harer KN. Irritable bowel syndrome and eating disorders: a burgeoning concern in gastrointestinal clinics. Gastroenterol Clin 2021;50:595–610.
5. Simons M, Taft TH, Doerfler B, et al. Narrative review: Risk of eating disorders and nutritional deficiencies with dietary therapies for irritable bowel syndrome. Neurogastroenterol Motil 2021;34(1):e14188.
6. Chey WD, Hashash JG, Manning L, et al. AGA clinical practice update on the role of diet in irritable bowel syndrome: expert review. Gastroenterology 2022.
7. Burton Murray H, Riddle M, Rao F, et al. Eating disorder symptoms, including avoidant/restrictive food intake disorder, in patients with disorders of gut-brain interaction. Neurogastroenterol Motil 2021;24:e14258.
8. Burton Murray H, Kuo B, Eddy KT, et al. Disorders of gut-brain interaction common among outpatients with eating disorders including avoidant/restrictive food intake disorder. Int J Eat Disord 2021;54:952–8.
9. Burton Murray H, Jehangir A, Silvernale CJ, et al. Avoidant/restrictive food intake disorder symptoms are frequent in patients presenting for symptoms of gastroparesis. Neurogastroenterol Motil 2020;32:e13931.
10. Burton Murray H, Bailey AP, Keshishian AC, et al. Prevalence and characteristics of avoidant/restrictive food intake disorder in adult neurogastroenterology patients. Clin Gastroenterol Hepatol 2020;18:1995–2002. e1.

11. Burton Murray H, Rao FU, Baker C, et al. Prevalence and characteristics of avoidant/restrictive food intake disorder in pediatric neurogastroenterology patients. J Pediatr Gastroenterol Nutr Press 2022;74:588–92.

12. Harer K, Baker J, Reister N, et al. Avoidant/restrictive food intake disorder in the adult gastroenterology population: an under-recognized diagnosis? American College of Gastroenterology Annual Meeting. October 5-10, Philadelphia, PA2018.

13. Nicholas JK, van Tilburg MAL, Pilato I, et al. The diagnosis of avoidant restrictive food intake disorder in the presence of gastrointestinal disorders: Opportunities to define shared mechanisms of symptom expression. Int J Eat Disord 2021; 54:995–1008.

14. Satherley R, Howard R, Higgs S. Disordered eating practices in gastrointestinal disorders. Appetite 2015;84:240–50.

15. Gibson D, Watters A, Mehler PS. The intersect of gastrointestinal symptoms and malnutrition associated with anorexia nervosa and avoidant/restrictive food intake disorder: Functional or pathophysiologic?-A systematic review. Int J Eat Disord 2021;54:1019–54.

16. Kiss A, Bergmann H, Abatzi TA, et al. Oesophageal and gastric motor activity in patients with bulimia nervosa. Gut 1990;31:259–65.

17. Chun AB, Sokol MS, Kaye WH, et al. Colonic and anorectal function in constipated patients with anorexia nervosa. Am J Gastroenterol 1997;92:1879–83.

18. Kamal N, Chami T, Andersen A, et al. Delayed gastrointestinal transit times in anorexia nervosa and bulimia nervosa. Gastroenterology 1991;101:1320–4.

19. Benini L, Todesco T, Frulloni L, et al. Esophageal motility and symptoms in restricting and binge-eating/purging anorexia. Dig Liver Dis 2010;42:767–72.

20. Riedlinger C, Schmidt G, Weiland A, et al. Which symptoms, complaints and complications of the gastrointestinal tract occur in patients with eating disorders? a systematic review and quantitative analysis. Front Psychiatry 2020;11:195.

21. West M, McMaster CM, Staudacher HM, et al. Gastrointestinal symptoms following treatment for anorexia nervosa: a systematic literature review. Int J Eat Disord 2021.

22. Boyd C, Abraham S, Kellow J. Appearance and disappearance of functional gastrointestinal disorders in patients with eating disorders. Neurogastroenterol Motil 2010;22:1279–83.

23. Atkins M, Zar-Kessler C, Madva E, et al. Prevalence of exclusion diets and relationship with avoidant/restrictive food intake disorder in adult and pediatric neurogastroenterology patients. Poster presentation at Digestive Disease Week; 2022, San Diego, CA.

24. Burton Murray H, Doerfler B, Harer K, et al. Psychological considerations in the dietary management of patients with DGBI. Am J Gastroenterol 2022;117(6): 985–94, epub ahead of print.

25. Yelencich E, Truong E, Widaman AM, et al. Avoidant restrictive food intake disorder prevalent among patients with inflammatory bowel disease. Clin Gastroenterol Hepatol 2021;20(6):1282–9.e1.

26. Fink M, Simons M, Tomasino K, et al. When is patient behavior indicative of avoidant restrictive food intake disorder (ARFID) Vs reasonable response to digestive disease? Clin Gastroenterol Hepatol 2021;20(6):1241–50.

27. Stein K, Warne N, Heron J, et al. Do children with recurrent abdominal pain grow up to become adolescents who control their weight by fasting? Results from a UK population-based cohort. Int J Eat Disord 2021;54:915–24.

28. Hedman A, Breithaupt L, Hübel C, et al. Bidirectional relationship between eating disorders and autoimmune diseases. J Child Psychol Psychiatry 2019;60:803–12.
29. Burton Murray H, Flanagan R, Banashefski B, et al. Frequency of eating disorder pathology among patients with chronic constipation and contribution of gastrointestinal-specific anxiety. Clin Gastroenterol Hepatol 2020;18:2471–8.
30. Vanheel H, Carbone F, Valvekens L, et al. Pathophysiological abnormalities in functional dyspepsia subgroups according to the Rome III criteria. Am J Gastroenterol 2017;112:132–40.
31. Kim D-Y, Delgado-Aros S, Camilleri M, et al. Noninvasive measurement of gastric accommodation in patients with idiopathic nonulcer dyspepsia. Am J Gastroenterol 2001;96:3099–105.
32. Burton Murray H, Staller K. When Food Moves From Friend to Foe: Why Avoidant/Restrictive Food Intake Matters in Irritable Bowel Syndrome. Clin Gastroenterol Hepatol 2021.
33. Eating disorders: a guide to medical care. Academy for Eating Disorders; 2021. Available at. https://higherlogicdownload.s3.amazonaws.com/AEDWEB/27a3b6 9a-8aae-45b2-a04c-2a078d02145d/UploadedImages/Publications_Slider/2120_ AED_Medical_Care_4th_Ed_FINAL.pdf. Accessed December 1, 2021.
34. Schaumberg K, Welch E, Breithaupt L, et al. The science behind the academy for eating disorders' nine truths about eating disorders. Eur Eat Disord Rev 2017;25: 432–50.
35. Lemly DC, Dreier MJ, Birnbaum S, et al. Caring for Adults With Eating Disorders in Primary Care. Prim Care Companion CNS Disord 2022;24.
36. Waller G. Brief, intensive CBT for normal weight eating-disordered outpatients: What can one achieve in just ten sessions? International Conference on Eating Disorders. October 5-10, San Francisco, CA, 2016.
37. Lock J, Le Grange D. Treatment manual for anorexia nervosa: a family-based approach. New York, NY: Guilford Publications; 2015.
38. Thomas JJ, Eddy K. Cognitive-behavioral therapy for avoidant/restrictive food intake disorder: children, adolescents, and adults. Cambridge: UK: Cambridge University Press; 2019.
39. Thomas JJ, Becker KR, Kuhnle MC, et al. Cognitive-behavioral therapy for avoidant/restrictive food intake disorder: Feasibility, acceptability, and proof-of-concept for children and adolescents. Int J Eat Disord 2020;53:1636–46.
40. Lock J, Sadeh-Sharvit S, L'Insalata A. Feasibility of conducting a randomized clinical trial using family-based treatment for avoidant/restrictive food intake disorder. Int J Eat Disord 2019;52:746–51.

Psychosocial Aspects of Metabolic and Bariatric Surgeries and Endoscopic Therapies

Sara H. Marchese, PhD[a], Anjali U. Pandit, PhD MPH[b],*

KEYWORDS

- Metabolic and bariatric surgery (MBS)
- Endoscopic bariatric and metabolic therapies (EBMT)
- Preoperative psychosocial evaluation
- Psychosocial considerations for endoscopic therapies

KEY POINTS

- Preoperative psychosocial evaluation and ongoing monitoring is helpful in identifying patients most at-risk for poorer outcomes after metabolic and bariatric surgery (MBS) or endoscopic bariatric and metabolic therapies (EBMT).
- There are specific recommendations for mental health and substance use screening in MBS.
- Very little is known about psychosocial considerations for EBMT.

INTRODUCTION: PROBLEM OF OBESITY, DIABETES AND NONALCOHOLIC FATTY LIVER DISEASE

Obesity (ie, having a body mass index (BMI) $\geq$30 kg/m^2)[1] remains a pervasive public health problem with ever-increasing prevalence.[2] As of most recent estimates, approximately 42% of adults in the United States have obesity, with 9% having "severe obesity" (BMI $\geq$40 kg/m^2).[3,4] Persons with overweight (ie, BMI of 25–29.9 kg/m^2) comprise an additional 31% of US adults.[3] Obesity is often comorbid with type 2 diabetes (T2DM), nonalcoholic fatty liver disease (NAFLD), and other chronic health conditions, and is predictive of all-cause mortality.[5,6]

[a] Department of Psychiatry & Behavioral Sciences, Section of Bariatric & Outpatient Psychotherapy, Rush University Medical Center, 1645 W. Jackson Boulevard, Suite 400, Chicago, IL 60618, USA; [b] Division of Gastroenterology and Hepatology & Psychiatry, Northwestern University Feinberg School of Medicine, 676 N. St. Clair Street, 14th Floor, Chicago, IL 60611, USA
* Corresponding author.
E-mail address: a-pandit@northwestern.edu

Gastroenterol Clin N Am 51 (2022) 785–798
https://doi.org/10.1016/j.gtc.2022.07.005
0889-8553/22/© 2022 Elsevier Inc. All rights reserved.

T2DM is a condition closely linked with obesity, in which patients develop insulin resistance and a resulting rise in blood sugar.[7] Ninety percent of patients with T2DM also have overweight or obesity.[8] Left un- or under-treated, T2DM can result in long-term complications like diabetic neuropathy, cardiovascular disease, and blindness.[9] Obesity and T2DM are also implicated in the development of NAFLD,[10] characterized by a concentration of fat on the liver. Estimates suggest over 90% of patients with obesity also have NAFLD.[10]

Several levels of intervention exist for obesity including lifestyle change, antiobesity medication, endoscopic therapies, and surgical intervention. More and more, patients with obesity and difficulty maintaining weight loss are referred for bariatric surgery, which is the most efficacious treatment and linked to improvement in associated chronic conditions[11,12] Endoscopic therapies are growing in number and may have a unique value in the range of obesity treatment options.

SURGICAL PROCEDURES

Metabolic and bariatric surgeries (MBS) come in several forms, with the primary goal of addressing obesity and metabolic processes. Five surgical procedures are endorsed by the American Society for Metabolic and Bariatric Surgery (ASMBS)[13]; these include the Roux-en-Y Gastric Bypass (RYGB), Laparoscopic Sleeve Gastrectomy (SG), adjustable gastric banding (AGB), Biliopancreatic Diversion with Duodenal Switch (BPD/DS) and Single Anastomosis Duodenal-Ileal Bypass with Sleeve Gastrectomy (SADI-S).[13] See **Table 1** for an overview of each procedure.

Table 1 MBS procedures endorsed by ASMBS	
Roux-en-Y Gastric Bypass (RYGB)	The Stomach is transected, and ingested nutrients are diverted from the stomach to a Roux-en-Y Gastrojejunostomy. As a result, gastric capacity is reduced, and nutrients are hypoabsorbed.
Sleeve Gastrectomy (SG)	In this procedure, approximately 80% of the stomach is resected, which changes the shape of the organ into a tube or sleeve shape. As a result of this procedure, gastric capacity is reduced, and gastric emptying is enhanced.
Biliopancreatic Diversion with Duodenal Switch (BPD/DS)	Following the creation of an SG, nutrients are diverted from the stomach to a duodenoileostomy, then an additional enteroenterostomy is performed between the biliopancreatic and common limbs.[83,84] This results in significant hypoabsorption of nutrients, secondary to the gastric restriction from the SG.
Adjustable Gastric Banding (AGB)	An adjustable band is placed over the proximal stomach, which constricts the size of the gastric pouch and reduces emptying time. The band can be adjusted by a medical provider through a subcutaneous port. The popularity of AGB has declined over time, in part due to known complications of the procedure (eg, band slippage and need for follow-up band adjustments), as well as lower rates of postoperative weight loss compared with RYGB and SG.[8]
Single Anastomosis Duodeno Ileal Bypass with Sleeve Gastrectomy (SADI-S)	The SADI-S procedure is similar to the BPD/DS, though ultimately simpler and with fewer risks due to the creation of a single duodenoileostomy following the formation of an SG.[84] This procedure leads to gastric restriction and hypoabsorption of nutrients.

Clinical practice guidelines recommend MBS be considered in patients with a BMI ≥ 40 kg/m^2 without co-existing medical conditions or excessive risk, patients with a BMI ≥ 35 kg/m^2 with one or more obesity-related conditions which can be improved with weight loss, or for patients with BMI 30 to 34.9 kg/m^2 and T2DM with inadequate glycemic control despite intervention.[14]

Psychosocial Considerations for Metabolic and Bariatric Surgery

The psychological evaluation is required for surgical centers following the Metabolic and Bariatric Surgery Accreditation and Quality Improvement Program (MBSAQIP) standards[15] and for insurance coverage in most US states. This typically involves a combination of objective assessment measures and a structured interview.[16,17] Several pre- and postoperative psychosocial considerations exist for MBS patients to ensure optimal postsurgical weight loss and preservation of mental health and quality of life.[17] Of note, owing to its evaluative nature, there is a risk for presentation bias in the interview, so the prevalence and severity of various psychosocial concerns may be higher and of greater concern than suggested in the extant literature.

Mental Health

Overall, psychiatric diagnoses are more prevalent for patients seeking MBS as compared with the general population. Outside of substance use and eating disorders (see below), anxiety disorders and affective disorders (eg, depression) are the most commonly reported psychiatric diagnoses current and lifetime for MBS patients,[18,19] with a recent review suggesting approximately 32% of patients presenting for MBS have a diagnosable mood disorder.[17] In the Longitudinal Assessment of Bariatric Surgery-3 (LABS-3) study,[18] lifetime experience of a mood disorder at baseline was almost 70%, whereas anxiety disorders of any kind were the most common current mental health diagnosis (18%). A recent preoperative study with a racially and ethnically diverse sample using a structured diagnostic assessment found that 25% of presenting patients currently met the criteria for an anxiety disorder, and 44% of patients had a lifetime diagnosis of major depressive disorder (MDD).[19]

Predictably, the risk of experiencing any mental health concern postsurgery is also higher for those who have a history of these concerns presurgery.[16] Weight loss trajectories after surgery are also tempered for patients with a history of mental health symptoms.[17] It is rarer that patients without mental health concerns presurgery develop new concerns and/or newly use mental health resources postoperatively, with one population-cohort study noting that of patients without preexisting mental health concerns, approximately 7% accessed mental health resources for the first time postoperatively.[20–22,] As such, any current psychiatric symptoms and their impact on function should be thoroughly assessed in the presurgical evaluation.

When considering severe mental illnesses, untreated bipolar disorder, psychosis, and recent suicide attempts are contraindications for surgery for safety reasons. Severe mental illness should be monitored throughout the surgical process but is not itself a contraindication to surgery if patients are properly treated. One study assessing patients with bipolar disorder and schizophrenia who underwent MBS found no difference in weight loss compared with the rest of the surgical population; however, all study patients experienced symptom exacerbation in the postoperative period.[23] Similarly, symptoms of hypomania as measured by the MMPI-2 have been associated with higher postoperative BMIs and slower weight loss trajectories.[24] With respect to suicidality, of particular concern are findings that completed suicide, suicide attempt, and nonsuicidal self-injury (NSSI) risk increases after MBS, though the event rate is small.[23,25] For patients who have a history of suicide attempts or NSSI, it is recommended to establish with a general therapist before MBS. Ongoing postoperative monitoring is also warranted, and it is recommended that patients not move forward with surgery until at least a year after their last suicide attempt or inpatient psychiatric hospitalization.[16]

Trauma exposure is not uncommon among presurgical MBS patients. One study reported two-thirds of female and nearly half of male patients had exposure to any form of trauma (physical, emotional, or sexual) in childhood, which was associated with an increased prevalence of psychiatric diagnoses in female patients.[26] Patients who have experienced abuse do not appear to have poorer postoperative weight loss trajectories compared with those without an abuse history.[16,27–29] However, some studies suggest patients with trauma exposure and/or trauma-related diagnoses (eg, post-traumatic stress disorder (PTSD), MDD) might experience worsening symptoms or challenges adapting to life after surgery.[16] As such, patients with a history of significant trauma and/or a diagnosis of PTSD should be monitored closely postoperatively by mental health providers to ensure no worsening of symptoms.

Personality pathology alone is also not a contraindication for surgery, as literature is still mixed as to its association with postsurgical outcomes.[16] Although the exact prevalence of personality disorders in MBS patients is unknown, it is estimated to be higher than the general population at 20% to 30%.[16] Of notable importance for psychologists: studies have shown traits implicated in borderline personality disorder (BPD) and other externalizing disorders, such as problems with identity, difficulty in relationships, and impulsivity, are associated with less weight loss and higher BMIs postoperatively.[24,30]

Cognitive Impairment

Other psychosocial considerations for surgery include the presence of cognitive impairments or learning disabilities. There is an association between obesity and suboptimal neurocognitive outcomes, particularly in the realm of executive function.[31,32] Within the LABS bariatric surgery cohort, 53.8% of patients met the criteria for mild cognitive impairment before surgery.[33] Promisingly, it seems that bariatric surgery and its associated weight loss does help to improve cognitive concerns in this patient population.[34] Given the elective nature of MBS, it is critical that providers assess cognitive function and a patient's ability to consent to not only the surgical procedure itself, but the extensive lifestyle changes required in the lifetime after surgery.

Eating Disorders and Maladaptive Eating Patterns

Binge eating disorder (BED) is the most prevalent eating disorder diagnosed in MBS patients, with a comprehensive longitudinal cohort study (LABS-3) finding that 12.1% of RYGB patients and 14.6% of SG patients met the criteria for BED presurgery.[35] A diagnosis of BED presurgery is associated with higher BMI after surgery, as well as greater weight regain than those without BED.[24,35,36] Current severe BED is a contraindication for surgery; this requires initial treatment and a reassessment by the team as symptoms improve. Mild-to-moderate binge eating can be improved with brief presurgical psychological treatment (eg, CBT, behavioral changes to dietary patterns, developing adaptive coping strategies).

Loss of control eating (LOC), or the feeling of being unable to stop eating once started, is a hallmark symptom of BED, but can occur independently as well. LOC is a common symptom of disordered eating in patients seeking surgery, with prevalence rates of approximately 10% to 16% observed in one sample depending on surgery type.[17,37] For patients with LOC presurgery, therapy should focus on building skills, as LOC occurring postoperatively is associated with both suboptimal weight loss and weight regain after surgery.[37,38] Notably, LOC occurring postoperatively is postulated to be a more significant problem for MBS patients than BED presurgery, because although the amount of food patients can consume postsurgery changes (ie, an "objective" binge episode may not be present), the LOC mechanism may not.[37,39–41]

MBS patients often report other maladaptive eating patterns that may not rise to the level of a diagnosable eating disorder, the most common of which are emotional eating (EE) and grazing. EE occurs when eating is used as a way to cope with feeling states, like sadness or boredom.[42,43] Poorly treated EE represents challenges for postoperative patients, who may eat instead of using other coping strategies.[16] This puts MBS patients at risk for GI distress (eg, nausea, vomiting, diarrhea, dumping syndrome), particularly as foods high in fat and sugar are more commonly chosen in EE.[44,45] Grazing, or the tendency to nibble and pick at foods over long periods, represents a particular problem if not treated before surgery.[16,46] Regardless of surgery type, patients are often unable to tolerate large portions of food after surgery given the reduction in stomach size. However, patients who engage in grazing after surgery are effectively able to unintentionally take in more calories than they intend. Grazing and EE are both associated with weight regain postsurgery.[17,40,42,46,47]

Substance Use

The use of substances before and following MBS has the potential to affect perioperative risks and longer-term psychosocial outcomes.

It is well-established that smoking in the perioperative period can have a significant impact on risks and complications.[48] Smokers are more likely to require ED visits and inpatient readmissions in the first 30 days postoperatively for both RYGB and SG.[49] Smokers undergoing RYGB are additionally more likely to need interventions and re-operations in the month following surgery.[49] Rates of Electronic Nicotine Delivery Systems (ENDS) are also rising, especially in younger patients,[50,51] but no literature has directly assessed for risks of ENDS in MBS patients.[52] There is no consistent relationship between smoking and weight loss postoperatively; however, due to known increases in mortality, long-term smoking cessation is encouraged.[52,53]

With legalization in many states, both recreational and medical cannabis use is rising.[54] Evidence suggests cannabis use and overuse is increasing in medical settings, with a recent study of surgical admissions showing diagnoses of cannabis use disorder growing over 3 fold between 2006 to 2015.[55] Prolonged use of cannabis is associated with increased surgical risk for myocardial infarction[55] and other cardiac and pulmonary complications.[56] Regarding MBS, patients using cannabis 1+ times per month used significantly higher opioid medication in the perioperative period.[57] Outcomes regarding weight loss are mixed,[58] although there may be a higher disposition for disordered eating, like eating with LOC.[59] There continues to be a lack of reliable evidence about cannabis use in MBS; as the mode of ingestion has historically not been assessed or tracked and especially before legalization, disclosure of substance use may be minimized in presurgical evaluations.

The longitudinal LABS-2 cohort provides the most comprehensive data about the rates of alcohol use in MBS patients. Preoperative alcohol use and alcohol use disorder (AUD) symptoms are estimated at 59% and 7.8%, respectively.[60] Postoperative AUD symptoms are estimated between 2.3% to 28.4%.[61] LABS-2 data indicate rates of alcohol use and AUD symptoms rise as years from surgery pass.[60] The previously assumed "addiction transfer" theory has fallen out of favor for mechanisms related to pharmacokinetic and hormonal changes impacting reward neurocircuitry in the brain.[61]

Opioid use is at epidemic levels in the United States. The relationship between obesity and pain is longstanding and self-reinforcing,[62] and contributes to the high rates of opioid use in patients seeking MBS, estimated at 12%.[63] Opioid use is associated with surgical risks, like longer lengths of stay and higher complication rates.[64] Alarmingly, opioid naïve patients are developing new persistent opioid use at a rate of 6% following MBS.[63] LABS-2 data show opioid use after MBS rises, in contrast to assumptions it would decrease with weight (and presumably pain).[65]

Social Support

The relationship between social support and weight loss is strong in both the MBS and behavioral weight loss literature.[66–68] For MBS patients, providers should consider how different forms of social support might impact the postoperative experience. Patients may find certain loved ones can provide emotional support (eg, cheering on patients in lifestyle change), whereas others provide instrumental support (eg, driving to appointments, cooking bariatric-friendly meals).[69] It is important that providers also determine the influence of a patient's support network on their home food environment. Providers should incorporate loved ones into conversations around bariatric dietary guidelines; for one, given the spread of obesity within close social networks,[70,71] it is not unlikely that a patient's loved ones also have obesity. Even if loved ones do not have obesity themselves, their adjustment to a patient's dietary needs increases the patient's chances of postoperative success. At minimum, providers should ensure patients have a loved one(s) available in the weeks following surgery to help with any medical needs, like commuting to postoperative appointments. Providers should also consider referral to MBS support groups, as evidence suggests attending support groups increases weight loss after surgery.[68,72,73]

ENDOSCOPIC BARIATRIC AND METABOLIC THERAPIES

Gaining popularity are endoscopic bariatric and metabolic therapies (EBMTs), which are a collection of devices and nonsurgical procedures for weight loss (**Table 2**). These therapies aim to reduce gastric volume by using space-occupying devices,

Table 2 Selected EBMT procedures	
Endoscopy Sleeve Gastroplasty	In this procedure, an endoscopic suturing device to create apposition of the anterior, greater curvature, and posterior wall of the gastric body. This results in delayed gastric emptying and restricted gastric volumes. Specific potential risks include peritoneal adhesions and gastric imbrication.[85] Meta-analysis found at 12-mo, patients lost an average of 16% of TBW.[86]
Intragastric balloons (IGB)	Several devices have been designed to take up gastric space to reduce appetite and increase satiety and consequently reduce caloric intake. These devices have to this point taken the form of balloons which are placed endoscopically for a span of 6 mo, intended as a temporary treatment during which time a patient may be able to shift lifestyle habits. Risks may include esophageal and gastric perforation and small bowel obstruction because of migration of the device.[85] Patients may be able to lose 15% of TBW over 32 wk.[76]
Aspiration therapy (AT)	An aspiration device is an endoscopically placed A tube inserted into the stomach with a valve adhered to the outside of the abdomen. Using this device, the patient has the opportunity to empty the stomach contents following meals. Patients may be able to lose approximately 12% of TBW over the course of 1 year.[77]

endoscopic suturing or plication of the stomach, and through aspiration of stomach contents.[14] Typically, these therapies are recommended to fill the gap of needed interventions for patients with Class II or III Obesity who are not eligible or interested in surgery. In addition, there are advantages related to the reversibility and repeatability of these therapies. According to the American Society of Gastrointestinal Endoscopy (ASGE),[74] some EBMTs are recommended to achieve a mean of >5% total body weight (TBW) loss and >25% excess weight loss (EWL)[74]; however, these data are not available for all therapies and there continue to be unknowns about risks, efficacy, and metabolic effects.

Psychosocial Considerations for Endoscopic Bariatric and Metabolic Therapies

Psychosocial considerations for EBMTs are currently limited, likely because these procedures are typically paid for out-of-pocket and therefore do not come with an insurance requirement for a psychological preoperative evaluation. However, patients entering into clinical trials for these therapies were excluded if currently endorsing eating disorders, uncontrolled psychiatric symptoms, and substance abuse per self-reported questionnaires and staff interviews.[75,76] Endoscopists now performing these procedures may choose to connect with an existing MBS or nonsurgical weight loss program and leverage embedded resources and providers, particularly for patients that show potential to have adverse psychosocial outcomes known to MBS populations.[75] As specific guidelines do not currently exist, it is assumed psychosocial providers follow a similar protocol preprocedure as they do for MBS.

Importantly, EBMTs are proposed as adjunctive to lifestyle change and, in many cases, placed on a limited time frame ($\sim$6–12 months), during which patients will benefit most from consistent lifestyle and behavioral changes to compliment the anatomic changes. Frequent contact with the support team (ie, RDs and psychologists) is therefore valuable in the ongoing monitoring of patients.[75,76] Evidence suggests patients who undergo AT plus lifestyle counseling are more successful with weight loss compared with lifestyle change alone.[76] AT requires a significant daily commitment to work properly; specifically, patients must chew their food thoroughly and wait approximately 20 to 30 min after eating before they can aspirate. It can be reasonably assumed that greater adherence to these procedures increases weight loss results and minimizes risk.

Gastrointestinal Considerations for Metabolic and Bariatric Surgery and Endoscopic Bariatric and Metabolic Therapies

All the procedures discussed in this paper have implications for gastrointestinal (GI) tract functioning, as they each intend to alter its performance and carry risk for longer-term consequences. Given patients often pursue these surgeries or therapies to reduce the burden of medical conditions and improve quality of life, it is important that patients are made aware of the possibility of developing a longer-term GI consequence and the potential impact on satisfaction with the surgery or therapy. See for examples **Box 1**.

DISCUSSION

Obesity rates are rising, and the risks of chronic obesity are numerous. The need for viable and accessible treatment options for long-term obesity management is critical. In addition to antiobesity medications, MB surgeries are being refined and less invasive endoscopic therapies are developed and approved by the FDA yearly. Only 1.1% of eligible patients undergo MBS,[78] so if EBMTs become covered by insurance,

---

Box 1
Long-term GI complications after MBS or EBMT with potential psychosocial impact

- Gastroesophageal reflux disease (GERD), either that persists after surgery or is new[87]
- Sleeve stenosis, or a narrowing of the new stomach[88,89]
- Gastrointestinal leakage, more common in SG than RYGB[90]
- Small bowel obstruction in RYGB[88]
- Dumping Syndrome in RYGB, occurring with highly processed and/or sugary foods and resulting in "early" symptoms like nausea/vomiting, abdominal cramps, bloating, and diarrhea in the first 30 min postmeal, as well as "late" symptoms occurring several hours after a meal, like sweating, heart racing, feeling shaky/jittery)[91]
- Anastomotic stenosis in RYGB, or the narrowing between where the new stomach pouch and intestines connect[88]
- Esophageal perforation in endoscopically placed devices like balloons and shuttles[92,93]
- Permanent gastroabdominal fistula in AT[86]
- Nausea/vomiting in all procedures[88]
- Ulcers[91]
- Abdominal pain[91]

---

it is possible their use will rise dramatically. These options are important given the progressive and relapsing nature of obesity, and the understanding that often multiple or sequential interventions are needed to control the disease. Although not all those who seek MBS or EBMT will be approved candidates, the benefits of these procedures often outweigh the risks as it relates to both physical and mental health functioning.

Clinically significant weight loss through MBS and EBMTs is coupled with a significant adjustment to both physiologic and psychological states. The preoperative psychosocial evaluation is most well studied in MBS because of the well-established understanding that some disorders have the potential to harm the patient or impact outcomes if not adequately treated before surgery. Areas of particular concern include mental health, substance use, and eating disorders. New evidence suggests findings from the presurgical evaluation are predictive of mental health and body image concerns 5+ years after surgery,[79] further emphasizing its value. With the rise of EBMTs, continuous evolution of the science will be needed as there will be an increased need to develop formalized patient pathways and assessment protocols.

There are relevant areas for further research which have not yet been extensively studied. For example, factors related to health literacy and numeracy have the potential to impact patient's ability to comprehend and consent to MBS and EBMT and subsequently may affect adherence to recommendations.[80] In addition, as much of the outcomes related to surgery hinge on dietary adherence, reliable access to food and products needed postoperatively may be important to formally screen for preoperatively, as the emerging research in this area indicates around 30% of MBS patients experience food insecurity.[81,82] Another future area of study is the role of weight loss as a trigger for the increase in trauma-related symptoms; this is particularly relevant if trauma was in any way related to a patient's weight (eg, an assault that occurred at a certain body weight), as returning to the body shape or size akin to the time one experienced trauma may be challenging.

In sum, MBS and EBMT procedures are available to patients with obesity as permanent or temporary weight loss options; given their complexity, providers must consider

psychosocial considerations alongside potential weight loss and GI-related consequences, which may impact the likelihood for patient success, quality of life and satisfaction with the surgery or therapy. Both preprocedure and longitudinal psychiatric
and medical monitoring is critical to understanding psychosocial challenges patients
may face after surgery.

CLINICS CARE POINTS

- Obesity is a chronic disease and ongoing public health concern that is challenging to treat.
  Bariatric surgery represents the best long-term treatment option for weight loss and
  maintenance for patients with obesity, though it is not without physical (eg, gastrointestinal
  [GI] concerns) or mental health risks.

- Mental health professionals should screen for cognitive status, psychiatric symptoms, eating
  disorders, substance abuse, and social support before metabolic and bariatric surgery (MBS)
  and be available for ongoing monitoring postoperatively.

- In many cases, preoperative psychological evaluation is not required for endoscopic bariatric
  and metabolic therapies (EBMT), but could be useful to optimize results. Interface with a
  multidisciplinary care team, including registered dietitians, mental health professionals, and
  physical therapy may be needed.

- GI functioning is permanently or temporarily altered in MBS and EBMT, respectively, and can
  impact psychosocial outcomes. Monitoring for GI risks and longer-term quality of life impact
  is recommended.

DISCLOSURE

The authors have nothing to disclose.

REFERENCES

1. Centers for Disease Control and Prevention. Defining Adult Overweight and
   Obesity. Defining Adult Overweight and Obesity. 2021. Available at: https://
   www.cdc.gov/obesity/adult/defining.html. Accessed March 25, 2022.
2. Hales CM, Carroll MD, Fryar CD, et al. Prevalence of Obesity Among Adults and
   Youth: United States, 2015-2016. NCHS Data Brief 2017;288:1–8.
3. Hales CM, Carroll MD, Fryar CD, et al. Prevalence of Obesity and Severe Obesity
   Among Adults: United States, 2017-2018. NCHS Data Brief 2020;360:1–8.
4. Fryar CD, Carroll MD, Afful J. Prevalence of Overweight, Obesity, and Extreme
   Obesity Among Adults Aged 20 and Over: United States, 1960–1962 Through
   2017–2018. NCHS Health E-Stats 2020. Available at: https://www.cdc.gov/nchs/
   data/hestat/obesity-adult-17-18/obesity-adult.htm. Accessed March 25, 2022.
5. Aune D, Sen A, Prasad M, et al. BMI and all cause mortality: systematic review
   and non-linear dose-response meta-analysis of 230 cohort studies with 3.74
   million deaths among 30.3 million participants. BMJ 2016;353:i2156. https://doi.
   org/10.1136/bmj.i2156.
6. Angelantonio ED, Bhupathiraju SN, Wormser D, et al. Body-mass index and all-
   cause mortality: individual-participant-data meta-analysis of 239 prospective
   studies in four continents. Lancet 2016;388(10046):776–86.
7. Centers for Disease Control and Prevention. Type 2 Diabetes. Type 2 Diabetes.
   Available at: https://www.cdc.gov/diabetes/basics/type2.html. Accessed March
   25, 2022.

8. American Society for Metabolic, Surgery Bariatric. Type 2 Diabetes and Metabolic Surgery | ASMBS. Available at: https://asmbs.org/resources/type-2-diabetes-and-metabolic-surgery-fact-sheet. Accessed March 25, 2022.

9. Zheng Y, Ley SH, Hu FB. Global aetiology and epidemiology of type 2 diabetes mellitus and its complications. Nat Rev Endocrinol 2018;14(2):88–98.

10. Cotter TG, Rinella M. Nonalcoholic fatty liver disease 2020: the state of the disease. Gastroenterology 2020;158(7):1851–64.

11. American Society for Metabolic and Bariatric Surgery. Metabolic and Bariatric Surgery Fact Sheet | ASMBS. Metabolic and Bariatric Surgery Fact Sheet | ASMBS. Available at: https://asmbs.org/resources/metabolic-and-bariatric-surgery. Accessed March 25, 2022.

12. Chang SH, Stoll CRT, Song J, et al. Bariatric surgery: an updated systematic review and meta-analysis, 2003–2012. JAMA Surg 2014;149(3):275–87. https://doi.org/10.1001/jamasurg.2013.3654.

13. American Society for Metabolic and Bariatric Surgery. Bariatric Surgery Procedures | ASMBS. Bariatric Surgery Procedures. Available at: https://asmbs.org/patients/bariatric-surgery-procedures. Accessed March 25, 2022.

14. Mechanick JI, Apovian C, Brethauer S, et al. Clinical Practice Guidelines for the Perioperative Nutrition, Metabolic, and Nonsurgical Support of Patients Undergoing Bariatric Procedures – 2019 Update: Cosponsored by American Association of Clinical Endocrinologists/American College of Endocrinology, The Obesity Society, American Society for Metabolic and Bariatric Surgery, Obesity Medicine Association, and American Society of Anesthesiologists. Obesity 2020;28(4):O1–58.

15. Available at: 2019_mbsaqip_standards_manual.pdf https://www.facs.org/-/media/files/quality-programs/bariatric/2019_mbsaqip_standards_manual.ashx. Accessed March 26, 2022.

16. Sogg S, Lauretti J, West-Smith L. Recommendations for the presurgical psychosocial evaluation of bariatric surgery patients. Surg Obes Relat Dis 2016;12(4):731–49.

17. Sarwer DB, Heinberg LJ. A review of the psychosocial aspects of clinically severe obesity and bariatric surgery. Am Psychol 2020;75(2):252–64.

18. Mitchell JE, Selzer F, Kalarchian MA, et al. Psychopathology prior to surgery in the longitudinal assessment of bariatric surgery-3 (LABS-3) psychosocial study. Surg Obes Relat Dis 2012;8(5):533–41.

19. Sarwer DB, Wadden TA, Ashare R, et al. Psychopathology, disordered eating, and impulsivity in patients seeking bariatric surgery. Surg Obes Relat Dis 2021;17(3):516–24.

20. Morgan DJR, Ho KM, Platell C. Incidence and determinants of mental health service use after bariatric surgery. JAMA Psychiatry 2020;77(1):60–7.

21. King WC, Chen JY, Mitchell JE, et al. Prevalence of alcohol use disorders before and after bariatric surgery. JAMA 2012;307(23):2516–25.

22. Arhi CS, Dudley R, Moussa O, et al. The complex association between bariatric surgery and depression: a national nested-control study. OBES SURG 2021;31(5):1994–2001.

23. Shelby SR, Labott S, Stout RA. Bariatric surgery: a viable treatment option for patients with severe mental illness. Surg Obes Relat Dis 2015;11(6):1342–8.

24. Marek RJ, Ben-Porath YS, van Dulmen MHM, et al. Using the presurgical psychological evaluation to predict 5-year weight loss outcomes in bariatric surgery patients. Surg Obes Relat Dis 2017;13(3):514–21.

25. Castaneda D, Popov VB, Wander P, et al. Risk of suicide and self-harm is increased after bariatric surgery—a systematic review and meta-analysis. OBES SURG 2019;29(1):322–33.
26. Orcutt M, King WC, Kalarchian MA, et al. The relationship between childhood maltreatment and psychopathology in adults undergoing bariatric surgery. Surg Obes Relat Dis 2019;15(2):295–303.
27. Gorrell S, Mahoney CT, Lent M, et al. Interpersonal abuse and long-term outcomes following bariatric surgery. Obes Surg 2019;29(5):1528–33.
28. King WC, Hinerman A, Kalarchian MA, et al. The impact of childhood trauma on change in depressive symptoms, eating pathology and weight following Roux-en-Y gastric bypass. Surg Obes Relat Dis 2019;15(7):1080–8.
29. Shinagawa A, Ahrendt AJ, Epstein EM, et al. The association between adverse childhood experiences (aces) and postoperative bariatric surgery weight loss outcomes. Obes Surg 2020;30(11):4258–66.
30. Oltmanns JR, Rivera Rivera J, Cole J, et al. Personality psychopathology: Longitudinal prediction of change in body mass index and weight post-bariatric surgery. Health Psychol 2020;39(3):245.
31. Morledge MD, Pories WJ. Bariatric surgery and cognitive impairment. Obesity 2021;29(8):1239–41. https://doi.org/10.1002/oby.23187.
32. Yang Y, Shields GS, Guo C, et al. Executive function performance in obesity and overweight individuals: A meta-analysis and review. Neurosci Biobehav Rev 2018;84:225–44.
33. Rochette AD, Spitznagel MB, Strain G, et al. Mild cognitive impairment is prevalent in persons with severe obesity. Obesity (Silver Spring) 2016;24(7):1427–9.
34. Spitznagel MB, Hawkins M, Alosco M, et al. Neurocognitive Effects of Obesity and Bariatric Surgery. Eur Eat Disord Rev 2015;23(6):488–95. https://doi.org/10.1002/erv.2393.
35. Smith KE, Orcutt M, Steffen KJ, et al. Loss of control eating and binge eating in the seven years following bariatric surgery. Obes Surg 2019;29(6):1773–80.
36. Chao AM, Wadden TA, Faulconbridge LF, et al. Binge eating disorder and the outcome of bariatric surgery in a prospective, observational study: two year results. Obesity (Silver Spring) 2016;24(11):2327–33.
37. Devlin MJ, King WC, Kalarchian MA, et al. Eating pathology and associations with long-term changes in weight and quality of life in the longitudinal assessment of bariatric surgery study. Int J Eat Disord 2018;51(12):1322–30.
38. White MA, Kalarchian MA, Masheb RM, et al. Loss of control over eating predicts outcomes in bariatric surgery: a prospective 24-month follow-up study. J Clin Psychiatry 2010;71(2):175–84.
39. Grilo CM, Ivezaj V, Duffy AJ, et al. Randomized controlled trial of treatments for loss-of-control eating following bariatric surgery. Obesity 2021;29(4):689–97.
40. Ivezaj V, Lydecker JA, Wiedemann AA, et al. Does bariatric binge-eating size matter? conceptual model and empirical support. Obesity 2020;28(9):1645–51.
41. Goldschmidt AB, Conceição EM, Thomas JG, et al. Conceptualizing and studying binge and loss of control eating in bariatric surgery patients—Time for a paradigm shift? Surg Obes Relat Dis 2016;12(8):1622–5.
42. Wiedemann AA, Ivezaj V, Grilo C. An examination of emotional and loss-of-control eating after Sleeve Gastrectomy surgery. Eat Behav 2018;31:48–52.
43. Koenders PG, van Strien T. Emotional Eating, rather than lifestyle behavior, drives weight gain in a prospective study in 1562 employees. J Occup Environ Med 2011;53(11):1287–93.

44. Nguyen-Michel ST, Unger JB, Spruijt-Metz D. Dietary correlates of emotional eating in adolescence. Appetite 2007;49(2):494–9. https://doi.org/10.1016/j.appet.2007.03.005.

45. Tomiyama JA, Finch LE, Cummings JR. Did That Brownie Do Its Job? Stress, Eating, and the Biobehavioral Effects of Comfort Food. In: Emerging Trends in the social and behavioral sciences. John Wiley & Sons, Ltd; 2015. p. 1–15. https://doi.org/10.1002/9781118900772.etrds0324.

46. Colles SL, Dixon JB, O'Brien PE. Grazing and Loss of Control Related to Eating: Two High-risk Factors Following Bariatric Surgery. Obesity 2008;16(3):615–22. https://doi.org/10.1038/oby.2007.101.

47. Cooper TC, Simmons EB, Webb K, et al. Trends in Weight Regain Following Roux-en-Y Gastric Bypass (RYGB) Bariatric Surgery. Obes Surg 2015;25(8):1474–81. https://doi.org/10.1007/s11695-014-1560-z.

48. Grønkjær M, Eliasen M, Skov-Ettrup LS, et al. Preoperative Smoking Status and Postoperative Complications: A Systematic Review and Meta-analysis. Ann Surg 2014;259(1):52–71. https://doi.org/10.1097/SLA.0b013e3182911913.

49. Janik MR, Aryaie AH. The effect of smoking on bariatric surgical 30-day outcomes: propensity-score-matched analysis of the MBSAQIP. Surg Endosc 2021;35(7):3905–14. https://doi.org/10.1007/s00464-020-07838-4.

50. Evans-Polce R, Veliz P, Boyd CJ, et al. Trends in E-Cigarette, Cigarette, Cigar, and Smokeless Tobacco Use Among US Adolescent Cohorts, 2014–2018. Am J Public Health 2020;110(2):163–5.

51. E-cigarettes, Vapes, JUUL. What parents should know. Available at: https://www.lung.org/quit-smoking/e-cigarettes-vaping/e-cigarettes-parents. Accessed March 26, 2022.

52. Srikanth N, Xie L, Morales-Marroquin E, et al. Intersection of smoking, e-cigarette use, obesity, and metabolic and bariatric surgery: a systematic review of the current state of evidence. J Addict Dis 2021;39(3):331–46.

53. Mohan S, Samaan JS, Samakar K. Impact of smoking on weight loss outcomes after bariatric surgery: a literature review. Surg Endosc 2021;35(11):5936–52.

54. Data and Statistics. Available at: https://www.cdc.gov/marijuana/data-statistics.htm. Accessed March 26, 2022.

55. Goel A, McGuinness B, Jivraj NK, et al. Cannabis use disorder and perioperative outcomes in major elective surgeries. Anesthesiology 2020;132(4):625–35. https://doi.org/10.1097/ALN.0000000000003067.

56. Echeverria-Villalobos M, Todeschini AB, Stoicea N, et al. Perioperative care of cannabis users: A comprehensive review of pharmacological and anesthetic considerations. J Clin Anesth 2019;57:41–9. https://doi.org/10.1016/j.jclinane.2019.03.011.

57. Bauer F. Marijuana's influence on pain scores, initial weight loss, and other bariatric surgical outcomes. Permj 2018. https://doi.org/10.7812/TPP/18-002.

58. Shockcor N, Adnan SM, Siegel A, et al. Marijuana use does not affect the outcomes of bariatric surgery. Surg Endosc 2021;35(3):1264–8. https://doi.org/10.1007/s00464-020-07497-5.

59. Vidot DC, Prado G, De La Cruz-Munoz N, et al. Postoperative marijuana use and disordered eating among bariatric surgery patients. Surg Obes Relat Dis 2016;12(1):171–8. https://doi.org/10.1016/j.soard.2015.06.007.

60. King WC, Chen JY, Courcoulas AP, et al. Alcohol and other substance use after bariatric surgery: prospective evidence from a U.S. multicenter cohort study. Surg Obes Relat Dis 2017;13(8):1392–402. https://doi.org/10.1016/j.soard.2017.03.021.

61. Ivezaj V, Benoit SC, Davis J, et al. Changes in Alcohol Use after Metabolic and Bariatric Surgery: Predictors and Mechanisms. Curr Psychiatry Rep 2019; 21(9):85.
62. McVinnie DS. Obesity and pain. Br J Pain 2013;7(4):163–70.
63. Tian C, Maeda A, Okrainec A, et al. Impact of preoperative opioid use on health outcomes after bariatric surgery. Surg Obes Relat Dis 2020;16(6):768–76.
64. Brummett CM, Waljee JF, Goesling J, et al. New persistent opioid use after minor and major surgical procedures in US adults. JAMA Surg 2017;152(6):e170504.
65. King WC, Chen JY, Belle SH, et al. Use of prescribed opioids before and after bariatric surgery: prospective evidence from a U.S. multicenter cohort study. Surg Obes Relat Dis 2017;13(8):1337–46.
66. Wing RR, Jeffery RW. Benefits of recruiting participants with friends and increasing social support for weight loss and maintenance. J Consulting Clin Psychol 1999;67(1):132–8.
67. Funk LM, Grubber JM, McVay MA, et al. Patient predictors of weight loss following a behavioral weight management intervention among U.S. Veterans with severe obesity. Eat Weight Disord 2018;23(5):587–95.
68. Ufholz K. Peer Support Groups for Weight Loss. Curr Cardiovasc Risk Rep 2020; 14(10):19.
69. House JS, Umberson D, Landis KR. Structures and processes of social support. Annu Rev Sociol 1988;14(1):293–318.
70. Christakis NA, Fowler JH. The Spread of Obesity in a Large Social Network over 32 Years. New Engl J Med 2007;357(4):370–9. https://doi.org/10.1056/NEJMsa066082.
71. Smith NR, Zivich PN, Frerichs L. Social influences on obesity: current knowledge, emerging methods, and directions for future research and practice. Curr Nutr Rep 2020;9(1):31–41. https://doi.org/10.1007/s13668-020-00302-8.
72. Andreu A, Jimenez A, Vidal J, et al. Bariatric support groups predicts long-term weight loss. Obes Surg 2020;30(6):2118–23. https://doi.org/10.1007/s11695-020-04434-2.
73. Livhits M, Mercado C, Yermilov I, et al. Is social support associated with greater weight loss after bariatric surgery?: a systematic review. Obes Rev 2011;12(2): 142–8.
74. Abu Dayyeh BK, Kumar N, Edmundowicz SA, et al. ASGE Bariatric Endoscopy Task Force systematic review and meta-analysis assessing the ASGE PIVI thresholds for adopting endoscopic bariatric therapies. Gastrointest Endosc 2015; 82(3):425–38. https://doi.org/10.1016/j.gie.2015.03.1964, e5.
75. Sullivan S, Kumar N, Edmundowicz SA, et al. ASGE position statement on endoscopic bariatric therapies in clinical practice. Gastrointest Endosc 2015;82(5): 767–72.
76. Abu Dayyeh BK, Maselli DB, Rapaka B, et al. Adjustable intragastric balloon for treatment of obesity: a multicentre, open-label, randomised clinical trial. Lancet 2021;398(10315):1965–73.
77. Thompson CC, Abu Dayyeh BK, Kushner R, et al. Percutaneous Gastrostomy Device for the Treatment of Class II and Class III Obesity: Results of a Randomized Controlled Trial. Am J Gastroenterol 2017;112(3):447–57.
78. English WJ, DeMaria EJ, Hutter MM, et al. American Society for Metabolic and Bariatric Surgery 2018 estimate of metabolic and bariatric procedures performed in the United States. Surg Obes Relat Dis 2020;16(4):457–63.

79. Martin-Fernandez KW, Marek RJ, Heinberg LJ, et al. Six-year bariatric surgery outcomes: the predictive and incremental validity of presurgical psychological testing. Surg Obes Relat Dis 2021;17(5):1008–16.

80. Hecht L, Cain S, Clark-Sienkiewicz SM, et al. Health literacy, health numeracy, and cognitive functioning among bariatric surgery candidates. OBES SURG 2019;29(12):4138–41.

81. Lin D, Zickgraf H, Butt M, et al. Food insecurity is linked to poorer dietary quality in prebariatric surgery patients. Surg Obes Relat Dis 2021;17(2):263–70.

82. Brown CL, Skelton JA, Palakshappa D, et al. High prevalence of food insecurity in participants attending weight management and bariatric surgery programs. OBES SURG 2020;30(9):3634–7.

83. Wolfe BM, Kvach E, Eckel RH. Treatment of Obesity: Weight Loss and Bariatric Surgery. Circ Res 2016;118(11):1844–55.

84. Pereira SS, Guimarães M, Almeida R, et al. Biliopancreatic diversion with duodenal switch (BPD-DS) and single-anastomosis duodeno-ileal bypass with sleeve gastrectomy (SADI-S) result in distinct post-prandial hormone profiles. Int J Obes 2019;43(12):2518–27.

85. Brunaldi VO, Neto MG. Endoscopic Procedures for Weight Loss. Curr Obes Rep 2021;10(3):290–300.

86. Li P, Ma B, Gong S, et al. Efficacy and safety of endoscopic sleeve gastroplasty for obesity patients: a meta-analysis. Surg Endosc 2020;34(3):1253–60.

87. Yeung KTD, Penney N, Ashrafian L, et al. Does sleeve gastrectomy expose the distal esophagus to severe reflux?: a systematic review and meta-analysis. Ann Surg 2020;271(2):257–65.

88. Ma IT, Madura JA. Gastrointestinal complications after bariatric surgery. Gastroenterol Hepatol (N Y) 2015;11(8):526–35.

89. Iannelli A, Treacy P, Sebastianelli L, et al. Perioperative complications of sleeve gastrectomy: Review of the literature. J Minim Access Surg 2019;15(1):1–7.

90. Chang SH, Freeman NLB, Lee JA, et al. Early major complications after bariatric surgery in the USA, 2003–2014: a systematic review and meta-analysis. Obes Rev 2018;19(4):529–37.

91. Schulman AR, Thompson CC. Complications of bariatric surgery: what you can expect to see in your GI practice. ACG 2017;112(11):1640–55.

92. Castro M, Guerron AD. Bariatric endoscopy: current primary therapies and endoscopic management of complications and other related conditions. Mini-invasive Surg 2020;4:47.

93. Jirapinyo P, Kumar N, Saumoy M, et al. Association for Bariatric Endoscopy systematic review and meta-analysis assessing the American Society for Gastrointestinal Endoscopy Preservation and Incorporation of Valuable Endoscopic Innovations thresholds for aspiration therapy. Gastrointest Endosc 2021;93(2):334–42.e1. https://doi.org/10.1016/j.gie.2020.09.021.

Psychological Evaluation and Management of Chronic Pancreatitis

Brooke Palmer, PhD, Megan Petrik, PhD*

KEYWORDS

- Chronic pancreatitis • Pain • Psychogastroenterology
- Total pancreatectomy islet auto transplant

KEY POINTS

- Chronic pancreatitis is associated with a high disease burden and negatively affects the quality of life and psychological health.
- Psychosocial and behavioral factors are important considerations in disease management, health care utilization and expenditures, and quality of life for chronic pancreatitis.
- Multidisciplinary care that includes a behavioral health provider is a best practice recommendation for chronic pancreatitis.
- Psychological treatment may improve pain, anxiety, depressive symptoms, and disease management in chronic pancreatitis.
- Identifying psychosocial risk factors may improve outcomes following surgical treatment of chronic pancreatitis.

BACKGROUND

Chronic pancreatitis (CP) is a chronic digestive disorder defined as a "pathologic fibro-inflammatory syndrome of the pancreas" in which the hallmark feature is upper abdominal pain that radiates to the back.[1,2] A range of other symptoms can also occur in CP such as nausea, vomiting, diarrhea, greasy stools, and glucose intolerance. Prevalence rate is 41.76 per 100,000[3] and it is more common in male individuals and in Black individuals as compared with White individuals.[3,4] Health disparities are of note in CP as Black individuals are twice as likely to have severe, constant pain and higher levels of disability.[5] Although approximately half of CP cases are associated with alcohol misuse,[3] the other half are composed of a diverse range of factors such as idiopathic etiologies, genetic mutations, hereditary factors, autoimmune disorders, episodes of acute recurrent pancreatitis, and obstructive causes.[6]

Department of Medicine, Division of General Internal Medicine, University of Minnesota Medical School, MMC 741, 420 Delaware Street Southeast, Minneapolis, MN 55455, USA
* Corresponding author.
E-mail address: mlpetrik@umn.edu

Gastroenterol Clin N Am 51 (2022) 799–813
https://doi.org/10.1016/j.gtc.2022.07.006
0889-8553/22/© 2022 Elsevier Inc. All rights reserved.

CP is associated with high societal costs, disease burden, and morbidity. As a leading cause of hospitalization for digestive disorders,[7] the direct and indirect costs associated with CP are substantial.[8] Estimates of treating chronic pain associated with CP alone are $638 million annually.[8] Patients with CP report significant impairments in health-related quality of life.[9] Severity and chronicity of pain are major contributors to poor quality of life, yet health behaviors (eg, smoking) and cognitive factors (eg, perceived pain intensity and perceived self-blame) also impact the quality of life.[10,11]

CP has a significant negative impact on psychological health. In one cross-sectional study,[12] a large portion of individuals with CP present with clinically significant levels of anxiety (46.8%) and depression (38.6%) as well as the overlap between the two (29%). Those with anxiety or depression show greater pain-related distress and interference as well as poorer functionality.[12] Outside of the bidirectional relationship between pain and psychological distress, other aspects of the illness itself can contribute to depression and anxiety such as worry about disease progression, worry about surgery, grief related to loss of roles, etc. Diagnosis of CP is associated with an increased risk of psychiatric disorder or even suicide attempts.[13-15] Genetic evidence of the link between those at risk for depression, anxiety, and more severe pain experiences has been emerging in the CP population.[16,17] Psychological health is important to address because depression, psychosis, and drug abuse can increase readmission risk after inpatient medical admissions for CP.[18]

Abdominal pain is present in the vast majority (85%–90%) of patients with CP and is a key predictor of quality of life and disability.[19] Pain in CP is complex and may present in different patterns. For example, Type A pain is defined as short, relapsing pain episodes with pain-free periods in between flares whereas Type B pain is constant or prolonged episodes of pain.[20] These patterns require differing medical and behavioral interventions. From an antiquated biomedical perspective, it was thought that CP pain was limited to changes in the morphology of the pancreas but recent research shows that patient reports of pain symptoms do not correlate with results from imaging and other biological markers as would be predicted.[21] Current understanding of CP pain acknowledges that pain is diverse and is related to multiple mechanisms such as central sensitization and "pancreatic neuroplasticity."[22]

THERAPEUTIC OPTIONS

The primary target for managing CP is to alleviate pain and treat related issues such as endocrine or nutritional issues.[2] However, due to the multifactorial nature of pain and subsequent impact on psychological health, it behooves providers to use a biopsychosocial approach to CP management by following a multidisciplinary care model.[23] A multidisciplinary care model includes collaboration between professionals from multiple specialties and disciplines including a gastroenterologist, surgeon, endocrinologist, nurse, dietician, pain specialist, psychologist, and psychiatrist.[24] This is consistent with guidelines to address pain management for those with CP from a working group for the International Consensus Guidelines for Chronic Pancreatitis[23]; however, it is not yet detailed in the American College of Gastroenterology Clinical Guidelines.[2]

There is significant empirical support for integrating psychological care into multidisciplinary treatment for chronic pain[25-28] but little empirical evidence currently exists for this model of care in CP management. Despite the scarcity of published data, the limited results are promising. Two specific models have shown that including programmatic psychological interventions in CP treatment and/or involving psychologists in care lead to improvements in health care utilization (length of stay for inpatient admissions decreased significantly and cost savings) and clinical outcomes (improvement in quality of life and pain ratings and reductions in opioid use).[29,30]

When a psychologist is integrated into the care of patients with CP, it is recommended that they target assessment and intervention to match the needs of the patients and take a broad approach. Assessment of psychosocial needs may include, but is not limited to, assessment of the pain experience and management, adjustment to illness, medical and surgical history, psychiatric history, and current psychiatric functioning including suicide risk, substance abuse, social history, and social supports. **Table 1** highlights relevant domains of psychosocial functioning to assess and select assessment tools; information gathered from these tools may be used to guide treatment for patients with CP. Psychologists can provide support to patients by providing psychoeducation about pain management and mental health challenges, adjusting unhelpful thinking styles about pain or CP, and supporting patients in behavioral interventions such as relaxation training, activity pacing, etc., to name a few.[24]

Given the importance of pain management, psychological interventions for chronic pain are highly indicated for patients with CP. Cognitive behavioral therapy (CBT) is a first-line behavioral intervention for chronic pain and other empirically supported psychological interventions include acceptance- and mindfulness-based interventions and hypnosis.[31,32] In addition to improvements in patient reports of pain, psychological interventions can improve symptoms of depression, anxiety, and quality of life.[31,33–35] Despite strong evidence for CBT and other psychological interventions to treat chronic pain, there are few studies looking at these interventions to treat chronic pain in those with CP. One randomized controlled trial (RCT) has compared outcomes of internet-based CBT on various aspects of pain for patients with CP and results showed greater numbers of treatment responders, or those with greater than 30% of improvement in areas of pain interference, intensity, and quality of life for those who participated in CBT versus the control group.[36]

Evidence-based psychological interventions are strongly encouraged to improve the management of gastrointestinal (GI) illness.[37] CBT has received empirical support in the management of other GI conditions[38] and can help CP patients challenge unhelpful thinking and behavioral patterns that maintain symptoms of depression and anxiety. Mindfulness and acceptance-based interventions are also useful in helping patients cope with emotional distress and improve physical functioning when living with chronic illness.[39,40]

Given the severity of chronic pain in patients with CP, there is an increased risk of suicide attempts or death by suicide.[14,41] Additional risk factors for suicide in this population include abdominal pain in particular and using high doses of opioid medications.[42–44] Recommendations for reducing suicide risk in the CP population are to effectively treat the chronic pain. Psychologists can monitor risk over time and use interventions to reduce risk and engage in safety planning.

Alcohol misuse is associated with roughly half of all CP cases but is likely not the sole cause of symptoms.[3,6] However, complete abstinence from alcohol is necessary for CP management. In some cases, chemical dependency treatment may be necessary. In addition to abstinence from alcohol, tobacco cessation is also recommended as tobacco use is a predictor of quality of life for those with CP, it exacerbates the toxic effects of alcohol on the pancreas, and even when used alone, tobacco is associated with an increased risk for pancreatitis.[45,46] Tobacco cessation can be achieved with pharmacologic agents and nonpharmacologic interventions.

EVALUATION

When CP is refractory to medical, endoscopic, or other surgical interventions and results in high functional impairment, total pancreatectomy with islet autotransplantation

Table 1
Psychosocial assessments relevant for chronic pancreatitis care

Test	Considerations for Use
Health-related quality of life	
36-Item Short Form Health Survey (SF-36)[62]	• No cost to use • Good validity and reliability for a range of medical populations • Contains 8 scales and two subscales highlighting mental and physical components of quality of life • Validated in chronic pancreatitis populations[63]
12-Item Short Form Health Survey (SF-32)[64]	• No cost to use • Same scales and subscales as SF-36 with fewer questions • Also validated in chronic pancreatitis population[65]
EuroQol-5 Dimension (EQ-5D)[66]	• No cost to use after registering • Assesses health-related quality of life over five domains: mobility, self-care, usual activities, pain/discomfort, and anxiety/depression • Valid and reliable in a wide range of populations • Comprehensive catalog of scores based on a range of disease, including digestive disease[67]
Pancreatitis Quality of Life Instrument (PANQOLI)[68]	• Available for use from published article • 18-item instrument developed specifically for patients with chronic pancreatitis • Four subscales: emotional function scale, role function scale, physical function scale, and "self-worth" scale • Excellent reliability and construct validity • Good correlation with SF-12
Psychiatric functioning	
Hospital Anxiety and Depression Scale (HADS)[69]	• 14-item tool developed for measurement of depressive and anxiety symptoms in medical populations • Has been used to assess psychiatric functioning in other pain[70] and GI populations[71] • Does not include an item assessing suicidal thoughts or behaviors
Patient Health Questionnaire-9 (PHQ-9)[72]	• 9-item tool to measure depressive symptoms • Strong psychometric data across large samples in medical settings[73] • No validated normative data with a CP population • Includes an item assessing suicidal ideation • No cost for use • Widely used in research examining psychiatric functioning in digestive disorders
Generalized Anxiety Disorder-7 (GAD-7)[74]	• Valid 7-item tool to assess general anxiety in medical settings[74] • No validated normative data with a CP population • No cost for use • Assesses general anxiety but does not capture disease- or GI-specific anxiety

(continued on next page)

Test	Considerations for Use
Table 1 (*continued*)	
Minnesota Multiphasic Personality Inventory-2-Restructured Form (MMPI-2-RF)[75]	• Originally validated with psychiatric populations and results with medical populations should be taken into context of medical diagnoses • No specific normative data pertaining to CP • Established use in presurgical evaluations and behavioral medicine settings[76] • Consider MMPI-2-RF results in presurgical evaluations as only one data point to be considered in the context of all other information gathered
Pain	
Pain Catastrophizing Scale[77]	• 13-item self-report measure that assesses catastrophic thinking related to pain • Psychometric properties validated across a wide number of pain conditions, yet not with CP[78] • May inform targets for cognitive behavioral therapy for pain in patients with CP
Brief Pain inventory[79]	• Measures pain intensity and interference in daily functioning available in short and long form • Used in a wide range of research for pain conditions; strong psychometric properties • Used in outcomes studies for psychological treatment with patients with CP[36] • Short form available for increased usability in clinical practice
Comprehensive pain assessment tool (COMPAT)[80]	• Validated pain assessment tool for CP • Accounts for complexity in types of pain in CP • Preliminary validation data suggests good face validity and high patient acceptance • Short form available for increased usability in clinical practice
Substance use	
Alcohol Use Disorders Identification Test (AUDIT)[81]	• 10-item scale assessing alcohol intake, dependence, and adverse consequences • Available with no cost • Originally developed for use in primary care settings • Strong reliability and validity to identify harmful use, abuse, and dependence in a range of illness and community populations • Brief version with three items—AUDIT-C
CAGE Adapted to Include Drugs Questionnaire (CAGE-AID)[82]	• Four-item screening assessment of alcohol and drug misuse • Valid for use in medical settings[83] • Good sensitivity and specificity for substance use disorder • Validated for chronic pain patients
Opioid Risk Tool (ORT)[84]	• Brief screening tool designed to predict aberrant opioid use • Developed for use in predicting likelihood of future opioid misuse in primary care patients with chronic pain • This measure may be more reflective of suboptimal management of refractory pain in CP rather than opioid abuse in patients with TPIAT[54]

(continued on next page)

Table 1 (continued)	
Test	**Considerations for Use**
Suicidal thoughts and behaviors	
Suicidal Behaviors Questionnaire[85]	• Four-item screening questionnaire assessing historical, current, and future-oriented suicidal thinking and behaviors • No cost for use • Recommended in clinical and nonclinical settings
Columbia-Suicide Severity Rating Scale[86]	• Interview risk assessment with multiple versions ranging from risk assessment checklist to more complete lifetime history of suicidal ideation/behavior • Can be useful to monitor treatment outcomes • No cost for use • Effective for clinicians and researchers

(TPIAT) offers a surgical treatment approach. This section will focus on presurgical psychological evaluation in patients undergoing TPIAT. The primary goal of TPIAT is to alleviate pain and improve quality of life via resection of the pancreas, whereas the islet autotransplantation helps to achieve a secondary goal of minimizing the risk of insulin-dependent diabetes that would naturally occur following pancreatectomy alone.[47] The majority of patients experience improvement or resolution of pain (85%) and are able to cease use of opioids (59%) within 2 years of surgery.[48] Results are durable with pain relief maintained for 82% of patients at 10 years.[49]

TPIAT is a complex surgical intervention with a long postoperative recovery period as full recovery is estimated to take 6 to 12 months. It also has high demands for self-management of health behaviors to ensure optimal outcomes. The surgery is appropriate only if patients are willing to accept noteworthy postoperative management considerations such as lifelong use of pancreatic enzyme replacement therapy and possible insulin-dependent diabetes.[47] Medical complications in the postoperative period can result in or exacerbate adjustment challenges. Behavioral goals of recovery include weaning opioid medications, returning to work or school, increasing functioning, and ensuring adherence to health behavior goals like diet or substance use support recovery. Pain burden remains unchanged for 15% of patients following TPIAT,[48] with central sensitization and gastrointestinal dysmotility associated with suboptimal pain relief.[50] Thus, patient selection for TPIAT requires consideration of psychosocial factors that may impact outcomes.

Medical literature indicates that psychosocial contraindications to TPIAT include the presence of an active alcohol use disorder or current illegal drug use (abstinence for 6 months required before being considered for surgery), uncontrolled psychiatric illness, or other psychosocial factors that could be expected to impair one's ability to adhere to a complicated postoperative medical management regimen.[51] It has also been shown that the etiology of the disease may an important consideration as CP because of genetic mutations as compared with alcoholic etiologies is associated with improved postoperative pain.[52,53] Interestingly, one study found that higher preoperative scores on a measure of opioid misuse predicted larger improvements in physical quality of life following TPIAT as compared with patients without opioid misuse behaviors.[54] This may suggest that instruments assessing opioid misuse may indicate challenges with refractory pain in this population as compared with traditional opioid misuse. In addition, preliminary evidence suggests that preoperative depression and a history of suicide attempts or substance abuse may heighten risk for post-TPIAT death by suicide or accidental overdose.[55] Little else is known about specific psychosocial predictors of TPIAT outcomes.

Presurgical psychological evaluation in general aims to identify risk factors that would contribute to poor surgical outcomes and identify factors that mitigate risks to offer recommendations to enhance surgical results.[56] Currently, there are no best practice guidelines to conduct a presurgical psychological evaluation for TPIAT. Thus, a model for TPIAT presurgical psychological evaluation may be informed by literature pertinent to other surgeries aimed at improving chronic pain (eg, spinal cord stimulator implantation) and transplantation.

Regarding predictors of spinal cord stimulator implantation and lumbar surgeries, higher presurgical depression, anxiety, emotional dysfunction, somatic complaints, cognitive complaints, and interpersonal problems were related to poorer pain outcomes and patient satisfaction.[57] Other factors associated with poorer outcomes following transplant include presurgical treatment nonadherence, depression, and suboptimal social support.[58] A systematic review and meta-analysis implicates state and trait anxiety, depression, catastrophic thinking patterns, pain self-efficacy, and kinesiophobia as psychological predictors of chronic postoperative pain more generally.[59]

Components of the presurgical TPIAT psychological evaluation include a review of medical records, clinical interview, and a combination of broadband and narrowband assessments. Collateral information from family/caregivers may be obtained, if relevant, with patient consent. The clinical interview focuses on understanding the patient's history with CP, pain history, knowledge and expectations about the surgical procedure, as well as review of medical, psychiatric, substance use, educational, social, and occupational histories. Ensuring that the patient has strong knowledge about TPIAT and realistic expectations about the postoperative impacts is essential given the lengthy recovery and notable self-management requirements. It is essential that the behavioral health provider conducting this assessment is well informed about TPIAT to accurately assess patient knowledge and expectations.

Broadband and narrowband instruments may be used to obtain data about functioning across a range of psychological domains (see **Table 1**). It is recommended that assessments are selected to evaluate psychiatric functioning, pain, health-related quality of life, and substance misuse. A testing battery ultimately depends on cost, psychometric properties of the instrument, patient language and reading level, and mode of administering tests (eg, in-person vs telemedicine).

The selection of TPIAT candidates is recommended to occur through discussion among a multidisciplinary team that combines surgical, medical, and psychological team members.[47,51] A psychologist can help the team weigh the medical benefits against the risk that psychosocial factors would impair surgical outcomes or result in psychiatric decompensation. The presence of psychosocial risk factors or psychiatric comorbidity does not exclude a patient from TPIAT if their risk factors can be stabilized before surgery.[24] Patients will have close postoperative follow-up plans with their medical providers (eg, endocrinology, gastroenterology) and it is encouraged that postoperative mental health follow-up plans are created before surgery. Identification of patients with high-risk features such as previous suicide attempts or a history of substance abuse may especially benefit from being followed by a health psychologist for postoperative follow-up.[55]

Postoperative psychological support could be helpful to address the following therapeutic topics: optimizing pain management, cessation or lowering dose of opioid medications in conjunction with medical recommendations, diabetes management, adjustment challenges, and management of comorbid psychiatric conditions or suicide risk. Psychological quality of life has been found to improve more slowly than the physical quality of life, suggesting that mental recovery from long periods of chronic illness is a process that takes time.[60] Emotional challenges may arise when complications or delays in progress happen, further reinforcing the need for psychological support in a multidisciplinary team. As TPIAT is only routinely offered at a small number of institutions nationally, patients often travel far distances for destination medical care. Ensuring proper psychological follow-up of patients in their local area once they return to their initial place of residence is an important consideration for ethical psychological care.[61] The advent of telemedicine allows for follow-up remotely but interstate jurisdictional issues are to be considered. Appropriate local referrals must include providers well versed in CP, digestive illness, or chronic pain.

DISCUSSION

The literature regarding the psychosocial impacts of CP and psychological care for these patients is growing. However, there are current limitations in our knowledge base and future research would be beneficial to address these gaps. First, most of our knowledge regarding psychosocial factors that impact the quality of life and pain/disease management in CP pertains to substance misuse. By focusing on alcohol, tobacco, or opioid misuse, there is a large segment of patients with CP for whom we do not fully understand which psychosocial factors impact their illness trajectories. It would be beneficial for the literature to further understand more nuanced psychosocial risk factors, such as cognitions and behaviors related to pain, trauma history, or current social support, as potential mediators of disease. Second, there is a lack of established norms or validation of psychological measures for patients with CP. This is a limitation in providing psychological care for these patients, especially when using psychological measures to understand a patient's candidacy for TPIAT. It is recommended that future research may examine how these measures perform in patients with CP as compared with other patients with chronic pain or other chronic digestive illness. In addition, there is preliminary evidence that CBT interventions can be effectively applied in this patient population.[36] More work is needed to evaluate psychological treatments for improving pain, depression/anxiety, quality of life and ability of the presurgical assessment to predict surgical outcomes. Although best practice guidelines and psychological literature predicting outcomes for pain-focused surgical procedures and transplantation may provide a preliminary guide to patient readiness for surgery, it is not to replace future research identifying psychosocial predictors of TPIAT outcomes. Finally, it is recommended that future research examine health disparities in CP to promote health equity in this patient population. **Box 1** summarizes future directions for psychosocial research for patients with CP.

SUMMARY

The present state of the literature on managing psychological and behavioral aspects of CP is nascent. The majority of empirical research speaks to the psychological burden that CP and chronic pain have on patients by highlighting connections between CP symptoms and outcomes such as health-related quality of life, comorbid depression and anxiety, and functional limitations. Research on CP and substance use also clearly identifies the role of individuals' behaviors in exacerbating or alleviating symptoms. Although there are substantial data supporting significant psychosocial challenges living with CP, there is much less information about empirically supported psychological and behavioral interventions for this patient population despite clear intervention targets such as chronic pain, maladaptive thinking patterns

---

Box 1
Future directions for psychosocial research for patients with chronic pancreatitis

Understand psychosocial risk factors that impact quality of life, pain, and disease management for people with chronic pancreatitis (ie, cognitions and behaviors related to pain, trauma history, and social support)

Examine how assessment measures perform in patients with chronic pancreatitis as compared with other patients with chronic pain or other chronic digestive illnesses

Assess efficacy and effectiveness of psychological treatments targeting pain management, depression, anxiety, and quality of life, and the ability of presurgical assessment to predict surgical outcomes in patients with chronic pancreatitis

Understand psychosocial predictors of outcomes post-TPIAT

Investigate health disparities in chronic pancreatitis to promote health equity

---

about disease, substance use, and self-management of living with CP or post-TPIAT. The peer-reviewed data that does exist aligns with existing research and recommendations for support patients in managing chronic pain, such as the importance of integrating psychological and behavioral interventions, or a psychologist, into CP treatment[29,30] and using CBT for chronic pain in CP patients.[36] Similarly, when patients with CP pursue TPIAT, there are very little data about psychological and behavioral factors that predict long-term surgical outcomes.

Based on the state of the literature, our care recommendations are designed to address broad symptom and behavioral categories while acknowledging that additional research is necessary, as mentioned above, to further identify relevant assessments and interventions for patients with CP. Recommendations for care, as displayed in **Fig. 1**, include (1) use a multidisciplinary treatment team that includes behavioral health to support patients with CP; (2) recommend incorporating evidence-based psychological interventions into a patient's treatment plan (eg, CBT) to address needs such as chronic pain or depressive symptoms; (3) consider additional psychological interventions such as mindfulness- and acceptance-based interventions to also augment the quality of life and psychological health; and (4) integrate psychological assessment into the pre-TPIAT process to prepare patients for surgery and optimize long-term outcomes.

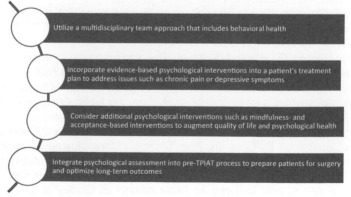

Fig. 1. Care recommendations for working with patients with chronic pancreatitis.

CLINICS CARE POINTS

- Accurate psychological assessment is crucial to understanding pain and comorbid psychosocial impacts of chronic pancreatitis
- Consistent with recommendations for managing chronic pain, multidisciplinary care with teams that includes psychologists is more effective for the management of pain and mental health symptoms and can improve health care utilization
- Psychosocial risk factors for suboptimal outcomes following total pancreatectomy with islet autotransplantation can be mitigated and optimized using a preoperative psychological assessment

DISCLOSURE

M. Petrik serves as a consultant for Mahana Therapeutics. There are no other disclosures.

REFERENCES

1. Whitcomb DC, Frulloni L, Garg P, et al. Chronic pancreatitis: An international draft consensus proposal for a new mechanistic definition. Pancreatology 2016;16(2): 218–24.
2. Gardner TB, Adler DG, Forsmark CE, et al. ACG Clinical Guideline: Chronic Pancreatitis. Am J Gastroenterol 2020;115(3):322–39.
3. Yadav D, Timmons L, Benson JT, et al. Incidence, prevalence, and survival of chronic pancreatitis: a population-based study. Am J Gastroenterol 2011; 106(12):2192–9.
4. Yang AL, Vadhavkar S, Singh G, et al. Epidemiology of Alcohol-Related Liver and Pancreatic Disease in the United States. Arch Intern Med 2008;168(6):649–56.
5. Wilcox CM, Sandhu BS, Singh V, et al. Racial Differences in the Clinical Profile, Causes, and Outcome of Chronic Pancreatitis. Am J Gastroenterol 2016;111(10):1488–96.
6. Kalivarathan J, Yadav K, Bataller W, et al. Etiopathogenesis and pathophysiology of chronic pancreatitis. In: Orlando G, Piemonti L, Ricordi C, et al, editors. Transplantation, bioengineering, and regeneration of the endocrine pancreas, vol. 2. Cambridge, MA8: Academic Press; 2019. p. 5–32.
7. Peery AF, Crockett SD, Murphy CC, et al. Burden and Cost of Gastrointestinal, Liver, and Pancreatic Diseases in the United States: Update 2018. Gastroenterology 2019;156(1):254–72, e11.
8. Hall TC, Garcea G, Webb MA, et al. The socio-economic impact of chronic pancreatitis: a systematic review. J Eval Clin Pract 2014;20(3):203–7.
9. Amann ST, Yadav D, Barmada MM, et al. Physical and mental quality of life in chronic pancreatitis: a case-control study from the North American Pancreatitis Study 2 cohort. Pancreas 2013;42(2):293–300.
10. Machicado JD, Amann ST, Anderson MA, et al. Quality of Life in Chronic Pancreatitis is Determined by Constant Pain, Disability/Unemployment, Current Smoking, and Associated Co-Morbidities. Am J Gastroenterol 2017;112(4):633–42.
11. Keller CE, Mel Wilcox C, Gudleski GD, et al. Beyond Abdominal Pain: Pain Beliefs, Pain Affect, and Distress as Determinants of Quality of Life in Patients with Chronic Pancreatitis. J Clin Gastroenterol 2018;52(6):563–8.

12. Phillips AE, Faghih M, Drewes AM, et al. Psychiatric Comorbidity in Patients With Chronic Pancreatitis Associates With Pain and Reduced Quality of Life. Am J Gastroenterol 2020;115(12):2077–85.

13. Cho J, Walia M, Scragg R, et al. Frequency and risk factors for mental disorders following pancreatitis: a nationwide cohort study. Curr Med Res Opin 2019;35(7): 1157–64.

14. Chen CH, Lin CL, Hsu CY, et al. A Retrospective Administrative Database Analysis of Suicide Attempts and Completed Suicide in Patients With Chronic Pancreatitis. Front Psychiatry 2018;9:147.

15. Alkhayyat M, Abou Saleh M, Coronado W, et al. Increasing Prevalence of Anxiety and Depression Disorders After Diagnosis of Chronic Pancreatitis: A 5-Year Population-Based Study. Pancreas 2021;50(2):153–9.

16. Dunbar EK, Saloman JL, Phillips AE, et al. Severe Pain in Chronic Pancreatitis Patients: Considering Mental Health and Associated Genetic Factors. J Pain Res 2021;14:773–84.

17. Dunbar E, Greer PJ, Melhem N, et al. Constant-severe pain in chronic pancreatitis is associated with genetic loci for major depression in the NAPS2 cohort. J Gastroenterol 2020;55(10):1000–9.

18. Shah R, Haydek C, Mulki R, et al. Incidence and predictors of 30-day readmissions in patients hospitalized with chronic pancreatitis: A nationwide analysis. Pancreatology 2018;18(4):386–93.

19. Drewes AM, Krarup AL, Detlefsen S, et al. Pain in chronic pancreatitis: the role of neuropathic pain mechanisms. Gut 2008;57(11):1616–27.

20. Ammann RW, Muellhaupt B. The natural history of pain in alcoholic chronic pancreatitis. Gastroenterology 1999;116(5):1132–40.

21. Wilcox CM, Yadav D, Ye T, et al. Chronic pancreatitis pain pattern and severity are independent of abdominal imaging findings. Clin Gastroenterol Hepatol 2015; 13(3):552–60 [quiz: e28–9].

22. Muthulingam J, Olesen SS, Hansen TM, et al. Progression of Structural Brain Changes in Patients With Chronic Pancreatitis and Its Association to Chronic Pain: A 7-Year Longitudinal Follow-up Study. Pancreas 2018;47(10):1267–76.

23. Drewes AM, Bouwense SAW, Campbell CM, et al. Guidelines for the understanding and management of pain in chronic pancreatitis. Pancreatology 2017;17(5): 720–31.

24. Petrik ML, Freeman ML, Trikudanathan G. Multidisciplinary Care for Adults With Chronic Pancreatitis: Incorporating Psychological Therapies to Optimize Outcomes. Pancreas 2022;51(1):4–12.

25. Adams LM, Turk DC. Central sensitization and the biopsychosocial approach to understanding pain. J Appl Biobehav Res 2018;23(2):e12125.

26. Gatchel RJ, Peng YB, Peters ML, et al. The biopsychosocial approach to chronic pain: scientific advances and future directions. Psychol Bull 2007;133(4): 581–624.

27. Gatchel RJ, McGeary DD, McGeary CA, et al. Interdisciplinary chronic pain management: past, present, and future. Am Psychol 2014;69(2):119–30.

28. Oslund S, Robinson RC, Clark TC, et al. Long-term effectiveness of a comprehensive pain management program: strengthening the case for interdisciplinary care. Proc Bayl Univ Med Cent 2009;22(3):211–4.

29. Madan A, Borckardt JJ, Barth KS, et al. Interprofessional collaborative care reduces excess service utilization among individuals with chronic pancreatitis. J Healthc Qual 2013;35(5):41–6.

30. Mavilakandy A, Oyebola T, Boyce R, et al. Pilot study examining the impact of a specialist multidisciplinary team clinic for patients with chronic pancreatitis. Pancreatology 2020;20(8):1661–6.
31. Ehde DM, Dillworth TM, Turner JA. Cognitive-behavioral therapy for individuals with chronic pain: efficacy, innovations, and directions for research. Am Psychol 2014;69(2):153–66.
32. Skinner M, Wilson HD, Turk DC. Cognitive-behavioral perspective and cognitive-behavioral therapy for people with chronic pain: Distinctions, outcomes, and innovations. J Cogn Psychother 2012;26(2):93–113.
33. Hilton L, Hempel S, Ewing BA, et al. Mindfulness Meditation for Chronic Pain: Systematic Review and Meta-analysis. Ann Behav Med 2017;51(2):199–213.
34. Veehof MM, Trompetter HR, Bohlmeijer ET, et al. Acceptance- and mindfulness-based interventions for the treatment of chronic pain: a meta-analytic review. Cogn Behav Ther 2016;45(1):5–31.
35. Thompson T, Terhune DB, Oram C, et al. The effectiveness of hypnosis for pain relief: A systematic review and meta-analysis of 85 controlled experimental trials. Neurosci Biobehav Rev 2019;99:298–310.
36. Palermo TM, Law EF, Topazian MD, et al. Internet Cognitive-Behavioral Therapy for Painful Chronic Pancreatitis: A Pilot Feasibility Randomized Controlled Trial. Clin Transl Gastroenterol 2021;12(6):e00373.
37. Keefer L, Palsson OS, Pandolfino JE. Best Practice Update: Incorporating Psychogastroenterology Into Management of Digestive Disorders. Gastroenterology 2018;154(5):1249–57.
38. Ballou S, Keefer L. Psychological Interventions for Irritable Bowel Syndrome and Inflammatory Bowel Diseases. Clin Transl Gastroenterol 2017;8(1):e214.
39. Graham CD, Gouick J, Krahé C, et al. A systematic review of the use of Acceptance and Commitment Therapy (ACT) in chronic disease and long-term conditions. Clin Psychol Rev 2016;46:46–58.
40. Niazi AK, Niazi SK. Mindfulness-based stress reduction: a non-pharmacological approach for chronic illnesses. North Am J Med Sci 2011;3(1):20–3.
41. Petrosky E, Harpaz R, Fowler KA, et al. Chronic Pain Among Suicide Decedents, 2003 to 2014: Findings From the National Violent Death Reporting System. Ann Intern Med 2018;169(7):448–55.
42. Ilgen M. Pain, Opioids, and Suicide Mortality in the United States. Ann Intern Med 2018;169(7):498–9.
43. Ilgen MA, Bohnert ASB, Ganoczy D, et al. Opioid dose and risk of suicide. Pain 2016;157(5):1079–84.
44. Smith MT, Edwards RR, Robinson RC, et al. Suicidal ideation, plans, and attempts in chronic pain patients: factors associated with increased risk. Pain 2004; 111(1–2):201–8.
45. Edderkaoui M, Thrower E. Smoking and Pancreatic Disease. J Cancer Ther 2013; 4(10A):34–40.
46. Aune D, Mahamat-Saleh Y, Norat T, et al. Tobacco smoking and the risk of pancreatitis: A systematic review and meta-analysis of prospective studies. Pancreatology 2019;19(8):1009–22.
47. Bellin MD, Gelrud A, Arreaza-Rubin G, et al. Total pancreatectomy with islet autotransplantation: summary of a National Institute of Diabetes and Digestive and Kidney diseases workshop. Pancreas 2014;43(8):1163–71.
48. Sutherland DER, Radosevich DM, Bellin MD, et al. Total pancreatectomy and islet autotransplantation for chronic pancreatitis. J Am Coll Surg 2012;214(4):409–24 [discussion: 424–6].

49. Bellin MD, Beilman GJ, Sutherland DE, et al. How Durable Is Total Pancreatectomy and Intraportal Islet Cell Transplantation for Treatment of Chronic Pancreatitis? J Am Coll Surg 2019;228(4):329–39.

50. McEachron KR, Bellin MD. Total pancreatectomy and islet autotransplantion for chronic and recurrent acute pancreatitis. Curr Opin Gastroenterol 2018;34(5): 367–73.

51. Abu-El-Haija M, Anazawa T, Beilman GJ, et al. The role of total pancreatectomy with islet autotransplantation in the treatment of chronic pancreatitis: A report from the International Consensus Guidelines in chronic pancreatitis. Pancreatology 2020;20(4):762–71.

52. Chinnakotla S, Radosevich DM, Dunn TB, et al. Long-term outcomes of total pancreatectomy and islet auto transplantation for hereditary/genetic pancreatitis. J Am Coll Surg 2014;218(4):530–43.

53. Dunderdale J, McAuliffe JC, McNeal SF, et al. Should pancreatectomy with islet cell autotransplantation in patients with chronic alcoholic pancreatitis be abandoned? J Am Coll Surg 2013;216(4):591–6 [discussion: 596–8].

54. Moran RA, Klapheke R, John GK, et al. Prevalence and predictors of pain and opioid analgesic use following total pancreatectomy with islet autotransplantation for pancreatitis. Pancreatology 2017;17(5):732–7.

55. McEachron KR, Melton M, Beilman GJ, et al. Psychiatric Comorbidities in Patients Undergoing Total Pancreatectomy With Islet Cell Autotransplantation and Associated Mortality. Pancreas 2018;47(4):e16.

56. Block AR, Marek RJ. Presurgical Psychological Evaluation: Risk Factor Identification and Mitigation. J Clin Psychol Med Settings 2020;27(2):396–405.

57. Celestin J, Edwards RR, Jamison RN. Pretreatment Psychosocial Variables as Predictors of Outcomes Following Lumbar Surgery and Spinal Cord Stimulation: A Systematic Review and Literature Synthesis. Pain Med 2009;10(4):639–53.

58. Bailey P, Vergis N, Allison M, et al. Psychosocial Evaluation of Candidates for Solid Organ Transplantation. Transplantation 2021;105(12):e292–302.

59. Giusti EM, Lacerenza M, Manzoni GM, et al. Psychological and psychosocial predictors of chronic postsurgical pain: a systematic review and meta-analysis. PAIN 2021;162(1):10–30.

60. Morgan KA, Borckardt J, Balliet W, et al. How are select chronic pancreatitis patients selected for total pancreatectomy with islet autotransplantation? Are there psychometric predictors? J Am Coll Surg 2015;220(4):693–8.

61. Ashton K, Sullivan A. Ethics and confidentiality for psychologists in academic health centers. J Clin Psychol Med Settings 2018;25(3):240–9.

62. Ware JE, Sherbourne CD. The MOS 36-item short-form health survey (SF-36). I. Conceptual framework and item selection. Med Care 1992;30(6):473–83.

63. Wehler M, Reulbach U, Nichterlein R, et al. Health-related quality of life in chronic pancreatitis: a psychometric assessment. Scand J Gastroenterol 2003;38(10): 1083–9.

64. Ware J, Kosinski M, Keller SD. A 12-Item Short-Form Health Survey: construction of scales and preliminary tests of reliability and validity. Med Care 1996;34(3): 220–33.

65. Pezzilli R, Morselli-Labate AM, Frulloni L, et al. The quality of life in patients with chronic pancreatitis evaluated using the SF-12 questionnaire: A comparative study with the SF-36 questionnaire. Dig Liver Dis 2006;38(2):109–15.

66. Rabin R, de Charro F. EQ-5D: a measure of health status from the EuroQol Group. Ann Med 2001;33(5):337–43.

67. Van Wilder L, Rammant E, Clays E, et al. A comprehensive catalogue of EQ-5D scores in chronic disease: results of a systematic review. Qual Life Res 2019; 28(12):3153–61.

68. Wassef W, DeWitt J, McGreevy K, et al. Pancreatitis Quality of Life Instrument: A Psychometric Evaluation. Am J Gastroenterol 2016;111(8):1177–86.

69. Zigmond AS, Snaith RP. The hospital anxiety and depression scale. Acta Psychiatr Scand 1983;67(6):361–70.

70. Trudeau J, Turk D, Dworkin R, et al. Validation of the Hospital Anxiety and Depression Scale (HADS) in patients with acute low back pain. J Pain 2012;13(4):S24.

71. Avinir A, Dar S, Taler M, et al. Keeping it simple: mental health assessment in the Gastroenterology Department – using the Hospital Anxiety and Depression Scale (HADS) for IBD patients in Israel. Ther Adv Gastroenterol 2022;15. 17562848211066440.

72. Kroenke K, Spitzer RL, Williams JB. The PHQ-9: validity of a brief depression severity measure. J Gen Intern Med 2001;16(9):606–13.

73. Kroenke K, Spitzer RL, Williams JBW, et al. The Patient Health Questionnaire Somatic, Anxiety, and Depressive Symptom Scales: a systematic review. Gen Hosp Psychiatry 2010;32(4):345–59.

74. Spitzer RL, Kroenke K, Williams JBW, et al. A brief measure for assessing generalized anxiety disorder: the GAD-7. Arch Intern Med 2006;166(10):1092–7.

75. Tellegen A, Ben-Porath YS. Minnesota multiphasic personality inventory-2-restructured form (MMPI-2-RF). Minneapolis, MN: University of Minnesota Press; 2011.

76. Marek RJ, Ben-Porath YS. Using the Minnesota Multiphasic Personality Inventory-2-Restructured Form (MMPI-2-RF) in behavioral medicine settings. In: Mariusch M, editor. Handbook of psychological assessment in primary care Settings. 2nd edition. Oxfordshire, England, UK: Routledge/Taylor & Francis Group; 2017. p. 631–62.

77. Sullivan MJL, Bishop SR, Pivik J. The Pain Catastrophizing Scale: Development and validation. Psychol Assess 1995;7(4):524–32.

78. Wheeler CHB, Williams AC de C, Morley SJ. Meta-analysis of the psychometric properties of the Pain Catastrophizing Scale and associations with participant characteristics. Pain 2019;160(9):1946–53.

79. Cleeland CS, Ryan KM. Pain assessment: global use of the Brief Pain Inventory. Ann Acad Med Singapore 1994;23(2):129–38.

80. Kuhlmann L, Teo K, Olesen SS, et al. Development of the Comprehensive Pain Assessment Tool Short Form for Chronic Pancreatitis: Validity and Reliability Testing. Clin Gastroenterol Hepatol 2022;20(4):e770–83.

81. Saunders JB, Aasland OG, Babor TF, et al. Development of the Alcohol Use Disorders Identification Test (AUDIT): WHO Collaborative Project on Early Detection of Persons with Harmful Alcohol Consumption–II. Addict Abingdon Engl 1993; 88(6):791–804.

82. Brown RL, Rounds LA. Conjoint screening questionnaires for alcohol and other drug abuse: criterion validity in a primary care practice. Wis Med J 1995;94(3): 135–40.

83. Dhalla S, Kopec JA. The CAGE questionnaire for alcohol misuse: a review of reliability and validity studies. Clin Investig Med Med Clin Exp 2007;30(1):33–41.

84. Webster LR, Webster RM. Predicting aberrant behaviors in opioid-treated patients: preliminary validation of the Opioid Risk Tool. Pain Med Malden Mass 2005;6(6):432–42.

85. Osman A, Bagge CL, Gutierrez PM, et al. The Suicidal Behaviors Questionnaire-Revised (SBQ-R):Validation with Clinical and Nonclinical Samples. Assessment 2001;8(4):443–54.
86. Posner K, Brown GK, Stanley B, et al. The Columbia–Suicide Severity Rating Scale: Initial Validity and Internal Consistency Findings From Three Multisite Studies With Adolescents and Adults. Am J Psychiatry 2011;168(12):1266–77.

Management of Sexual Dysfunction in Gastrointestinal Disorders

Alyse Bedell, PhD[a],*, Alana Friedlander, MA[a,b]

KEYWORDS

- Sexual dysfunction • Sexual functioning • Sex therapy • Gastrointestinal disorders
- Inflammatory bowel disease • Irritable bowel syndrome • Sexual medicine

INTRODUCTION

Sexual dysfunction (SD) refers to problems that occur during any stage of the sexual response cycle (**Fig. 1**) that interfere with a person's sexual satisfaction. Patients with gastrointestinal (GI) disorders are at an increased risk of SD.[1–3] **Table 1** shows the list of common sexual problems and **Fig. 2** shows the relevant terminology.

Sexual Dysfunction in Patients with Gastrointestinal Disorders

The vast majority of research on SD in patients with GI is within inflammatory bowel disease (IBD). SD is significantly higher in IBD than in healthy controls, and can vary based on gender.[1,2,4–7] In women with IBD, rates of SD range from 49% to 97%[1,2,5,7] compared to 19% to 28% in healthy controls.[2,8] Specifically, female patients report experiencing sexual fear, guilt, distress, low interest, low arousal, poor body image, and abstinence as a result of their IBD diagnosis.[9] In men with IBD, rates of SD range from 14% to 39.1%[1,2,10] compared to a rate of 7% in healthy controls.[1,2] In one study, 38% percent of men with IBD reported that their IBD negatively affected their libido, 27% reported that it prevented sexual activity, and 18% reported that it caused problems during sexual activity.[11]

Irritable bowel syndrome (IBS) has been shown to have a negative impact on sexual relationships.[12,13] Prevalence of SD in patients with IBS ranges from 26% to 83%.[1,13–16] Across studies, female patients with IBS report higher SD rates than male patients with IBS, ranging from 44.9% to 77% and 26.4% to 39.4%, respectively.[1,14] Women most commonly report decreased desire and dyspareunia[14] while men report decreased desire and erectile dysfunction (ED).[1,14] One study found that 54.7% of men with IBS experienced ED, compared to only 12.5% of healthy controls.[1]

a Department of Psychiatry & Behavioral Neuroscience, The University of Chicago, 5841 South Maryland Avenue, MC 3077, Chicago, IL 60637, USA; b Department of Psychology, Roosevelt University, 430 South Michigan Avenue, Chicago, IL 60605, USA
* Corresponding author.
E-mail address: alysebedell@gmail.com
Twitter: @DrAlyseBedell (A.B.)

Gastroenterol Clin N Am 51 (2022) 815–828
https://doi.org/10.1016/j.gtc.2022.06.012
0889-8553/22/© 2022 Elsevier Inc. All rights reserved.

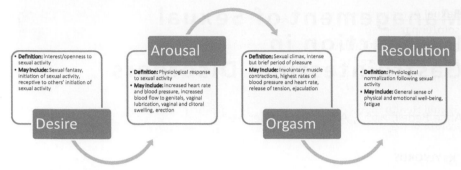

Fig. 1. The sexual response cycle.

Fass and colleagues[14] found that SD was positively correlated with symptom severity while Eugenio and colleagues[13] reported SD was the same regardless of the severity of IBS symptoms.

Though research is limited, SD has also been shown in a variety of other GI disorders. SD has been documented in GERD, dyspepsia, globus, chest pain, and aerophagia.[3,17] Lovino and colleagues[18] found that 21.7% of patients with GERD (vs 0% of the HC) reported difficulty achieving orgasm and 14.4% of patients with GERD (vs 0% of HC) experienced painful intercourse. Fass and colleagues found the prevalence of SD in patients with nonulcer dyspepsia to be 38.8%. SD is also found in patients with conditions in the lower GI tract, including celiac disease, functional abdominal pain, constipation, diarrhea, and bloating. For information on SD and colorectal cancer, please refer to a systematic review by Traa and colleagues.[19]

APPLYING THE BIOPSYCHOSOCIAL MODEL TO SEXUAL DYSFUNCTION IN GASTROINTESTINAL DISORDERS

When addressing sexual functioning in patients with GI disorders, it is important to highlight the role that biopsychosocial factors play in its etiology, perpetuation, and

Table 1 Common sexual problems		
Sexual Problems	**Definition**	**Sex**
Low desire/libido	Lack of interest or desire for sexual activity	Men or women
Erectile dysfunction	Difficulty achieving or maintain an erection	Men
Premature (early) ejaculation	Ejaculating earlier than desired	Men
Delayed ejaculation	Requiring an extended period of time or being unable to ejaculate at all	Men
Anorgasmia	Difficulty or inability in reaching orgasm after sufficient stimulation	Women
Vulvodynia	Chronic pain or discomfort of the vulva	Women
Dyspareunia	Pain associated with intercourse	Women
Vaginismus	An automatic reaction for which the vaginal muscles contract when penetration is attempted	Women

Sexual Activity: Activity that is associated with sexual arousal. This may include solo/unpartnered sexual activity (i.e., masturbation) or partnered activity such as manual or oral stimulation, anal or vaginal intercourse. Sexual activity is sometimes referred to as simply "sex", though we recommend against use of this term as it can be misinterpreted as referring to intercourse only.

Sexual Health: Rather than simply the absence of disease or dysfunction, refers to a state of physical, mental, emotional, and social *well-being* related to sexuality.[1]

Emotional Intimacy: An experience of comfort and closeness between people that can be expressed verbally or non-verbally. We recommend use of this term when discussing broader relationship interactions. Though "intimacy" is often used as a euphemism for sexual activity, we recommend against use of this term when the intended meaning is sexual activity.

Fig. 2. Relevant terminology.

treatment (**Fig. 3**). If it is unclear which specific factors are contributing, patients should be referred for evaluation by their primary care physician or a sexual medicine specialist.

Biomedical Factors

Pelvic floor dysfunction
The muscles of the pelvic floor are responsible for urination, defecation, and sexual function. As such, pelvic floor dysfunction may sometimes serve as a shared cause of GI and sexual symptoms. Pelvic floor dysfunction is common among patients with lower GI conditions, such as IBS[20,21] and constipation.[22]

Medications and other substances
With the exception of corticosteroids and methotrexate,[1] most medications prescribed for GI concerns do not directly contribute to SD. The use of suppositories, enemas, or foams can indirectly contribute to SD by limiting sexual spontaneity and desexualizing the genitalia. Non-GI medications, including antihypertensives and psychotropics, as well as recreational substances including alcohol, tobacco, and amphetamines can contribute to SD. The impact of cannabis use on sexual function is in its early stages and results are mixed.[23–25]

Medical factors
Non-GI medical conditions can drive SD in patients with GI disorders, such as uncontrolled diabetes, hypertension, obesity, age-related factors, and neurological causes (eg, stroke, spinal cord injury). Menopause can also be a common contributor to SD in women, contributing to symptoms such as decreased desire and arousal, and painful intercourse.

Surgery and active disease
GI surgeries and active disease can directly cause SD due to anatomical and physiological changes. They can indirectly contribute to SD through changes in body image, pain, or fatigue.

GI-related surgeries vary in their impact on sexual functioning. In some studies, patients that underwent ileal pouch-anal anastomosis[26,27] and restorative proctocolectomy[28] demonstrated improvements in sexual functioning, while others

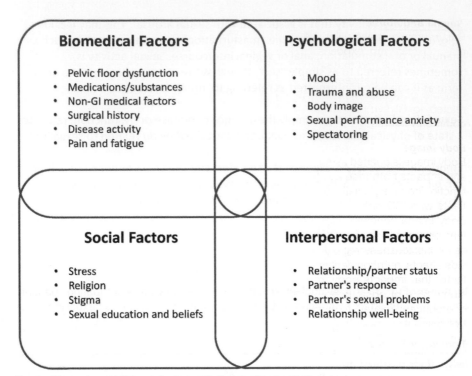

Biomedical Factors

- Pelvic floor dysfunction
- Medications/substances
- Non-GI medical factors
- Surgical history
- Disease activity
- Pain and fatigue

Psychological Factors

- Mood
- Trauma and abuse
- Body image
- Sexual performance anxiety
- Spectatoring

Social Factors

- Stress
- Religion
- Stigma
- Sexual education and beliefs

Interpersonal Factors

- Relationship/partner status
- Partner's response
- Partner's sexual problems
- Relationship well-being

Fig. 3. Biopsychosocial model of sexual dysfunction in GI disorders.

demonstrated increased SD.[29] Though lacking empirical data, it is important to consider that a variety of individuals engage in sexual stimulation in and around the rectum, and as such, the surgical removal of the rectum or inflammation of the rectum result in a significant loss of sexual pleasure.

Pain and fatigue
Both pain and fatigue are well-known disruptors in the sexual response cycle that should be considered as potential factors for many patients with GI disorders. In a 2013 study of patients with IBD, 38% were shown to have chronic pain.[30] IBS, in and of itself a pain condition, commonly cooccurs with chronic pelvic pain.[31,32] Fatigue is a commonly reported extra-intestinal symptom among patients with GI conditions[33,34] and was ranked the number one cited cause of worsened sex life in a study of 355 participants with IBD.[2]

Psychological Factors

Mood
Studies have found that mood disorders, especially depression, are highly correlated with both SD[35,36] and GI disorders.[37,38] A systematic review by Mikocka-Walus and colleagues[38] demonstrated significantly higher rates of depression and anxiety compared to healthy controls. Increased rates of mood and anxiety disorders among patients with GI disorders may, in part, result from the impact of the GI concerns themselves, such as adjusting to a diagnosis, coping with unpredictable symptoms, and impacts on social activities. Recent research has found that mood disorders are the mediating variable and/or risk factor for SD in patients with GI disorders.[1,11,39–41]

Trauma and abuse

Posttraumatic stress disorder (PTSD) refers to a constellation of symptoms that can develop following exposure to the threat of life, injury, and/or violence (DSM-5). Research has found that sexual processes operate along similar networks as PTSD, leading to a link between trauma and SD in both men and women.[42] In some cases, patients may experience symptoms of posttraumatic stress due to experiences related to GI symptoms and treatment.[43,44] Trauma, SD, and GI functioning can commonly intersect and benefit from multidisciplinary treatment.

Body image

Body image is defined as the attitudes and perceptions one has toward their own body and impacts both men and women.[45] The impact of body image concerns on sexual functioning is especially great among women.[46] Seventy-five percent of female patients with IBD and 50% of male patients with IBD report body image concerns.[47] Body image concerns in patients with GI disorders vary widely, but can pertain to fear or embarrassment about passing gas or urgency during sexual situations, or self-consciousness regarding weight and shape changes resulting from medication side effects, nutrition deficits, or abdominal distention. Postsurgical scarring is another factor that impacts body image and the sexual function of patients with GI. In one study, 86% of postsurgery anal and rectal cancer female patients reported at least one concern related to body image. In the same study, the authors found that in this population, poor body image was significantly correlated with poor sexual functioning across all domains, except for pain.[48] Patients with ostomies reported lower body image and poorer sexual functioning.[49] Perianal disease has an effect on body image and sexual functioning in patients with GI disorders and is especially common among patients with setons, fistulas, and drainage.

Cognitive factors

Cognitive distractions during sexual activity play a role in SD, specifically at the point of arousal and desire.[35] Masters and Johnson were the first to introduce this concept and coined the term spectatoring.[50] Spectatoring is the process of being hyperaware of and highly judgmental of oneself during a sexual encounter. Spectatoring causes a distraction from the sexual experience and contributes to SD.

Sexual performance anxiety is defined as thoughts and concerns related to satisfactory sexual performance, and are a key factor in the development and maintenance of SD in both men and women.[51] Sexual performance anxiety is often a concern of patients with IBD,[5] especially among women[52] and among patients with ostomies.[53]

Social Factors

Stress

Though research on whether acute stressors facilitate or inhibit sexual function is mixed,[54,55] data are more consistent in the deleterious effect of chronic stress on sexual function.[56,57] Clinicians should consider that patients suffering from ongoing stress related to family, work, or GI illness are at risk of negative sexual health outcomes.

Cultural and societal factors

An individual's cultural background, including attitudes related to sexual activity, sexuality, gender, and relationships, can cause conflict for the individual. One common example includes individuals raised in religious or other cultural traditions in which sexuality is considered "sinful," and may include specific guidelines (eg, only for procreation, only for male pleasure). Individuals with GI conditions and sexual problems may experience shame or embarrassment twofold, as both GI symptoms and sexual concerns are associated with a high degree of stigma in most societies.

Sexual education and beliefs

An individual's level of understanding regarding sexual anatomy, the sexual response cycle, and basic information regarding sexual norms can significantly contribute to their ability to improve their sexual problem as well as understand reasonable expectations for progress. Many people are surprised by the common duration of vaginal intercourse (5.4 minutes[58]) that 1/3 of women require clitoral stimulation to orgasm during intercourse,[59] or the average length of an erect penis (between 5.1 and 5.5 inches[60]). Understanding a person's beliefs and correcting misinformation can be very helpful in differentiating normal or abnormal sexual phenomena, reducing anxiety, and setting appropriate treatment goals.

Interpersonal Factors

Partner factors

Patients who are single and patients who are partnered can both experience SD due to their GI symptoms. Unpartnered and partnered individuals may also engage in masturbation. When considering an individual's sexual problem, it is especially relevant to consider how his or her partner responds to the sexual problem, such as whether they are frustrated, supportive, and open to participating in the intervention. When an individual is in a sexual relationship, it is important to recognize that the partner's sexual desire and sexual function play an important role in the sexual experiences of the identified patient.

Intimacy and relationship well-being

Intimacy can be expressed in a variety of ways, such as through deep conversation, spending time in leisure activities together, celebrating each other's victories, and supporting each other through life's challenges. Engaging in sexual activity is one way to be intimate with a partner and desiring intimacy and emotional connectedness is a strong motivator for sex in humans.[61]

ASSESSMENT OF SEXUAL FUNCTION

Despite the high rate of SD in patients with GI disorders, no guidelines exist that directly address how GI physicians should assess for and treat SD in patients.[62] While 93% of gastroenterologists believe that they should discuss sexual concerns with their patients, only 16% actually do; reasons cited for avoiding the topic include lack of knowledge (45%), fears of upsetting the patient (29%), and personal embarrassment (18.8%).[63]

Even though only 16% of physicians address sexual functioning with their patients with GI, 64% of women and 50% of men would prefer that their physicians provide them with information on the relationship between their disease and their sexual functioning.[2] Two separate studies indicate that two-thirds of women[9] and 78%[11] of men feel comfortable discussing the topic of sexual functioning with their GI provider, but are often waiting for their provider to initiate the conversation.

Gastroenterologists can fill this gap by developing systematically screening for their patients for SD. The use of self-report measures can be a helpful tool, and recommended measures are listed in **Table 2**. However, assessing sexual functioning with a clinical interview can be quickly and easily integrated with questions assessing a patient's emotional well-being and quality of life.

Table 2 Assessment tools	
Sexual Function Screening Measures	
General Measures	
Female Sexual Function Index (FSFI)[68]	• Gold standard measure of female sexual functioning • Measures female sexual functioning across 6 domains: desire, arousal, orgasm, lubrication, satisfaction, and pain • 19 items
International Index of Erectile Function (IIEF)[69]	• Gold standard measure of male sexual functioning • Measures male sexual functioning across 5 domains: erectile function, orgasm function, desire, intercourse satisfaction, and overall satisfaction • 15 items
Single-Item Screener for Self-Reporting Sexual Problems[70]	• Clinical screener to capture common sexual problems in men and women • 1 item with 9 "check all that apply" choices
GI-Specific Measures	
IBD-specific Female Sexual Dysfunction Scale (IBD-FSDS)[9]	• Measures sexual dysfunction in women with IBD • 15 items
IBD-specific Male Sexual Dysfunction Scale (IBD-MSDS)[11]	• Measures sexual dysfunction in men with IBD • 10 items
Irritable Bowel Syndrome Quality of Life Instrument (IBS-QOL)[71]	• Measures 8 factors that affect QOL in patients with IBS, including 2 items that screen for SD • 34 items

The PLISSIT Model

The PLISSIT Model is a tool to help health care providers initiate conversations about sexual health, assess for potential SD, and provide referrals to the most appropriate provider. It consists of 4 steps, beginning with initiating the conversation and ending with a treatment plan or referral.[64] The first stage of this model is "Permission." This stage represents a foundational expectation for which the provider opens a conversation and all patients are given the opportunity to talk about their sexual health with their health care provider. In this stage, it is important that the provider validates the patient's concerns and communicates care and understanding. "Limited Information," the second stage, refers to providing patients with basic education, such as the role of psychosocial factors in sexual function and the effect that GI disease has on sexual function. Providers should have the basic knowledge to address patients' questions and resources they can supply. In the third step, "Specific Suggestions," information and guidance are tailored to the patient, such as prescribing medication or referring them to a sexual medicine, sex therapy, or physical therapy colleague for further evaluation. "Intensive Therapy," the fourth step, is required by fewer patients and involves a comprehensive sexual health intervention (eg, sex therapy) by a skilled provider. By following the PLISSIT model, and being thoughtful regarding the stages of the model

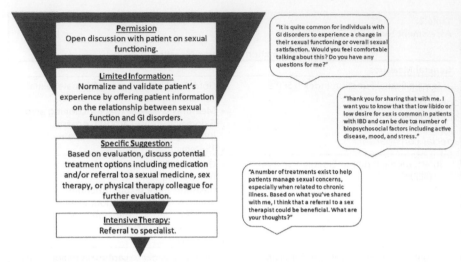

Fig. 4. The PLISSIT model.

that they themselves can provide, health care providers are able to address the sensitive topic of sexual functioning and provide suggestions and treatment where indicated. See **Fig. 4** for a depiction of the PLISSIT model with suggestions regarding helpful language.

PSYCHOSOCIAL TREATMENT OF SEXUAL DYSFUNCTION
Sex Therapy

Sex therapy is a type of psychotherapy for which the primary goals of treatment are related to sexual function and sexual well-being. Sex therapists are mental health professionals with expertise in sexual health; the term *certified* sex therapists (CSTs) refers to a select pool of professionals that have undergone rigorous sexual health education and clinical training to be certified and registered. A directory of CSTs is available at https://www.aasect.org/referral-directory. While sex therapy can include brief, targeted interventions for a sexual problem, sex therapists also provide more comprehensive psychotherapy for longer courses of treatment when clinically indicated. Sex therapy can be with one individual only or with couples (with the couple itself as the "identified patient" or with the individual seeking treatment and their partner).

Psychoeducation is a key component of sex therapy, with topics such as the biopsychosocial model of sexual health, providing information, and correcting misinformation regarding male and female anatomy and the sexual response cycle.

Sex therapists use various psychotherapeutic orientations and treatment modalities as the basis for their work. This includes cognitive behavior therapy (CBT), psychodynamic therapies, and more recently, mindfulness-based therapies. Though treatment varies from provider to provider, it typically includes a psychosocial sexual evaluation to determine specific psychosocial variables that may be contributing to current sexual health concerns. Sex therapists will typically offer treatment to target these identified variables, though in some cases, may recommend that the patient see a provider with a more advanced skillset in a certain area (eg, trauma, substance use). Some interventions transcend theoretical orientation and are commonly employed by many sex therapists, the most notable of which is sensate focus. Sensate focus is a multiple-step intervention that is conducted between psychotherapy sessions that encourages couples to reduce anxiety, increase intimacy and improve communication through scaffolded touching exercises ranging from nonsexual to sexual.

Referrals to sex therapy often come from the medical provider. In some cases, patients may benefit from an assessment with a sexual medicine provider, such as a urologist or gynecologist, for a more comprehensive assessment to identify any biomedical factors that may be contributing to their symptoms.

Special considerations

Members of the LGBTQ + community are more likely to experience a number of risk factors associated with SD in patients with GI, including anxiety and depression, a lack of social support, stress, stigma, and trauma and abuse.[65] Nonbinary and transgender patients are also more likely to be mistreated, victimized, and discriminated against by medical professionals.[66] According to a study by Dibley and colleagues,[67] gay and lesbian individuals with IBD reported experiencing increased stress in the doctor's office and reported being treated differently by their health care team. Patients reported that neither doctors nor the literature provided to them at diagnosis addressed their sexual functioning concerns, specifically the implications of sexual restrictions following GI surgeries such as ileo-anal pouch formation.[67]

It is important to assess for SD and provide sexual health information to patients regardless of age, or perceptions of health status, ability, sexual orientation, or gender identity. GI providers should also provide a safe environment for their patients to disclose this information, rather than relying on their own assumptions.

DISCUSSION

Sexual health concerns are common among GI patient populations. Gastroenterologists and other members of the care team should routinely query their patients regarding sexual function and satisfaction through the use of the clinical interview or self-report measures and develop competency in discussing sexual health concerns, such as knowledge of common sexual problems, an understanding of bio-psychosocial factors contributing to sexual problems, and options for further evaluation and/or treatment. Perhaps most importantly, providers should take care to normalize the discussion of sexual health in a clinical setting and provide permission for the patient to discuss these concerns by initiating the conversation.

Many patients with GI disorders are ready to talk with their gastroenterologists about their sexual health. For those who are experiencing SD, this first conversation can be a first step in reducing stigma and instilling hope that with appropriate treatment, they can enhance their sexual well-being.

Though there is a large body of research documenting the prevalence of SD in IBD, there is a need to expand this research to other GI disorders. Finally, future research is warranted to evaluate the effectiveness of addressing sexual health within a GI setting.

CLINICS CARE POINTS

- Sexual dysfunction (SD) is highly prevalent in patients with GI disorders of both the upper and lower gastrointestinal (GI) tract.
- A number of biopsychosocial factors contribute to and exacerbate SD in patients with GI disorders.

- Patients desire information on the effect their GI condition may have on their sexual functioning, but rarely is the topic addressed between patient and provider.
- Gastroenterologists should routinely screen their patients for SD using clinical interviews and objective measures.
- GI providers should develop the knowledge necessary to discuss sexual health concerns, including SD and its associated factors, as well as provide resources, treatment, and referrals for sexual health management.

DISCLOSURE

The authors do not have any commercial or financial conflicts of interest, nor any funding sources to disclose.

REFERENCES

1. Rivière P, Zallot C, Desobry P, et al. Frequency of and factors associated with sexual dysfunction in patients with inflammatory bowel disease. J Crohns Colitis 2017;11(11):1347–52.
2. Marín L, Mañosa M, Garcia-Planella E, et al. Sexual function and patients' perceptions in inflammatory bowel disease: a case-control survey. J Gastroenterol 2013;48(6):713–20.
3. Romano L, Granata L, Fusco F, et al. Sexual dysfunction in patients with chronic gastrointestinal and liver diseases: a neglected issue. Sex Med Rev 2021. https://doi.org/10.1016/j.sxmr.2021.02.002.
4. Organization WH. Working Together for Health: The World Health Report. 2006.
5. Jedel S, Hood MM, Keshavarzian A. Getting personal: a review of sexual functioning, body image, and their impact on quality of life in patients with inflammatory bowel disease. Inflamm Bowel Dis 2015;21(4):923–38.
6. Zhao S, Wang J, Liu Y, et al. Inflammatory bowel diseases were associated with risk of sexual dysfunction in both sexes: a meta-analysis. Inflamm Bowel Dis 2019;25(4):699–707.
7. Shmidt E, Suárez-Fariñas M, Mallette M, et al. A longitudinal study of sexual function in women with newly diagnosed inflammatory bowel disease. Inflamm Bowel Dis 2019;25(7):1262–70.
8. Leenhardt R, Rivière P, Papazian P, et al. Sexual health and fertility for individuals with inflammatory bowel disease. World J Gastroenterol 2019;25(36):5423–33.
9. de Silva PS, O'Toole A, Marc LG, et al. Development of a sexual dysfunction scale for women with inflammatory bowel disease. Inflamm Bowel Dis 2018;24(11):2350–9.
10. Shmidt E, Suárez-Fariñas M, Mallette M, et al. Erectile dysfunction is highly prevalent in men with newly diagnosed inflammatory bowel disease. Inflamm Bowel Dis 2019;25(8):1408–16.
11. O'Toole A, de Silva PS, Marc LG, et al. Sexual dysfunction in men with inflammatory bowel disease: a new IBD-specific scale. Inflamm Bowel Dis 2018;24(2):310–6.
12. Sørensen J, Schantz Laursen B, Drewes AM, et al. The incidence of sexual dysfunction in patients with irritable bowel syndrome. Sex Med 2019;7(4):371–83.

13. Eugenio MD, Jun SE, Cain KC, et al. Comprehensive self-management reduces the negative impact of irritable bowel syndrome symptoms on sexual functioning. Dig Dis Sci 2012;57(6):1636–46.

14. Fass R, Fullerton S, Naliboff B, et al. Sexual dysfunction in patients with irritable bowel syndrome and non-ulcer dyspepsia. Digestion 1998;59(1):79–85.

15. Guthrie E, Creed FH, Whorwell PJ. Severe sexual dysfunction in women with the irritable bowel syndrome: comparison with inflammatory bowel disease and duodenal ulceration. Br Med J (Clin Res Ed) 1987;295(6598):577–8.

16. Sławik P, Szul M, Fuchs A, et al. Could problems in the bedroom come from our intestines? A preliminary study of IBS and its impact on female sexuality. Psychiatr Danub 2019;31(Suppl 3):561–7.

17. Bouchoucha M, Devroede G, Mary F, et al. Both men and women with functional gastrointestinal disorders suffer from a high incidence of sexual dysfunction. Clin Res Hepatol Gastroenterol 2017;41(6):e93–6.

18. Iovino P, Pascariello A, Limongelli P, et al. The prevalence of sexual behavior disorders in patients with treated and untreated gastroesophageal reflux disease. Surg Endosc 2007;21(7):1104–10.

19. Traa MJ, De Vries J, Roukema JA, et al. Sexual (dys)function and the quality of sexual life in patients with colorectal cancer: a systematic review. Ann Oncol 2012;23(1):19–27.

20. Prott G, Shim L, Hansen R, et al. Relationships between pelvic floor symptoms and function in irritable bowel syndrome. Neurogastroenterol Motil 2010;22(7): 764–9.

21. Suttor VP, Prott GM, Hansen RD, et al. Evidence for pelvic floor dyssynergia in patients with irritable bowel syndrome. Dis Colon Rectum 2010;53(2): 156–60.

22. Bharucha AE, Lacy BE. Mechanisms, evaluation, and management of chronic constipation. Gastroenterology 2020;158(5):1232–49.e3.

23. Kasman AM, Bhambhvani HP, Wilson-King G, et al. Assessment of the association of cannabis on female sexual function with the female sexual function index. Sex Med 2020;8(4):699–708.

24. Shiff B, Blankstein U, Hussaen J, et al. The impact of cannabis use on male sexual function: a 10-year, single-center experience. Can Urol Assoc J 2021;15(12): E652–7.

25. Wiebe E, Just A. How cannabis alters sexual experience: a survey of men and women. J Sex Med 2019;16(11):1758–62.

26. Davies RJ, O'Connor BI, Victor C, et al. A prospective evaluation of sexual function and quality of life after ileal pouch-anal anastomosis. Dis Colon Rectum 2008; 51(7):1032–5.

27. Wang JY, Hart SL, Wilkowski KS, et al. Gender-specific differences in pelvic organ function after proctectomy for inflammatory bowel disease. Dis Colon Rectum 2011;54(1):66–76.

28. Berndtsson I, Oresland T, Hultén L. Sexuality in patients with ulcerative colitis before and after restorative proctocolectomy: a prospective study. Scand J Gastroenterol 2004;39(4):374–9.

29. Hueting WE, Buskens E, van der Tweel I, et al. Results and complications after ileal pouch anal anastomosis: a meta-analysis of 43 observational studies comprising 9,317 patients. Dig Surg 2005;22(1–2):69–79.

30. Morrison G, Van Langenberg DR, Gibson SJ, et al. Chronic pain in inflammatory bowel disease: characteristics and associations of a hospital-based cohort. Inflamm Bowel Dis 2013;19(6):1210–7.

31. Choung RS, Herrick LM, Locke GR, et al. Irritable bowel syndrome and chronic pelvic pain: a population-based study. J Clin Gastroenterol 2010;44(10):696–701.
32. Williams RE, Hartmann KE, Sandler RS, et al. Prevalence and characteristics of irritable bowel syndrome among women with chronic pelvic pain. Obstet Gynecol 2004;104(3):452–8.
33. Han CJ, Yang GS. Fatigue in irritable bowel syndrome: a systematic review and meta-analysis of pooled frequency and severity of fatigue. review article. Asian Nurs Res 2016;10(1):1–10.
34. Nocerino A, Nguyen A, Agrawal M, et al. Fatigue in inflammatory bowel diseases: etiologies and management. Adv Ther 2020;37(1):97–112.
35. Brotto L, Atallah S, Johnson-Agbakwu C, et al. Psychological and interpersonal dimensions of sexual function and dysfunction. J Sex Med 2016;13(4):538–71.
36. Kendurkar A, Kaur B. Major depressive disorder, obsessive-compulsive disorder, and generalized anxiety disorder: do the sexual dysfunctions differ? Prim Care Companion J Clin Psychiatry 2008;10(4):299–305.
37. Shah E, Rezaie A, Riddle M, et al. Psychological disorders in gastrointestinal disease: epiphenomenon, cause or consequence? Ann Gastroenterol 2014;27(3): 224–30.
38. Mikocka-Walus A, Knowles SR, Keefer L, et al. Controversies revisited: a systematic review of the comorbidity of depression and anxiety with inflammatory bowel diseases. Inflamm Bowel Dis 2016;22(3):752–62.
39. Bel LG, Vollebregt AM, Van der Meulen-de Jong AE, et al. Sexual dysfunctions in men and women with inflammatory bowel disease: the influence of IBD-related clinical factors and depression on sexual function. J Sex Med 2015;12(7): 1557–67.
40. Timmer A, Bauer A, Dignass A, et al. Sexual function in persons with inflammatory bowel disease: a survey with matched controls. Clin Gastroenterol Hepatol 2007; 5(1):87–94.
41. Yanartas O, Kani HT, Bicakci E, et al. The effects of psychiatric treatment on depression, anxiety, quality of life, and sexual dysfunction in patients with inflammatory bowel disease. Neuropsychiatr Dis Treat 2016;12:673–83.
42. Yehuda R, Lehrner A, Rosenbaum TY. PTSD and sexual dysfunction in men and women. J Sex Med 2015;12(5):1107–19.
43. Taft TH, Bedell A, Craven MR, et al. Initial assessment of post-traumatic stress in a US cohort of inflammatory bowel disease patients. Inflamm Bowel Dis 2019; 25(9):1577–85.
44. Pothemont K, Quinton S, Jayoushe M, et al. Patient perspectives on medical trauma related to inflammatory bowel disease. J Clin Psychol Med Settings 2021. https://doi.org/10.1007/s10880-021-09805-0.
45. Ramseyer Winter V, O'Neill EA, Cook M, et al. Sexual function in hook-up culture: the role of body image. Body Image 2020;34:135–44.
46. Woertman L, van den Brink F. Body image and female sexual functioning and behavior: a review. J Sex Res 2012;49(2–3):184–211.
47. Muller KR, Prosser R, Bampton P, et al. Female gender and surgery impair relationships, body image, and sexuality in inflammatory bowel disease: patient perceptions. Inflamm Bowel Dis 2010;16(4):657–63.
48. Benedict C, Philip EJ, Baser RE, et al. Body image and sexual function in women after treatment for anal and rectal cancer. Psychooncology 2016;25(3):316–23.
49. Ayaz-Alkaya S. Overview of psychosocial problems in individuals with stoma: A review of literature. Int Wound J 2019;16(1):243–9.
50. Masters W, Johnson V. Human sexual inadequacy. Boston: Little, Brown; 1970.

51. McCabe MP, Connaughton C. Psychosocial factors associated with male sexual difficulties. J Sex Res 2014;51(1):31–42.

52. Maunder RG, de Rooy EC, Toner BB, et al. Health-related concerns of people who receive psychological support for inflammatory bowel disease. Can J Gastroenterol 1997;11(8):681–5.

53. Carlsson E, Berndtsson I, Hallén AM, et al. Concerns and quality of life before surgery and during the recovery period in patients with rectal cancer and an ostomy. J Wound Ostomy Continence Nurs 2010;37(6):654–61.

54. Palace EM, Gorzalka BB. Differential patterns of arousal in sexually functional and dysfunctional women: physiological and subjective components of sexual response. Arch Sex Behav 1992;21(2):135–59.

55. Ter Kuile MM, Vigeveno D, Laan E. Preliminary evidence that acute and chronic daily psychological stress affect sexual arousal in sexually functional women. Behav Res Ther 2007;45(9):2078–89.

56. Hamilton LD, Meston CM. Chronic stress and sexual function in women. J Sex Med 2013;10(10):2443–54.

57. Basson R. The recurrent pain and sexual sequelae of provoked vestibulodynia: a perpetuating cycle. J Sex Med 2012;9(8):2077–92.

58. Waldinger MD, Quinn P, Dilleen M, et al. A multinational population survey of intravaginal ejaculation latency time. J Sex Med 2005;2(4):492–7.

59. Herbenick D, Fu TJ, Arter J, et al. Women's experiences with genital touching, sexual pleasure, and orgasm: results from a U.S. probability sample of women ages 18 to 94. J Sex Marital Ther 2018;44(2):201–12.

60. King BM. Average-size erect penis: fiction, fact, and the need for counseling. J Sex Marital Ther 2021;47(1):80–9.

61. Meston CM, Buss DM. Why humans have sex. Arch Sex Behav 2007;36(4):477–507.

62. Perez de Arce E, Quera R, Ribeiro Barros J, et al. Sexual dysfunction in inflammatory bowel disease: what the specialist should know and ask. Int J Gen Med 2021;14:2003–15.

63. Rivière P, Poullenot F, Zerbib F, et al. Quality of sex life in patients with inflammatory bowel disease: the gastroenterologists' perspective. Inflamm Bowel Dis 2017;23(10):E51–2.

64. Annon J. The PLISSIT model: a proposed conceptual scheme for the behavioral treatment of sexual problems. J Sex Educ Ther 1976;2:1–15.

65. Hafeez H, Zeshan M, Tahir MA, et al. Health care disparities among lesbian, gay, bisexual, and transgender youth: a literature review. Cureus 2017;9(4):e1184.

66. Kattari SK, Bakko M, Langenderfer-Magruder L, et al. Transgender and nonbinary experiences of victimization in health care. J Interpers Violence 2021;36(23–24):NP13054–76.

67. Dibley L, Norton C, Schaub J, et al. Experiences of gay and lesbian patients with inflammatory bowel disease: a mixed methods study. Gastrointest Nurs 2014;12(6):19–30.

68. Rosen R, Brown C, Heiman J, et al. The Female Sexual Function Index (FSFI): a multidimensional self-report instrument for the assessment of female sexual function. J Sex Marital Ther 2000;26(2):191–208.

69. Rosen RC, Riley A, Wagner G, et al. The international index of erectile function (IIEF): a multidimensional scale for assessment of erectile dysfunction. Urology 1997;49(6):822–30.

70. Flynn KE, Lindau ST, Lin L, et al. Development and validation of a single-item screener for self-reporting sexual problems in U.S. adults. J Gen Intern Med 2015;30(10):1468–75.

71. Patrick DL, Drossman DA, Frederick IO, et al. Quality of life in persons with irritable bowel syndrome: development and validation of a new measure. Dig Dis Sci 1998;43(2):400–11.

Management of Sleep and Fatigue in Gastrointestinal Patients

Jessica K. Salwen-Deremer, PhD, DBSM[a],*, Michael Sun, PhD[b]

KEYWORDS

- Psychogastroenterology • Sleep disorders • Insomnia • Fatigue
- Irritable bowel syndrome • Inflammatory bowel disease • Behavioral sleep medicine

KEY POINTS

- Sleep complaints and fatigue are common in people with gastrointestinal (GI) conditions.
- Fatigue, sleep problems, and GI problems likely reinforce one another.
- There are evidence-based treatments for a variety of sleep problems.
- GI providers should assess sleep and fatigue with 1 to 2 simple questions and provide referrals if needed.

INTRODUCTION

You may be familiar with cases similar to the three below from your own clinic:

1. Alicia, a 28-year-old woman with irritable bowel syndrome (IBS) with diarrhea, comes in reporting that despite closely following pharmacologic and dietary recommendations, her symptoms are not well controlled. Lately, they have become particularly hard to manage. In recent months, she has been socializing and exercising less, because when she is out of the house she constantly worries about experiencing pain and needing to find a bathroom. She frequently monitors herself for symptoms and often thinks about what she might do in worst-case scenario situations, such as having an accident in public. When she gets to bed at night, she often thinks about how she will manage her symptoms the next day. She tells you she feels incredibly fatigued, that her symptoms are "ruining her life", and that she needs better treatment options.
2. George is a 45-year-old man with Crohn's disease. A recent colonoscopy indicated that his disease is mildly active, though his drug levels are therapeutic and he is

[a] Departments of Psychiatry and Medicine, Section of Gastroenterology & Hepatology, The Geisel School of Medicine at Dartmouth, Dartmouth-Hitchcock Medical Center, One Medical Center Drive, Lebanon, NH 03756, USA; [b] Department of Psychological and Brain Sciences, Dartmouth College, 3 Maynard Street, Hanover, NH 03755, USA
* Corresponding author.
E-mail address: Jessica.k.salwen-deremer@hitchcock.org

Gastroenterol Clin N Am 51 (2022) 829–847
https://doi.org/10.1016/j.gtc.2022.07.007
0889-8553/22/© 2022 Elsevier Inc. All rights reserved.

gastro.theclinics.com

adherent to his medication schedule. He reports that occasionally he has a bowel movement during the night and that abdominal pain can occur at any time, day or night. However, his biggest complaint is his fatigue. He understands it to be "par for the course" in Crohn's disease, but his fatigue is worsening, despite his other symptoms having been stable. His fatigue levels have been interfering with his ability to work and spend time with his family, resulting in an overall low mood.

3. Marco is a 58-year-old man with gastroesophageal reflux disease (GERD) who is stable on a proton pump inhibitor (PPI) regimen. Testing indicates that his GERD is well controlled. At a follow-up visit, he indicates that since being on a PPI, he has been thrilled that he is able to eat more, including foods he previously enjoyed such as chocolate ice cream and fried foods. He has gained 20 lbs. since the last visit 3 to 4 months ago and has begun to feel really sleepy during the day, even nodding off a few times at work. He has also started tossing and turning more during the night and waking up with headaches most mornings. He asks you if these problems (sleepiness and headaches) may be side effects of the PPI and expresses some worry that if he continues to fall asleep at work, he may lose his job.

What Alicia, George, and Marco share are complaints of fatigue, sleep disturbances, negative affect, and other daytime impairments. Sleep is critical for nearly all physiologic processes in the body, and problems with sleep can be both a cause and a consequence of other medical and psychiatric conditions.[1,2] The United States-based National Sleep Foundation recommends that healthy adults ages 18 to 64 need 7 to 9 h of sleep per night and adults 65 and older need approximately 7 to 8 h of sleep.[3] Although sleep duration decreases throughout adulthood, the time it takes a person to fall asleep generally remains stable and time spent awake during the night increases.[4] Unfortunately, many Americans do not get these recommended amounts; an estimated 28% to 40% of the United States population gets less than 7 h of sleep per 24-h period.[5–7] Further, nearly a quarter of Americans report poor sleep quality overall,[8] which may be attributable to sleep disorders, medical or psychiatric problems, and/or other ongoing difficulties (eg, social or family circumstances). This percentage increases to 60% to 75% in gastrointestinal (GI) patient populations.[9–12]

More recently, researchers have begun to probe the sleep-GI symptom relationship. In our own work, we have shown that people with inflammatory bowel disease (IBD) commonly report experiencing IBD-related sleep disruptions, including bowel movements at night, IBD-specific pain, feeling generally unwell, other kinds of pain, and worries about incontinence, among other things.[13] Others have found that in both IBD and IBS, poor sleep makes it more difficult to cope with GI symptoms and contributes significantly to reductions in quality of life.[14,15] Further, sleep disturbance may be a *driving* factor across GI conditions. In IBS it predicts next day abdominal pain and GI distress[16,17] and in IBD, it predicts a greater likelihood of disease flare 6 to 12 months later.[10,18] In addition, in IBD increased sleep fragmentation is positively associated with next-day abdominal pain.[19] Corroborating this viewpoint, in a longitudinal study on change in functional dyspepsia (FD) symptoms over 3 to 6 months, better baseline sleep (ie, lower severity of sleep disturbance) strongly predicted symptom improvement.[20]

Common Sleep Disorders and Prevalence Rates

Unfortunately, many sleep-related complaints and sleep disorders are more common in people with digestive disorders. Sleep disorders can also compound the difficulties of managing GI symptoms by increasing fatigue and pain. Three of the most common sleep disorders in the American population include insomnia, obstructive sleep apnea

(OSA), and restless leg syndrome (also called Willis–Ekbom disease); see **Table 1** for basic information on these three sleep disorders.

Insomnia is present in approximately 10% of the general population. It is characterized by difficulty falling asleep, staying asleep, or early morning awakening three times per week or more combined with daytime symptoms (eg, fatigue) and impairment (eg, impact on ability to function at work or as a caregiver).[21] Taking longer than 30 min to fall asleep or being awake for more than 30 min during the night are often considered by researchers to be clinically significant cut-points, although these experiences are not sufficiently diagnostic for insomnia.[22] Of all the sleep disorders, insomnia has been investigated most frequently in GI populations, with research suggesting there are elevated rates of insomnia in people with FD,[12] GERD (37%),[9,23] IBS (51%),[9] and both active and inactive IBD (63%–66% and 32%–33%, respectively).[13]

OSA is a sleep-related breathing disorder involving decreased airflow due to a block in the upper airway (usually from collapsed soft tissue in the throat). OSA is characterized by excessive daytime sleepiness, loud snoring, and gasping at night, though a diagnosis is made based on polysomnography. Based on recent definitions and trends, it is thought to affect 13% to 14% of men and 5% to 6% of women.[24] The risk for OSA increases moderately with age and dramatically with body mass index.[25,26] OSA and GERD may have a bidirectional relationship, and indeed risk for OSA is higher in people with GERD than in healthy controls.[11] Similarly, people with sleep-related breathing disorders have an increased risk for GERD.[27] Research on OSA and IBS has typically focused on the prevalence of IBS in people with OSA, and suggests a 2–4× increased risk of IBS in people with OSA compared with those without.[28,29] There is very limited research on OSA in IBD, though the existing data indicate there may be an elevation for OSA risk in people with active ulcerative colitis.[13]

Restless legs syndrome (RLS) centers around an evening urge to move one's legs often combined with an unpleasant, "creepy-crawly" feeling in the legs that may be relieved with movement. RLS has a prevalence of 8% to 10% in the general adult population.[30] Rates of RLS in people with IBD are similar to the general population,[13,31,32] though are three-fold the general population in people with IBS.[33]

Other sleep-related concerns. There are also several sleep-related phenomena that are associated with specific digestive disorders. First, humans follow a 24-h clock, with the majority of people having a natural sleep phase from about midnight to 8:00 AM [34] Having a *delayed* sleep phase or a biologically driven preference for a later bedtime and wake time (usually 2+ h later), appears to be more common in people with Crohn's disease.[13,35] Further, having a delayed sleep phase can increase the risk for insomnia and can significantly impact fatigue.[35,36] Second, trauma is common in GI disorders, with prevalence estimates of about 36%.[37] Both trauma and posttraumatic stress may increase the risk of developing IBS.[38,39] Thus, it is likely that GI providers will encounter patients who report complaints of nightmares (in addition to other trauma-related symptoms) which may worsen sleep quality, change sleep timing (eg, not wanting to sleep during the night), and increase overall hypervigilance and hyperarousal, thereby also worsening GI symptoms.

Fatigue

Fatigue is a common consequence of many sleep disorders, particularly as a result of insufficient, fragmented, or disturbed sleep.[40] However, fatigue may also be reported in the absence of sleep disorders or poor sleep quality. Although definitions of fatigue are highly variable as there is no gold standard measurement tool, it is general thought of as an "overwhelming sense of tiredness, lack of energy and a feeling of exhaustion,

Table 1
A brief description of the three most common sleep disorders

Sleep Disorder	Key Self-Reported Features	Prevalence
Insomnia	Difficulty falling asleep, staying asleep, and/or early morning awakening	10% of adults
Obstructive sleep apnea	Sleepiness, loud snoring, and gasping at night	13%–14% of men and 5%–6% of women
Restless legs syndrome	Evening urge to move legs combined with an unpleasant, "creepy-crawly" feeling	8%–10% of adults

associated with impaired physical and/or cognitive functioning" (pp. 70).[41] Overall, between 22% to 31% of US adults may experience significant or frequent fatigue,[42–44] and fatigue is more common in people with digestive diseases than the general population.[45] Prevalence rates for general fatigue in people with IBD are estimated to be as high as 86% when the disease is active and 41% to 52% when in remission.[46–48] Fatigue is also present in 54% of people with IBS and is significantly more common in patients seen in tertiary care settings.[49] Importantly, this experience of general fatigue is different from chronic fatigue syndrome/myalgic encephalomyelitis, a much more severe and debilitating illness with specific diagnostic criteria and a US population prevalence approximately .65%.[50]

Broadly, in people with GI conditions, fatigue may be related to a wide variety of factors, including, but not limited to, differences in immune system activation, physical deconditioning, pain, psychosocial/psychiatric issues (including sleep disorders), and disease-related stressors (eg, hospitalizations, medication use), among other things (**Fig. 1**).[45,51–54] Physiologically, sleep deprivation leads to increased levels of interleukin-6 (IL-6), a pro-inflammatory cytokine that can result in increased daytime fatigue.[55,56] Medications used to manage GI conditions may also increase fatigue and/or disrupt sleep quality.[57,58] Behaviorally, the complexities of managing day-to-day symptoms of digestive disorders combined with decreased physical activity and muscle mass may also contribute to fatigue.[52,59,60] The experience of fatigue may also result in changes in sleep quality, which may then further exacerbate fatigue.[40,58,61] Specific to IBD, longitudinal research suggests that disease activity, sleep quality, emotional distress, and psychological well-being are all independently associated with fatigue over time.[62] Further, Crohn's disease may be associated with subtle cognitive impairment, which can contribute to the experience of fatigue.[63]

METHODS FOR IMPROVING SLEEP AND TREATING SLEEP DISORDERS

Sleep hygiene, or engaging in behaviors and creating environmental conditions that facilitate sleep health, is generally thought to be important for everyone, although becomes more important if a person is prone to having difficulty with sleep. Although there is no overarching consensus on exactly what sleep hygiene is or how it is best implemented,[64] most guidelines tend to focus on:

- Avoiding or limiting alcohol, caffeine, and nicotine, particularly close to bedtime,
- Keeping the bedroom cool, dark, and quiet,
- Having wind-down time or a bedtime routine, and optimally one that doesn't include bright lights or electronics,
- Using one's bed for sleep and sex only, and

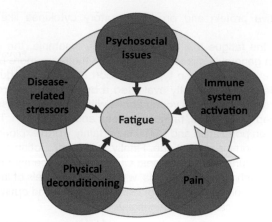

Fig. 1. Relevant contributions to fatigue.

- Going to bed and getting up at the same time every day, even on weekends and days off.[65–67]

It is also often recommended that people regulate meal times, which may be particularly important for people with GI conditions, and even more so in individuals with a circadian component to their symptoms. Specifically, people with GI conditions who also report sleep concerns should aware of not eating too late, not going to bed overly full or hungry, and eating regular meals spaced throughout the day. More sleep information may be found at https://sleepeducation.org/healthy-sleep/healthy-sleep-habits/

Importantly, improving sleep hygiene is not sufficient once insomnia has become chronic (ie, lasting longer than 3 months).[68,69]

Cognitive Behavioral Therapy for Insomnia (CBT-I) is the recommended first-line treatment for chronic insomnia disorder by the American College of Physicians. Compared with pharmacotherapy, it has comparable effectiveness, a lower side-effect profile, and improved durability.[70–72] Gold standard, multicomponent CBT-I typically involves sleep restriction (reducing time spent in bed to improve quality and depth of sleep), stimulus control (re-learning the relationship between the bed and sleep), sleep hygiene, relaxation skills, and cognitive therapy. CBT-I is typically administered over 4 to 8 visits with a specialist in behavioral sleep medicine, and improves sleep irrespective of physical or psychiatric comorbidities, age, and sleep medication use.[73–77] Remission rates are typically ~60% and CBT-I delivered via telehealth is as effective as in-person treatment.[69,78] Further, Brief Behavioral Treatment for Insomnia, 2 to 4 session insomnia treatment that excludes the cognitive components of CBT-I, is also quite effective and may be delivered by non-specialists.[79,80]

Not only is CBT-I highly effective for insomnia, it also may impact other comorbid or insomnia-maintaining processes such as pain, depression, and inflammation. CBT-I can show small but clinically significant and robust reductions in pain.[81–84] Some evidence points to having patients attain about 6.5 h of sleep for the improvement of pain.[85] Perhaps more importantly, CBT-I may improve pain interference, pain catastrophizing, pain-related disability, and pain coping.[86–89] In addition, insomnia is highly predictive of both initial episodes of major depressive disorder and relapses,[90–92] and research indicates that CBT-I is very effective in treating depression when it is comorbid with insomnia.[93,94] Finally, preliminary evidence suggests that CBT-I may lower levels of C-reactive protein and pro-inflammatory cytokines like IL-6 and TNF-alpha.[95–97]

With regard to the fatigue that may accompany insomnia, the evidence for the impact of CBT-I in general is mixed,[93,98,99] though there are more positive results in studies with cancer survivors, who typically report quite high fatigue.[100,101] Further, Hashash and colleagues[102] recently evaluated a brief behavioral treatment of sleep disturbance in 52 adolescents and young adults with Crohn's disease; they found improvements in sleep disturbance, fatigue, anxiety, and depression. Thus, results may be variable based on population and CBT-I is certainly worth exploring in people with GI conditions and insomnia and fatigue. Finally, it is worth noting that although napping is typically discouraged in traditional CBT-I, it has recently been incorporated in trials with people with multiple sclerosis, who have high levels of fatigue.[103] In those cases, patients are encouraged to nap for less than 30 min and optimally before lunch or as early in the day as can still be beneficial.

Fatigue Management

If a patient is experiencing fatigue in the context of another sleep disorder, treatment for that sleep disorder should take priority, as the fatigue may resolve or lessen significantly with adequate treatment.[104,105] If sleep disorders have either been ruled out or successfully treated, patients can be referred to behavioral health for CBT, which will address unhelpful thought and behavior patterns that may inadvertently be worsening fatigue, and/or to physical therapy for graded exercise therapy, in which the patient will gradually increase activity in order to improve overall functioning.[106,107] Both of these treatments have small to medium effects in chronic fatigue syndrome/myalgic encephalomyelitis (CFS/ME) and are likely appropriate for significant fatigue with or without a CFS/ME diagnosis. Referral to one treatment versus the other may be made based on severity of comorbidities. For example, if depression is present, the patient may benefit more from CBT, whereas if mobility concerns are present, the patient may benefit more from physical therapy. In addition, an occupational therapist may help the patient learn strategies to minimize energy use and maximize efficiency in everyday tasks.[108,109]

Other Relevant Sleep Treatments

In addition to providing treatment of insomnia and fatigue, psychologists specializing in behavioral sleep medicine are skilled in several other interventions. Briefly, for patients with trauma and nontrauma-based nightmares, the most efficacious treatment is imagery rehearsal therapy.[110] In this treatment patients are encouraged to practice positive imagery in their beds and develop alternative endings to their nightmares.[111] For patients with circadian rhythm sleep-wake phase disorders, appropriately timed melatonin and light therapy in combination with sleep hygiene is the recommended treatment.[112,113] For patients with RLS, providers may consider iron supplementation if iron deficiency is a known problem.[32,114] Finally, patients with OSA are most often recommended to use continuous positive airway pressure (CPAP); however, patients who cannot tolerate CPAP may benefit from motivational interviewing or exposure therapy to improve adherence or positional therapies to manage symptoms (eg, developing strategies to learn not to sleep on one's back).[115,116]

Referrals to Sleep Medicine

Typically, sleep medicine clinics can offer diagnosis and treatment for a wide range of sleep disorders and problems. Many sleep disorders require an in-lab and/or overnight sleep study for diagnosis, and these tests can be performed though sleep medicine. Patients suspected to have OSA, restless leg syndrome, or who express other significant complaints about their sleep timing, quality, or quantity would likely benefit from a referral to a sleep medicine clinic for further evaluation.

Preliminary Research on Sleep Treatments in Gastrointestinal Populations

Treatment of sleep disturbances in GI conditions is under active investigation through clinical trials. Although most of these trials are small and exploratory, they have consistently showed that sleep treatments may improve other aspects of health. In a single-arm pilot trial in 20 people with sleep disturbance and FD, Nakamura and colleagues[117] found that 4 weeks of pharmacotherapy targeting sleep disturbances also resulted in improvements in both quality of life and GI symptoms. Similarly, Ballou and colleagues[118] randomized 25 participants with IBS to either a four-session behavioral insomnia treatment or control condition. Participants in the intervention group evidenced significantly greater improvements in sleep (insomnia severity, sleep quality, sleep efficiency) and trends toward IBS symptom improvement as well. Salwen-Deremer and colleagues[119] have also showed that CBT-I is feasible and acceptable in people with active IBD, and that it may result not only in improvements in sleep quality and insomnia, but also in other aspects of physical and mental health. Finally, research also indicates that in people with both OSA and GERD, CPAP may substantially reduce the frequency of reflux events.[120]

There are also emerging data suggesting that when GI symptoms improve, some sleep disturbances may resolve as well. In IBD, longitudinal data indicate that use of biologics (both vedolizumab and anti-TNF medications) can result in improvements in sleep quality as early as 6 weeks after drug initiation, though patients with continued active disease are less likely to see improvements in sleep.[121] In IBS, a small pilot trial suggested that gut-directed hypnotherapy resulted not only in improved IBS-related quality of life, but also modest improvement in sleep quality.[122] In addition, small intestinal bacterial overgrowth (SIBO), often present in people with IBS,[123] is also common in RLS and preliminary data suggest that RLS symptoms may be responsive to rifaximin, a drug indicated for the treatment of SIBO.[124,125] In IBD and IBS, these data highlight the ways in which sleep and GI symptom experiences can potentially reinforce and maintain one another.

In people with silent reflux, insomnia, and frequent awakenings, one small pilot trial investigated the impact of 2 weeks of "aggressive" PPI treatment. Sixteen participants with minimal self-reported GERD symptoms were included and 4 evidenced silent reflux on 24-h pH monitoring. With PPI, 3 out of 4 participants experienced normalization of sleep efficiency.[126] In addition, there are now several large clinical trials indicating that 2 weeks of PPI treatment for GERD significantly and rapidly decreases GERD-related sleep disturbances and improved sleep quality.[127–129] Importantly, likely because of the bidirectional relationship between GI conditions and sleep problems, more frequent sleep disturbance at baseline was related to a lower likelihood of resolution of GERD symptoms.[128]

CASE EXAMPLES: TREATMENT PLANNING

For each of the above case examples, the provider should first ask some variant of the question, "how has your sleep been?" Follow-up questions or modifications could include:

- Have you found yourself lying in bed awake a lot recently?
- Are you waking up a lot during the night?
- Has anything about your sleep changed in recent weeks or months?

After the initial prompt about sleep, a discussion and recommendation for each of the above cases might proceed as follows:

1. Alicia indicates that although she has been really fatigued during the day, she does not feel like her sleep has changed much over the past few months. In recent weeks she started taking a little longer to fall asleep on occasion, and attributes this problem to worrying. When you ask if it is impacting her day-to-day health, she replies that difficulty falling asleep has not really caused her any major problems. However, the fatigue she feels is mentally tough for her to handle. Because Alicia's sleep has not changed very much and she reports a significant amount of worry about her GI symptoms, it is likely that her increases in catastrophizing (anticipating the worst case scenario) and hypervigilance (paying debilitating amounts of attention to symptoms) are driving her fatigue, not a sleep disorder. However, the arousal resulting from these cognitive and behavioral patterns has begun to affect her sleep and if untreated, could become acute and/or chronic insomnia.
   a. First, it will be important to help Alicia understand the role of the brain-gut connection in IBS, which would explain how her thought and behavior patterns influence her GI symptoms. She may or may not be aware that the ways in which she is thinking about symptoms, checking on her body, and avoiding people and places she once enjoyed are likely contributing to and worsening both her fatigue and her IBS. Keefer, Palsson, and Pandolfino's 2018 AGA Best Practice Update provides excellent examples of language to use for this patient discussion.[130]
   b. Second, Alicia would likely benefit most from a referral to a GI Psychologist who can provide CBT for IBS. CBT can target decreasing her avoidance behaviors and her checking/hypervigilance and help improve her ability to challenge catastrophic thinking patterns. However, not all practices have access to this resource. Other options could include referral to a mental health provider who has experience with CBT, evidence-based bibliotherapy/self-help books (eg, *Reclaim Your Life from IBS*[131]), or online/app-based programs (eg, *Zemedy*[132]).
2. George tells you that he feels like his sleep is terrible. Since being diagnosed with Crohn's disease nearly 20 years ago, his sleep has been up and down, and he has thought that not sleeping well and feeling tired all the time were part of the disease. However, recently, it feels like he can no longer "power through" the exhaustion. When he wakes up during the night with pain or a bowel movement, it can take him up to an hour to fall back asleep. After a bad night, he naps if he can, and if he cannot, he often finds himself irritable and unable to concentrate at work. He shares that he has started worrying about not being able to sleep—when he gets in bed at night, he will "try hard" to fall asleep, but often winds up just feeling frustrated and more awake.
   a. Although fatigue and nighttime awakenings for bowel movements can commonly occur in people with Crohn's disease, this sleep problem sounds more significant. In particular, worrying about not being able to sleep and difficulty with both falling asleep and staying asleep, combined with clear daytime consequences, are likely reflective of insomnia disorder. Based on what George told you, it is likely that he has been suffering from insomnia for many years and has been assuming that these issues are part of his Crohn's disease as opposed to a sleep disorder.
   b. George would likely benefit from referral to a psychologist or similar provider who specializes in insomnia or behavioral sleep medicine and who can provide CBT-I. If the practice has a GI psychologist, they may be an appropriate referral,

as insomnia treatment is often part of training in behavioral medicine/health psychology. Otherwise, George's provider could consider reaching out to a sleep medicine clinic, which may know of local referrals, or searching for a local provider through the Society of Behavioral Sleep Medicine. The provider could also refer George to self-help books (eg, *Quiet Your Mind and Get to Sleep*) or to evidence-based online/app-based programs (eg, *Sleepio.com*,[98] *Somryst*,[133] and *Insomnia Coach*[134]).

3. Marco states that although he has usually been a "pretty good" sleeper, in the past couple of months he has noticed himself waking up during the night more often. When you ask if there is anything else different about his sleep, he shares that his wife has been complaining about his snoring being louder and more frequent recently.
   a. Based on Marco's reports of snoring, awakenings, sleepiness, and morning headaches, you ask if he has ever been evaluated for OSA. He indicates that he thinks he was tested for it many years ago, and that he was told it was not significant enough to do anything about at the time.
   b. It is possible that with Marco's recent weight gain, what was once mild OSA has increased in severity. This diagnosis should be made based on polysomnography (ie, sleep study), so Marco would likely be best served by a referral to a local sleep medicine center for further evaluation. If his OSA has in fact worsened since his testing many years ago, it is possible symptoms might resolve with modest weight loss. Thus, it would likely be valuable to talk with Marco about his dietary changes since starting the PPI and the ways that some of these high fat/high sugar foods can impact not only sleep and weight, but also other aspects of health. If he has difficulty making behavior changes on his own, he could benefit from referral to a dietician and/or a psychologist to address dietary choices, mindful eating, and behavioral weight loss strategies.

Cultural Considerations

Names such as Alicia, George, and Marco are popular across nations and cultures and the patients described above could be members of any number of different cultural, racial, or ethnic groups. Their backgrounds also likely have a substantial impact on their health care access and needs. High quality, patient-centered health care that is linguistically and culturally sensitive is a national health priority,[135] yet incredible disparities in care exist and persist for non-White Americans.[136] Minority groups in America may perceive more discrimination, exhibit lower levels of health literacy, may be distrusting toward physicians and subsequently be less adherent to medical regimens, and may have more difficulties obtaining referrals to specialists.[137-143]

Specific to sleep, only an estimated 64% of clinical trials for sleep disorders make cultural adaptations for their target populations, and many of these adaptations are only surface level (eg, setting, delivery mode).[144] These data are particularly concerning given the racial/ethnic disparities that exist across numerous areas of sleep.[145] For example, compared with non-Hispanic White adults, US adults from Asian, Black, Hispanic/Latinx, and Native Hawaiian and Pacific Islander backgrounds all get fewer hours of sleep on average. Asian, Black, and Hispanic/Latinx adults also report lower sleep quality. Further, there is also substantial variability in sleep practices across cultures and countries.[146] For example, briefly napping in the workplace is much more common in Japan and views on the *siesta* can differ significantly across parts of Spain.[147,148] In addition, children from predominantly Asian countries are more likely to share both a bedroom and a bed with their parent(s) than children from predominantly-White countries.[149]

These differences in sleep patterns and practices are likely to impact adherence to standard treatment protocols when interventionists do not make adaptations; when culturally appropriate adaptations to interventions are made, there are significant improvements in intervention effectiveness.[150] Specific to the practice of medicine, health care providers may provide "deep structure" changes, integrating culturally consonant concepts and metaphors (eg, the use of proverbs), incorporating sociocultural values (eg, *familismo*: the dedication, commitment, and loyalty to family), religion and spirituality, as well as understanding and being inclusive of family members' and family systems' roles in health behavior change.[151,152] Being attuned to cultural influences gives providers opportunities to validate patient experiences, build sustainable rapport, and enlist familial and community resources that can facilitate improved management of health conditions.

SUMMARY

Overall, poor sleep quality, sleep disorders, and fatigue are quite common in people with GI conditions, and many of these issues occur at higher rates than the general population. Emerging research suggests that although the sleep/GI relationship is likely bidirectional once enacted, sleep may be a driving factor. Thus, it is likely that many people presenting to GI clinics will be experiencing issues with their sleep, whether or not they report sleep issues or fatigue as a current problem. In order for patients to get the adequate treatment, it is important that providers probe for possible relationships among GI conditions, sleep disorders, and fatigue. Several evidence-based treatments exist for sleep disorders, and we highly encourage providers to support their patients in accessing these care resources, whether through a local sleep medicine clinic, their primary care provider, an embedded GI psychologist, other community resources, or online or app-based services.

CLINICS CARE POINTS

- People with gastrointestinal (GI) conditions are likely to also experience sleep concerns.
- Sleep disorders, fatigue, and GI conditions may worsen and maintain one another.
- When patients report that GI symptoms are interfering with sleep or causing fatigue, providers should ask follow-up questions and make appropriate referrals.
- Insomnia will likely be the most common sleep disorder encountered.
- Cognitive behavioral therapy for insomnia is the recommended first-line treatment of insomnia.
- Providers should consider cultural factors in their assessments and treatment recommendations.

DISCLOSURE

The authors have nothing to disclose.

REFERENCES

1. Worley SL. The extraordinary importance of sleep: the detrimental effects of inadequate sleep on health and public safety drive an explosion of sleep research. Pharm Ther 2018;43:758.

2. Freeman D, Sheaves B, Waite F, et al. Sleep disturbance and psychiatric disorders. Lancet Psychiatry 2020;7:628–37.
3. Hirshkowitz M, Whiton K, Albert SM, et al. National Sleep Foundation's sleep time duration recommendations: methodology and results summary. Sleep health 2015;1:40–3.
4. Ohayon MM, Carskadon MA, Guilleminault C, et al. Meta-analysis of quantitative sleep parameters from childhood to old age in healthy individuals: developing normative sleep values across the human lifespan. Sleep 2004;27:1255–73.
5. Liu Y, Wheaton AG, Chapman DP, et al. Prevalence of healthy sleep duration among adults—United States, 2014. MMWR Morb Mortal Wkly Rep 2016;65: 137–41.
6. Krueger PM, Friedman EM. Sleep duration in the United States: a cross-sectional population-based study. Am J Epidemiol 2009;169:1052–63.
7. Grandner MA, Chakravorty S, Perlis ML, et al. Habitual sleep duration associated with self-reported and objectively determined cardiometabolic risk factors. Sleep Med 2014;15:42–50.
8. Buman MP, Phillips BA, Youngstedt SD, et al. Does nighttime exercise really disturb sleep? Results from the 2013 National Sleep Foundation Sleep in America Poll. Sleep Med 2014;15:755–61.
9. Ballou S, Alhassan E, Hon E, et al. Sleep disturbances are commonly reported among patients presenting to a gastroenterology clinic. Dig Dis Sci 2018;63: 2983–91.
10. Ananthakrishnan AN, Long MD, Martin CF, et al. Sleep disturbance and risk of active disease in patients with Crohn's disease and ulcerative colitis. Clin Gastroenterol Hepatol 2013;11:965–71.
11. Vela MF, Kramer JR, Richardson PA, et al. Poor sleep quality and obstructive sleep apnea in patients with GERD and Barrett's esophagus. Neurogastroenterol Motil 2014;26:346–52.
12. Lacy BE, Everhart K, Crowell MD. Functional dyspepsia is associated with sleep disorders. Clin Gastroenterol Hepatol 2011;9:410–4.
13. Salwen-Deremer JK, Smith MT, Haskell HG, et al. Poor Sleep in Inflammatory Bowel Disease Is Reflective of Distinct Sleep Disorders. Dig Dis Sci 2021;1–12.
14. Keefer L, Stepanski EJ, Ranjbaran Z, et al. An initial report of sleep disturbance in inactive inflammatory bowel disease. J Clin Sleep Med 2006;2:409–16.
15. Ranjbaran Z, Keefer L, Farhadi A, et al. Impact of sleep disturbances in inflammatory bowel disease. J Gastroenterol Hepatol 2007;22:1748–53.
16. Patel A, Hasak S, Cassell B, et al. Effects of disturbed sleep on gastrointestinal and somatic pain symptoms in irritable bowel syndrome. Aliment Pharmacol Ther 2016;44:246–58.
17. Buchanan DT, Cain K, Heitkemper M, et al. Sleep measures predict next-day symptoms in women with irritable bowel syndrome. J Clin Sleep Med 2014; 10:1003–9.
18. Uemura R, Fujiwara Y, Iwakura N, et al. Sleep disturbances in Japanese patients with inflammatory bowel disease and their impact on disease flare. SpringerPlus 2016;5:1792.
19. Conley S, Jeon S, Lehner V, et al. Sleep Characteristics and Rest–Activity Rhythms Are Associated with Gastrointestinal Symptoms Among Adults with Inflammatory Bowel Disease. Dig Dis Sci 2020;1–9.
20. Singh P, Ballou S, Rangan V, et al. Clinical and Psychological Factors Predict Outcome in Patients With Functional Dyspepsia: A Prospective Study. Clin Gastroenterol Hepatol 2022;20(6):1251–8.e1.

21. Mai E, Buysse DJ. Insomnia: prevalence, impact, pathogenesis, differential diagnosis, and evaluation. Sleep Med Clin 2008;3:167–74.

22. Lichstein K, Durrence H, Taylor D, et al. Quantitative criteria for insomnia. Behav Res Ther 2003;41:427–45.

23. Jung H-k, Choung RS, Talley NJ. Gastroesophageal reflux disease and sleep disorders: evidence for a causal link and therapeutic implications. J Neurogastroenterol Motil 2010;16:22.

24. Peppard PE, Young T, Barnet JH, et al. Increased prevalence of sleep-disordered breathing in adults. Am J Epidemiol 2013;177:1006–14.

25. Punjabi NM. The epidemiology of adult obstructive sleep apnea. Proc Am Thorac Soc 2008;5:136–43.

26. Dong Z, Xu X, Wang C, et al. Association of overweight and obesity with obstructive sleep apnoea: a systematic review and meta-analysis. Obes Med 2020;17:100185.

27. Modolell I, Esteller E, Segarra F, et al. Proton-pump inhibitors in sleep-related breathing disorders: clinical response and predictive factors. Eur J Gastroenterol Hepatol 2011;23:852–8.

28. Al Momani L, Alomari M, Patel A, et al. 2875 The Prevalence of Irritable Bowel Syndrome in Patients With Obstructive Sleep Apnea: A Meta-Analysis and Systematic Review. Official J Am Coll Gastroenterol ACG 2019;114:S1576–7.

29. Ghiasi F, Amra B, Sebghatollahi V, et al. Association of irritable bowel syndrome and sleep apnea in patients referred to sleep laboratory. J Res Med Sci 2017; 22:72.

30. Ohayon MM. Epidemiological overview of sleep disorders in the general population. Sleep Med Res 2011;2:1–9.

31. Mosli MH, Bukhari LM, Khoja AA, et al. Inflammatory bowel disease and restless leg syndrome. Neurosciences (Riyadh, Saudi Arabia) 2020;25:301–7.

32. Becker J, Berger F, Schindlbeck KA, et al. Restless legs syndrome is a relevant comorbidity in patients with inflammatory bowel disease. Int J colorectal Dis 2018;33:955–62.

33. Guo J, Pei L, Chen L, et al. Bidirectional association between irritable bowel syndrome and restless legs syndrome: a systematic review and meta-analysis. Sleep Med 2021;77:104–11.

34. Abbott SM, Reid KJ, Zee PC. Circadian Disorders of the Sleep-Wake Cycle. In: Kryger M, Roth T, Dement WC, editors. Principles and practice of sleep medicine. 6th edition. Philadelphia: Elsevier; 2017. p. 414–23.

35. Chrobak AA, Nowakowski J, Zwolińska-Wcisło M, et al. Associations between chronotype, sleep disturbances and seasonality with fatigue and inflammatory bowel disease symptoms. Chronobiol Int 2018;35:1142–52.

36. Kivelä L, Papadopoulos MR, Antypa N. Chronotype and psychiatric disorders. Curr Sleep Med Rep 2018;4:94–103.

37. Glynn H, Möller SP, Wilding H, et al. Prevalence and Impact of Post-traumatic Stress Disorder in Gastrointestinal Conditions: A Systematic Review. Dig Dis Sci 2021;66:4109–19.

38. Park SH, Videlock EJ, Shih W, et al. Adverse childhood experiences are associated with irritable bowel syndrome and gastrointestinal symptom severity. Neurogastroenterol Motil 2016;28:1252–60.

39. Ng QX, Soh AYS, Loke W, et al. Systematic review with meta-analysis: The association between post-traumatic stress disorder and irritable bowel syndrome. J Gastroenterol Hepatol 2019;34:68–73.

40. Graff LA, Vincent N, Walker JR, et al. A population-based study of fatigue and sleep difficulties in inflammatory bowel disease. Inflamm Bowel Dis 2010;17: 1882–9.
41. Shen J, Barbera J, Shapiro CM. Distinguishing sleepiness and fatigue: focus on definition and measurement. Sleep Med Rev 2006;10:63–76.
42. Meng H, Hale L, Friedberg F. Prevalence and predictors of fatigue among middle-aged and older adults: evidence from the Health and Retirement study. J Am Geriatr Soc 2010;58:2033.
43. Bültmann U, Kant I, Kasl SV, et al. Fatigue and psychological distress in the working population: psychometrics, prevalence, and correlates. J Psychosom Res 2002;52:445–52.
44. Cullen W, Kearney Y, Bury G. Prevalence of fatigue in general practice. Irish J Med Sci 2002;171:10–2.
45. Simren M, Svedlund J, Posserud I, et al. Predictors of subjective fatigue in chronic gastrointestinal disease. Aliment Pharmacol Ther 2008;28:638–47.
46. Minderhoud IM, Samsom M, Oldenburg B. Crohn's disease, fatigue, and infliximab: is there a role for cytokines in the pathogenesis of fatigue? World J Gastroenterol 2007;13:2089.
47. Jelsness-Jørgensen L-P, Bernklev T, Henriksen M, et al. Chronic fatigue is more prevalent in patients with inflammatory bowel disease than in healthy controls. Inflamm Bowel Dis 2011;17:1564–72.
48. Van Langenberg D, Gibson PR. Systematic review: fatigue in inflammatory bowel disease. Aliment Pharmacol Ther 2010;32:131–43.
49. Han CJ, Yang GS. Fatigue in irritable bowel syndrome: a systematic review and meta-analysis of pooled frequency and severity of fatigue. Asian Nurs Res 2016; 10:1–10.
50. Lim E-J, Ahn Y-C, Jang E-S, et al. Systematic review and meta-analysis of the prevalence of chronic fatigue syndrome/myalgic encephalomyelitis (CFS/ME). J translational Med 2020;18:1–15.
51. Vogelaar L, de Haar C, Aerts BR, et al. Fatigue in patients with inflammatory bowel disease is associated with distinct differences in immune parameters. Clin Exp Gastroenterol 2017;10:83.
52. Van Langenberg D, Gatta PD, Hill B, et al. Delving into disability in Crohn's disease: dysregulation of molecular pathways may explain skeletal muscle loss in Crohn's disease. J Crohn's Colitis 2014;8:626–34.
53. Sweeney L, Moss-Morris R, Czuber-Dochan W, et al. 'It's about willpower in the end. You've got to keep going': a qualitative study exploring the experience of pain in inflammatory bowel disease. Br J pain 2019;13:201–13.
54. Han CJ, Jarrett ME, Heitkemper MM. Relationships between abdominal pain and fatigue with psychological distress as a mediator in women with irritable bowel syndrome. Gastroenterol Nurs 2020;43:28.
55. Ali T, Choe J, Awab A, et al. Sleep, immunity and inflammation in gastrointestinal disorders. World J Gastroenterol 2013;19:9231.
56. Irwin MR, Olmstead R, Carroll JE. Sleep disturbance, sleep duration, and inflammation: a systematic review and meta-analysis of cohort studies and experimental sleep deprivation. Biol Psychiatry 2016;80:40–52.
57. Vogelaar L, van't Spijker A, van Tilburg AJ, et al. Determinants of fatigue in Crohn's disease patients. Eur J Gastroenterol Hepatol 2013;25:246–51.
58. van Langenberg DR, Gibson PR. Factors associated with physical and cognitive fatigue in patients with Crohn's disease: a cross-sectional and longitudinal study. Inflamm Bowel Dis 2014;20:115–25.

59. Van Langenberg D, Papandony M, Gibson P. Sleep and physical activity measured by accelerometry in Crohn's disease. Aliment Pharmacol Ther 2015;41:991–1004.

60. Spiegel BM. The burden of IBS: looking at metrics. Curr Gastroenterol Rep 2009;11:265–9.

61. Banovic I, Gilibert D, Jebrane A, et al. Personality and fatigue perception in a sample of IBD outpatients in remission: A preliminary study. J Crohn's Colitis 2012;6:571–7.

62. Graff LA, Clara I, Walker JR, et al. Changes in fatigue over 2 years are associated with activity of inflammatory bowel disease and psychological factors. Clin Gastroenterol Hepatol 2013;11:1140–6.

63. van Langenberg DR, Yelland GW, Robinson SR, et al. Cognitive impairment in Crohn's disease is associated with systemic inflammation, symptom burden and sleep disturbance. United Eur Gastroenterol J 2017;5:579–87.

64. Stepanski EJ, Wyatt JK. Use of sleep hygiene in the treatment of insomnia. Sleep Med Rev 2003;7:215–25.

65. Irish LA, Kline CE, Gunn HE, et al. The role of sleep hygiene in promoting public health: A review of empirical evidence. Sleep Med Rev 2015;22:23–36.

66. Mastin DF, Bryson J, Corwyn R. Assessment of sleep hygiene using the Sleep Hygiene Index. J Behav Med 2006;29:223–7.

67. Chung K-F, Lee C-T, Yeung W-F, et al. Sleep hygiene education as a treatment of insomnia: a systematic review and meta-analysis. Fam Pract 2018;35:365–75.

68. Taylor DJ, Pruiksma KE. Cognitive and behavioural therapy for insomnia (CBT-I) in psychiatric populations: a systematic review. Int Rev Psychiatry 2014;26: 205–13.

69. Edinger JD, Arnedt JT, Bertisch SM, et al. Behavioral and psychological treatments for chronic insomnia disorder in adults: an American Academy of Sleep Medicine systematic review, meta-analysis and GRADE assessment. J Clin Sleep Med 2021;17(2):263–98.

70. Qaseem A, Kansagara D, Forciea MA, et al. Management of chronic insomnia disorder in adults: a clinical practice guideline from the American College of Physicians. Ann Intern Med 2016;165:125–33.

71. Jacobs GD, Pace-Schott EF, Stickgold R, et al. Cognitive behavior therapy and pharmacotherapy for insomnia: a randomized controlled trial and direct comparison. Arch Intern Med 2004;164:1888–96.

72. Smith MT, Perlis ML, Park A, et al. Comparative meta-analysis of pharmacotherapy and behavior therapy for persistent insomnia. Am J Psychiatry 2002; 159:5–11.

73. Finan PH, Buenaver LF, Runko VT, et al. Cognitive-Behavioral Therapy for Comorbid Insomnia and Chronic Pain. Sleep Mdicine Clin 2014;9:261–74.

74. Smith M, Huang M, Manber R. Cognitive behavior therapy for chronic insomnia occurring within the context of medical and psychiatric disorders. Clin Psychol Rev 2005;25:559–611.

75. Trauer JM, Qian MY, Doyle JS, et al. Cognitive behavioral therapy for chronic insomnia: a systematic review and meta-analysis. Ann Intern Med 2015;163: 191–204.

76. Irwin MR, Cole JC, Nicassio PM. Comparative meta-analysis of behavioral interventions for insomnia and their efficacy in middle-aged adults and in older adults 55+ years of age. Health Psychol 2006;25:3.

77. van Straten A, van der Zweerde T, Kleiboer A, et al. Cognitive and behavioral therapies in the treatment of insomnia: a meta-analysis. Sleep Med Rev 2018; 38:3–16.

78. Cavanagh RC, Mackey R, Bridges L, et al. The Use of Digital Health Technologies to Manage Insomnia in Military Populations. J Technology Behav Sci 2020; 5:61–9.

79. Gunn HE, Tutek J, Buysse DJ. Brief behavioral treatment of insomnia. Sleep Med Clin 2019;14:235–43.

80. Buysse DJ, Germain A, Moul DE, et al. Efficacy of brief behavioral treatment for chronic insomnia in older adults. Arch Intern Med 2011;171:887–95.

81. Tang NK, Lereya ST, Boulton H, et al. Nonpharmacological treatments of insomnia for long-term painful conditions: a systematic review and meta-analysis of patient-reported outcomes in randomized controlled trials. Sleep 2015;38:1751–64.

82. Smith MT, Finan PH, Buenaver LF, et al. Cognitive–behavioral therapy for insomnia in knee osteoarthritis: a randomized, double-blind, active placebo–controlled clinical trial. Arthritis Rheumatol 2015;67:1221–33.

83. Vitiello MV, Rybarczyk B, Von Korff M, et al. Cognitive behavioral therapy for insomnia improves sleep and decreases pain in older adults with co-morbid insomnia and osteoarthritis. J Clin Sleep Med 2009;5:355–62.

84. McCurry SM, Shortreed SM, Von Korff M, et al. Who benefits from CBT for insomnia in primary care? Important patient selection and trial design lessons from longitudinal results of the Lifestyles trial. Sleep 2014;37:299–308.

85. Salwen JK, Smith MT, Finan PH. Mid-treatment sleep duration predicts clinically significant knee osteoarthritis pain reduction at 6 months: effects from a behavioral sleep medicine clinical trial. Sleep 2017;40:zsw064.

86. Martínez MP, Miró E, Sánchez AI, et al. Cognitive-behavioral therapy for insomnia and sleep hygiene in fibromyalgia: a randomized controlled trial. J Behav Med 2014;37:683–97.

87. Jungquist CR, O'Brien C, Matteson-Rusby S, et al. The efficacy of cognitive-behavioral therapy for insomnia in patients with chronic pain. Sleep Med 2010;11:302–9.

88. Lerman SF, Finan PH, Smith MT, et al. Psychological interventions that target sleep reduce pain catastrophizing in knee osteoarthritis. Pain 2017;158: 2189–95.

89. Lami MJ, Martínez MP, Miró E, et al. Efficacy of combined cognitive-behavioral therapy for insomnia and pain in patients with fibromyalgia: a randomized controlled trial. Cogn Ther Res 2018;42:63–79.

90. Dombrovski AY, Cyranowski JM, Mulsant BH, et al. Which symptoms predict recurrence of depression in women treated with maintenance interpersonal psychotherapy? Depress anxiety 2008;25:1060–6.

91. Franzen PL, Buysse DJ. Sleep disturbances and depression: risk relationships for subsequent depression and therapeutic implications. Dialogues Clin Neurosci 2008;10:473.

92. Buysse DJ, Angst J, Gamma A, et al. Prevalence, course, and comorbidity of insomnia and depression in young adults. Sleep 2008;31:473–80.

93. Ballesio A, Aquino MRJV, Feige B, et al. The effectiveness of behavioural and cognitive behavioural therapies for insomnia on depressive and fatigue symptoms: a systematic review and network meta-analysis. Sleep Med Rev 2018; 37:114–29.

94. Cunningham JE, Shapiro CM. Cognitive Behavioural Therapy for Insomnia (CBT-I) to treat depression: A systematic review. J Psychosom Res 2018;106:1–12.

95. Irwin MR, Olmstead R, Carrillo C, et al. Cognitive behavioral therapy vs. Tai Chi for late life insomnia and inflammatory risk: a randomized controlled comparative efficacy trial. Sleep 2014;37:1543–52.

96. Heffner KL, France CR, Ashrafioun L, et al. Clinical pain-related outcomes and inflammatory cytokine response to pain following insomnia improvement in adults with knee osteoarthritis. Clin J Pain 2018;34:1133–40.

97. Irwin MR, Olmstead R, Breen EC, et al. Cognitive behavioral therapy and tai chi reverse cellular and genomic markers of inflammation in late-life insomnia: a randomized controlled trial. Biol Psychiatry 2015;78:721–9.

98. Selvanathan J, Pham C, Nagappa M, et al. Cognitive Behavioral Therapy for Insomnia in Patients with Chronic Pain-A Systematic Review and Meta-Analysis of Randomized Controlled Trials. Sleep Med Rev 2021;60:101460.

99. Benz F, Knoop T, Ballesio A, et al. The efficacy of cognitive and behavior therapies for insomnia on daytime symptoms: A systematic review and network meta-analysis. Clin Psychol Rev 2020;80:101873.

100. Squires LR, Rash JA, Fawcett J, et al. Systematic Review and Meta-Analysis of Cognitive-Behavioural Therapy for Insomnia on Subjective and Actigraphy-Measured Sleep and Comorbid Symptoms in Cancer Survivors. Sleep Med Rev 2022;63:101615.

101. Garland SN, Johnson JA, Savard J, et al. Sleeping well with cancer: a systematic review of cognitive behavioral therapy for insomnia in cancer patients. Neuropsychiatr Dis Treat 2014;10:1113–24.

102. Hashash JG, Knisely MR, Germain A, et al. Brief Behavioral Therapy and Bupropion for Sleep and Fatigue in Young Adults with Crohn's Disease: An Exploratory Open Trial Study. Clin Gastroenterol Hepatol 2022;20(1):96–104.

103. Siengsukon CF, Alshehri M, Williams C, et al. Feasibility and treatment effect of cognitive behavioral therapy for insomnia in individuals with multiple sclerosis: A pilot randomized controlled trial. Mult Scler Relat Disord 2020;40:101958.

104. Chotinaiwattarakul W, O'Brien LM, Fan L, et al. Fatigue, tiredness, and lack of energy improve with treatment for OSA. J Clin Sleep Med 2009;5:222–7.

105. Vitiello MV, McCurry SM, Shortreed SM, et al. Short-term improvement in insomnia symptoms predicts long-term improvements in sleep, pain, and fatigue in older adults with comorbid osteoarthritis and insomnia. Pain 2014; 155:1547–54.

106. Yancey JR, Thomas SM. Chronic fatigue syndrome: diagnosis and treatment. Am Fam Physician 2012;86:741–6.

107. Castell BD, Kazantzis N, Moss-Morris RE. Cognitive behavioral therapy and graded exercise for chronic fatigue syndrome: A meta-analysis. Clin Psychol Sci Pract 2011;18:311.

108. Van Heest KN, Mogush AR, Mathiowetz VG. Effects of a one-to-one fatigue management course for people with chronic conditions and fatigue. Am J Occup Ther 2017;71. 7104100020p1-p9.

109. Blikman LJ, Huisstede BM, Kooijmans H, et al. Effectiveness of energy conservation treatment in reducing fatigue in multiple sclerosis: a systematic review and meta-analysis. Arch Phys Med Rehabil 2013;94:1360–76.

110. Morgenthaler TI, Auerbach S, Casey KR, et al. Position paper for the treatment of nightmare disorder in adults: an American Academy of Sleep Medicine position paper. J Clin Sleep Med 2018;14:1041–55.

111. Krakow B, Zadra A. Clinical management of chronic nightmares: imagery rehearsal therapy. Behav Sleep Med 2006;4:45–70.
112. Duffy JF, Abbott SM, Burgess HJ, et al. Workshop report. Circadian rhythm sleep–wake disorders: gaps and opportunities. Sleep 2021;44:zsaa281.
113. Barion A, Zee PC. A clinical approach to circadian rhythm sleep disorders. Sleep Med 2007;8:566–77.
114. Trotti LM, Becker LA. Iron for the treatment of restless legs syndrome. Cochrane Database Syst Rev 2019;1(1):CD007834.
115. Patil SP, Ayappa IA, Caples SM, et al. Treatment of adult obstructive sleep apnea with positive airway pressure: an American Academy of Sleep Medicine clinical practice guideline. J Clin Sleep Med 2019;15:335–43.
116. Srijithesh P, Aghoram R, Goel A, et al. Positional therapy for obstructive sleep apnoea. Cochrane Database Syst Rev 2019;5(5):CD010990.
117. Nakamura F, Kuribayashi S, Tanaka F, et al. Impact of improvement of sleep disturbance on symptoms and quality of life in patients with functional dyspepsia. BMC Gastroenterol 2021;21:1–10.
118. Ballou S, Katon J, Rangan V, et al. Brief behavioral therapy for insomnia in patients with irritable bowel syndrome: a pilot study. Dig Dis Sci 2020;65:3260–70.
119. Salwen-Deremer JK, Smith MT, Aschbrenner KA, et al. A pilot feasibility trial of cognitive–behavioural therapy for insomnia in people with inflammatory bowel disease. BMJ Open Gastroenterol 2021;8:e000805.
120. Tawk M, Goodrich S, Kinasewitz G, et al. The effect of 1 week of continuous positive airway pressure treatment in obstructive sleep apnea patients with concomitant gastroesophageal reflux. Chest 2006;130:1003–8.
121. Stevens BW, Borren NZ, Velonias G, et al. Vedolizumab therapy is associated with an improvement in sleep quality and mood in inflammatory bowel diseases. Dig Dis Sci 2017;62:197–206.
122. Riehl ME, Stidham RW, Goldstein C, et al. Su1591-The Impact of a Gi-Specific Behavioral Intervention on Sleep Quality in Functional Bowel Disorder Patients. Gastroenterology 2018;154:S-539.
123. Chen B, Kim JJ-W, Zhang Y, et al. Prevalence and predictors of small intestinal bacterial overgrowth in irritable bowel syndrome: a systematic review and meta-analysis. J Gastroenterol 2018;53:807–18.
124. Weinstock LB, Walters AS. Restless legs syndrome is associated with irritable bowel syndrome and small intestinal bacterial overgrowth. Sleep Med 2011; 12:610–3.
125. Weinstock LB, Zeiss S. Rifaximin antibiotic treatment for restless legs syndrome: a double-blind, placebo-controlled study. Sleep Biol Rhythms 2012;10:145–53.
126. Shaheen NJ, Madanick RD, Alattar M, et al. Gastroesophageal reflux disease as an etiology of sleep disturbance in subjects with insomnia and minimal reflux symptoms: a pilot study of prevalence and response to therapy. Dig Dis Sci 2008;53:1493–9.
127. Johnson DA, Le Moigne A, Hugo V, et al. Rapid resolution of sleep disturbances related to frequent reflux: effect of esomeprazole 20 mg in two randomized, double-blind, controlled trials. Curr Med Res Opin 2015;31:243–50.
128. Johnson DA, Le Moigne A, Li J, et al. Analysis of clinical predictors of resolution of sleep disturbance related to frequent nighttime heartburn and acid regurgitation symptoms in individuals taking esomeprazole 20 mg or placebo. Clin Drug Invest 2016;36:531–8.

129. Aimi M, Komazawa Y, Hamamoto N, et al. Effects of omeprazole on sleep disturbance: randomized multicenter double-blind placebo-controlled trial. Clin Transl Gastroenterol 2014;5:e57.

130. Keefer L, Palsson OS, Pandolfino JE. Best practice update: incorporating psychogastroenterology into management of digestive disorders. Gastroenterology 2018;154:1249–57.

131. Hunt MG. Reclaim your life from IBS: a scientifically proven CBT plan for relief without restrictive diets. New York, NY: Routledge; 2016.

132. Hunt M, Miguez S, Dukas B, et al. Efficacy of Zemedy, a mobile digital therapeutic for the self-management of irritable bowel syndrome: crossover randomized controlled trial. JMIR mHealth and uHealth 2021;9:e26152.

133. Ritterband LM, Thorndike FP, Ingersoll KS, et al. Effect of a web-based cognitive behavior therapy for insomnia intervention with 1-year follow-up: a randomized clinical trial. JAMA Psychiatry 2017;74:68–75.

134. Kuhn E, Miller KE, Puran D, et al. A Pilot Randomized Controlled Trial of the Insomnia Coach Mobile App to Assess Its Feasibility, Acceptability, and Potential Efficacy. Behav Ther 2022;53(3):440–57.

135. AHRQ, 2021 National Healthcare Quality and Disparities Report. AHRQ: Rockville, MD, 2021.

136. Mateo CM, Williams DR. Racism: a fundamental driver of racial disparities in health-care quality. Nat Rev Dis Primers 2021;7:1–2.

137. Cheng P, Cuellar R, Johnson DA, et al. Racial discrimination as a mediator of racial disparities in insomnia disorder. Sleep health 2020;6:543–9.

138. Casagrande SS, Gary TL, LaVeist TA, et al. Perceived discrimination and adherence to medical care in a racially integrated community. J Gen Intern Med 2007; 22:389–95.

139. Tormey LK, Farraye FA, Paasche-Orlow MK. Understanding health literacy and its impact on delivering care to patients with inflammatory bowel disease. Inflamm Bowel Dis 2016;22:745–51.

140. Wright JP, Edwards GC, Goggins K, et al. Association of health literacy with postoperative outcomes in patients undergoing major abdominal surgery. JAMA Surg 2018;153:137–42.

141. Pugh M, Perrin PB, Rybarczyk B, et al. Racism, mental health, healthcare provider trust, and medication adherence among black patients in safety-net primary care. J Clin Psychol Med Settings 2021;28:181–90.

142. Sasegbon A, Vasant DH. Understanding racial disparities in the care of patients with irritable bowel syndrome: The need for a unified approach. Neurogastroenterol Motil 2021;33:e14152.

143. Nguyen GC, LaVeist TA, Harris ML, et al. Racial disparities in utilization of specialist care and medications in inflammatory bowel disease. Am J Gastroenterol 2010;105:2202.

144. Alcántara C, Cosenzo LG, McCullough E, et al. Cultural adaptations of psychological interventions for prevalent sleep disorders and sleep disturbances: A systematic review of randomized controlled trials in the United States. Sleep Med Rev 2021;56:101455.

145. Johnson DA, Jackson CL, Williams NJ, et al. Are sleep patterns influenced by race/ethnicity–a marker of relative advantage or disadvantage? Evidence to date. Nat Sci Sleep 2019;11:79.

146. Foundation NS. International bedroom poll. Washington, DC: National Sleep Foundation; 2013.

147. Alger SE, Brager AJ, Capaldi VF. Challenging the stigma of workplace napping. Sleep 2019;42:zsz097.
148. It's time to put the tired Spanish siesta stereotype to bed. BBC; 2017. https://www.bbc.com/worklife/article/20170609-its-time-to-put-the-tired-spanish-siesta-stereotype-to-bed.
149. Mindell JA, Sadeh A, Wiegand B, et al. Cross-cultural differences in infant and toddler sleep. Sleep Med 2010;11:274–80.
150. Hall GCN, Ibaraki AY, Huang ER, et al. A meta-analysis of cultural adaptations of psychological interventions. Behav Ther 2016;47:993–1014.
151. Barrera M Jr, Castro FG, Strycker LA, et al. Cultural adaptations of behavioral health interventions: a progress report. J Consult Clin Psychol 2013;81:196.
152. Bernal G, Jiménez-Chafey MI, Domenech Rodríguez MM. Cultural adaptation of treatments: A resource for considering culture in evidence-based practice. Prof Psychol Res Pract 2009;40:361.

Gastrointestinal Disorders in Adolescents and Young Adults

Preparing for a Smooth Transition to Adult-Centered Care

A. Natisha Nabbijohn, BSc, MA[a],
Sara Ahola Kohut, PhD, CPsych[b,c,d,*]

KEYWORDS

- Health care transition • Gastrointestinal disease • Inflammatory bowel disease
- Disorders of the gut–brain interaction • Emerging adults • Adolescence • Adulthood

KEY POINTS

- Health care transition is the purposeful and planned process for addressing the medical, psychosocial, sexual, and educational/vocational needs of adolescents and young adults as they move from child-centered to adult-oriented health care systems.
- Health care transition efforts are associated with positive psychosocial outcomes in young people with childhood-onset gastrointestinal disease.
- Barriers to health care transition include the lack of formal written transition policies, low transition readiness, knowledge, and self-management skills among patients on transfer, limited access to multidisciplinary care in adulthood, gaps in medical insurance, rigidity in the age of transfer, and patients' lack of trust in the adult health care system and professionals.
- Key aspects of good health care transition practices include: (1) assessing transition readiness; (2) equipping patients with knowledge of their condition and treatment; (3) fostering self-management skills and independence; (4) implementing a well-organized and comprehensive transfer of documents; and (5) uninterrupted, coordinated, developmentally appropriate, and responsive multidisciplinary care.

[a] Department of Psychology, University of Guelph, 50 Stone Road East, Guelph, Ontario N1G 2W1, Canada; [b] Department of Gastroenterology, Hepatology, and Nutrition, Hospital for Sick Children, Toronto, Canada; [c] Department of Psychiatry, University of Toronto, Toronto, Canada; [d] Child Health Evaluative Sciences, SickKids Research Institute, Toronto, Canada
* Corresponding author. 555 University Avenue, Toronto, Ontario M5V 1X8, Canada.
E-mail address: sara.aholakohut@sickkids.ca

Gastroenterol Clin N Am 51 (2022) 849–865
https://doi.org/10.1016/j.gtc.2022.07.008
0889-8553/22/© 2022 Elsevier Inc. All rights reserved.

INTRODUCTION

Chronic gastrointestinal disorders (GIDs) characterize problems within the digestive tract resulting in variable combinations of symptoms such as nausea, bloating, diarrhea, constipation, and chronic abdominal pain, that lasts for months, years, or even life-long. There are two categories of chronic GI conditions. Disorders of the gut–brain interaction (DGBI), such as irritable bowel syndrome (IBS), are broadly referred to conditions that, after appropriate medical evaluation, could not be explained by physical or biochemical abnormalities.[1,2] In contrast, structural GI diseases (SGIDs), such as inflammatory bowel diseases (IBD), are characterized by specific physical or biochemical abnormalities in the digestive tract.[3] Approximately 25% of youth in North America are diagnosed with at least one DGBI[4] or SGID,[5–7] with peak onset in adolescence. Of note, Canada is reported to have the highest and most rapidly growing rates of IBD in the world, increasing by 50% over the course of the last decade.[8]

High rates of pediatric GIDs are concerning because they are associated with a unique set of psychological, functional, social, academic, and economic challenges across development. For example, common daily stressors in youth with GIDs include embarrassment associated fecal incontinence, poor body image, and social anxiety related to school absences and a loss of social learning opportunities.[9,10] Missed school is expectedly also associated with lower grade point averages and, thus, lower levels of education and/or job attainment.[9–11] Youth with GIDs also show higher rates of internalizing symptoms, lower self-esteem, and lower health-related quality of life compared with peers.[12,13]

Psychosocial comorbidities and physical symptoms associated with pediatric GIDs are frequently exacerbated by life stressors and persist even after short-term evidence-based medical and psychological interventions.[14,15] As such, youth with GIDs are two to four times more likely to become adults with GIDs.[16] Given that individuals age out of the pediatric health care system between 18 and 21 year old (depending on geographic region and psychosocial needs),[17] emerging adults with childhood-onset GID are faced with challenges associated with seeking new health care professionals and adjusting to new policies/procedures. Specifically, transitioning from pediatric to adult care involves moving from family-centered and comprehensive services with a high degree of caregiver involvement to person- and disease-centered care, and that leaves the responsibility for making decisions and seeking multidisciplinary care to the patients.[18] Simultaneously, these patients are also faced with the inherent challenges of transitioning into adulthood such as coping with pubertal changes and establishing financial security, independence, new social networks, and other aspects of an adult identity.[19–21] When self-identity and stability are in flux, learning to autonomously manage a GID can be particularly challenging. Therefore, it is our responsibility as health care professionals to be aware of and address these challenges. A concerted effort by health care professionals to provide knowledge and ensure continuity of care is important for promoting positive outcomes post-transfer, such as prevention or reduction of physical, mental, and social disabilities, increased patient satisfaction, and reduced health care costs[22]

The purposeful, planned process for addressing the medical, psychosocial, sexual, and educational/vocational needs of adolescents and young adults as they move from child-centered to adult-oriented health care systems is referred to as health care transition (HCT).[23] HCT goes beyond simply moving a patient and their medical files from one provider to another (ie, transfer); it involves a holistic approach to reduce patient burden and facilitate changes in work, school, and community engagement. As

such, there are three key goals of HCT efforts[24,25]: (1) to increase knowledge, independence, and self-management skills; (2) to assess and respond to patients' psychological
maturity and transition readiness; and (3) to ensure the best possible health care in
adulthood which includes an effective transfer of information between pediatric and
adult health care provider(s), promoting the patient's confidence in their adult health
care provider(s), and limiting insurance gaps.[24,26] Good HCT policies/programs should
also support caregivers in transferring the role and responsibilities of health care utilization, decision-making, and self-management to the emerging young adult.[27]

To date, research on HCT within the subspecialty of gastroenterology has been
focused on youth with IBD. This research indicates that a wide range of HCT efforts
are associated with positive clinical outcomes, such as reductions in missed medical
appointments and hospital visits as well as increases in patients' confidence in health
care professionals/treatments, adherence to medication, self-efficacy, independence,
self-management skills, health care satisfaction, and disease knowledge.[28] These
positive outcomes are consistent with findings from studies on HCT for other childhood chronic illnesses such as arthritis, diabetes, and asthma.[23,29,30] However,
despite the evidence to support HCT, patients are continuing to be transferred. In
this article, we draw upon the research literature and our own clinical experiences
working within a North American context to describe potential barriers to HCT in
gastroenterology services. Current models for supporting HCT in the context of
childhood-onset GID will be summarized and used to inform recommendations for
overcoming potential barriers.

NATURE OF THE PROBLEM

In North America, health service use (ie, emergency department use, outpatient visits,
and laboratory investigations) has been found to increase substantially within 2 year of
transfer into adult care,[31] which has significant social and financial repercussions both
for individual patients and society. This increase may be attributed to increased disease severity, difficulty accessing nonurgent care, and/or poor sharing of health information between pediatric and adult health care professionals. Upon transfer to adult
gastroenterology services, emerging adults are often poorly prepared and overwhelmed by the demands placed on them for autonomously managing their condition.
Transition readiness is established when one masters relevant disease-related knowledge, self-management skills, and access to care.[32] One study found that only 5.6%
of patients with IBD transitioning to adult care were shown to meet the benchmark for
transition readiness on the Transition Readiness Assessment Questionnaire (TRAQ),
as established by an interdisciplinary, multi-institutional Transition Task Force.[33]
Low transition readiness was attributed to deficits in health care utilization/self-
advocacy (eg, understanding insurance, scheduling appointments/following up on referrals) and self-management (eg, filling/reordering prescriptions). Other studies within
Canada and the United States have found that youth with IBD often lack knowledge of
their date of diagnosis, diagnostic classification, insurance providers, and medication
names and doses.[34,35] In addition, most older adolescents (16–18 years) deferred the
responsibility of scheduling appointments and refilling medications to their caregivers.[35] Consistent with these results, 42% of pediatric and 79% of adult gastroenterologists in the United Kingdom identified inadequacies in the preparation of
young people with IBD for adult care in terms of a lack of knowledge about the condition and treatment, lack of self-advocacy, and difficulty coordinating one's own
care.[36] This research highlights difficulties with translating HCT research into clinical
practice worldwide, not only for IBD, but also for all GIDs.[37,38]

Barriers to successful HCT are summarized in **Fig. 1**. One potential barrier to HCT is that there is yet to be a standard written policy or framework to create and maintain HCT practices.[39] As such, the constellation of health care professionals and types of interventions provided is quite variable across health care centers and clinics. In Canada, only 40% of gastroenterologists reported using a formal HCT program that ranged from informal agreements between pediatric and adult care health care professionals to structured transition programs/clinics.[40] Although much has been written on how to optimize HCT, logistical barriers and limits to generalizability need to be taken into consideration. For instance, many published recommendations or frameworks for HCT relating to childhood-onset GIDs in North America are focused on IBD and are based in the United States. Studies with an emphasis on IBD provide limited insight into the unique strengths and challenges associated with HCT in youth with other SGIDs or DGBIs. For example, we have observed clinically that youth with DGBIs struggle to receive publicly funded multidisciplinary care in hospital settings and often face challenges associated with diagnostic uncertainty. There is also a greater emphasis on psychological and lifestyle interventions in treating DGBIs.[41] It is possible that the lack of access to hospital-based integrated care for youth with DGIBs mitigates some of the challenges with HCT if their caregivers have already been successful in setting them up with a multidisciplinary team of community health care professionals who are able to provide support over the lifespan. Alternatively, the lack of support within the pediatric health care system may place these youth at an even greater disadvantage for seeking care in adulthood, especially for youth disadvantaged by financial or geographic barriers to accessing care. The extent to which these differences in pediatric care impact HCT for youth with DGBIs compared with youth with SGIDs is unclear.

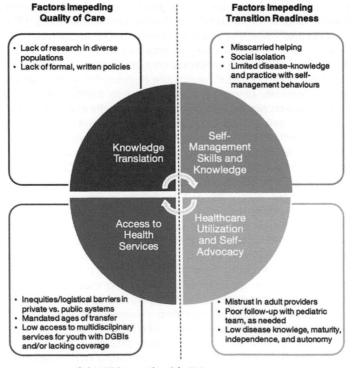

Factors Imepeding Quality of Care

- Lack of research in diverse populations
- Lack of formal, written policies

Factors Imepeding Transition Readiness

- Misscarried helping
- Social isolation
- Limited disease-knowledge and practice with self-management behaviours

Knowledge Translation

Self-Management Skills and Knowledge

Access to Health Services

Healthcare Utilization and Self-Advocacy

- Inequities/logistical barriers in private vs. public systems
- Mandated ages of transfer
- Low access to multidisciplinary services for youth with DGBIs and/or lacking coverage

- Mistrust in adult providers
- Poor follow-up with pediatric team, as needed
- Low disease knowlege, maturity, independence, and autonomy

Fig. 1. Barriers to successful HCT in youth with GIDs.

Another key aspect of multidisciplinary care is access to psychological services to provide biopsychosocial conceptualizations of the condition and offer interventions for navigating interpersonal challenges within the family, encouraging self-management skills, supporting identity formation and self-efficacy, promoting medical adherence, facilitating effective communication, promoting adaptive social, emotional, and school-related functioning, and addressing other psychosocial challenges associated with HCT. There is an abundance of evidence of gut and brain interactions that support biopsychosocial conceptualizations of GI conditions.[42] Likewise, there is a strong evidence base for the use of psychological interventions, such as cognitive-behavioral therapy, hypnosis, and mindfulness-based therapies, to effectively reduce symptoms of IBS; and a small but promising amount of literature to support the effectiveness of psychological intervention for supporting youth with IBD.[41] In response to this research evidence, various researchers and health professionals around the world have called for greater recognition of the roles of psychologists in treating pediatric GIDs, especially for more complex presentations.[43–45] However, the use of integrated care by medical professionals is seldom, especially in the context of SGIDs where the etiology and treatment have historically relied on the biomedical instead of the biopsychosocial model of care.[3] As such, despite the documented benefits of psychological treatment, the rate of referrals to mental health professionals and the follow-through on this referral from patients is generally low.[46] The underuse of psychogastroenterology services is even more likely in adulthood where there is reduced access to funding for integrated care and, therefore, the onus is on the patient to seek concomitant psychological services. More effective models of psychology integration and collaboration in gastroenterology settings are needed, especially in supporting youth transitioning into adult care.[43,45] Until then, physicians play a crucial role in setting the stage for greater buy-in and engagement from families toward seeking integrated biopsychosocial interventions by, for example, introducing a psychologist as a central member of the medical teams and/or providing more education about how psychosocial factors influence GI symptomology and offering referrals with regular follow-up.[3]

Moreover, a key distinction between the health care system in Canada compared with the United States is the publicly funded instead of privatized health care. Within both of these systems, factors such as high patient demand and variable funding can limit the amount of time to implement HCT programming. However, an advantage to privately funded systems is the consistency in billing for all health care professionals which may allow for greater flexibility in providing multidisciplinary services. Many adult gastroenterologists in Canada report lacking consistent access to a multidisciplinary team and affordable mental health care for patients.[40] One reason multidisciplinary care is seldom used in adulthood is because medications and allied health care services are generally no longer publicly funded for adult Canadians (with few exceptions for persons with disabilities). Given that young people with GIDs in Canada are not accustomed to independently seeking coverage and allied health care, this adds another layer of stress for young people at the time of transfer. In addition, many Canadian provinces have a mandated transfer of care at the age of 18 whereas some other countries such as the United States may extend care up until 21 years of age if beneficial to the young person.[17] Given that transition readiness tends to increase with age[47] and the brain is continuing to develop until 24 years of age,[48] this may require additional considerations for pediatric and adult health care professionals in preparing and receiving patients, respectively.

Barriers to successful HCT have also been hypothesized to vary across patients.[49] Increased psychological distress and functional disability among youth with GIDs tend to elicit and are exacerbated by protective and accommodative caregiver responses (eg, miscarried helping) across development.[50–52] As such, adolescents/young adults with GIDs are often accustomed to relying more heavily on caregivers when they should be becoming more independent. In addition, vulnerabilities to social isolation (due to socially embarrassing symptoms, fatigue, or chronic pain) and high levels of caregiver involvement can further impede developmental changes in autonomy, identity exploration, and cognitive maturation, which are important for developing self-management skills and adjusting to a new health care system.[52,53] Moreover, it is important to consider the emotional effects of terminating one's relationship with their pediatric health care professionals with whom they have likely known for an extended period and trust. It has also been observed clinically that families experience a gap in health care access between their last appointment with their pediatric provider(s) and intake appointment with their adult provider(s) even though they are often encouraged to reach out to the pediatric team during that time if needed. Part of the problem is the lack of comfort patients express regarding reaching out to pediatric health care professionals after undergoing the experience of termination. An initial lack of familiarity and trust in the adult medical team as well as a poor understanding and negative perceptions of adult health care can further disrupt HCT and access to care in early adulthood.[49]

GUIDELINES

Programs for HCT may take place as a formal transition clinic or informal practices between independent health care professionals.[40] Research suggests that structured/formalized transition care is associated with better economic, disease-specific, and developmental outcomes.[54–56] Although there remain no standard policies for HCT, it is widely agreed that a successful transition process involves providing health care that is uninterrupted, coordinated and developmentally appropriate, and psychologically sound both before and throughout the transfer into the adult system. Many models and recommendations for transition programming have been published.[18,28,39,49,57,58] However, the number of guidelines is truthfully overwhelming and challenging for clinics and health care professionals with limited resources and time to review and implement. This review set out to identify and summarize the most relevant recommendations for working with youth with GIDs to offer health care professionals a more concise and simplified toolbox for supporting HCT.

A guideline that is particularly relevant for guiding pediatric gastroenterology health care professionals in initiating early and developmentally appropriate conversations to facilitate HCT is the ON TRAC (Taking Responsibility for Adolescent/Adult Care) framework, which was developed in 1998 at the Children's and Women's Centre of British Columbia for supporting HCT for pediatric transplant patients[59] but was more recently adapted in the context of GID[58] (for a comprehensive clinical transition framework adapted to GIDs, see Pinzon and colleagues[58]). This framework was developed based on the belief that HCT is best facilitated by a multidisciplinary team consisting of physicians, nurses, psychologists, social workers, dieticians, occupational therapists, and physiotherapists, who have ideally supported the adolescent from birth because of established trust and knowledge. Recommendations, tools, and resources are provided in three stages: early transition (10–12 years), middle transition (13–15 years), and late transition (16–18 years). At each stage of the HCT process, it is recommended that health care professionals address concerns with self-advocacy, independent health behaviors, sexual health, social supports, lifestyle choices, and educational, vocational, and financial planning.[59]

The early transition stage is where the child and family can be introduced to the transition process and begin to participate in their own care, such as learning about their diagnosis (self-advocacy), choosing a method for remembering to take medications (independent behaviors), and discuss puberty changes and how they will be impacted by their GID and medication side-effects (sexual health).[58] The middle transition stage is for furthering the adolescent and family's understanding of the transition process through practicing skills and setting goals. For example, adolescents should be informed about their rights and responsibilities and the role of those involved in care (self-advocacy), plan and prepare for appointments (independent behaviors), and prepare for challenges that one's GID might cause for aspects of one's life such as driving or post-secondary education (lifestyle choices). Finally, the late transition stage might include, but is not limited to, reviewing one's GID and ways to stay informed (self-advocacy) and conversations about sexual capabilities and risks (sexual health), enrollment in GI support groups (social supports), future plans for insurance coverage (financial planning), and the importance of planning ahead for trips or moving away from home (health and lifestyle). During the late transition stage, it is especially important for health care professionals to assess for knowledge and successful demonstrations of self-management behaviors (eg, booking appointments, refilling prescriptions).

More recently, a national guideline for the transition from pediatric to adult care for youth with special health care needs was published by the Canadian Association of Pediatric Health Centers (CAPHC) to offer recommendations and tools for pediatric health care professionals.[57] Although this guideline is not specific to HCT in the context of GIDs, it summarizes the extensive literature on addressing HCT needs and effectively applies a systems approach to addressing youth's health and development. Specifically, recommendations were organized into three broad areas: (1) person-centered, holistic approaches; (2) clinical practices; and (3) system-level strategies. Within pediatric health settings, person-centered and holistic care recommendations include transition planning is youth-focused and family-centered, adaptable to the abilities and complexities of the youth's needs, and addresses youth's physical, developmental, psychosocial, mental health, educational, lifestyle, cultural and financial needs. Examples of clinical recommendations include assessing youth's readiness for adult care, individualized transition planning in the pediatric and community settings, education for youth and their families regarding transition, and all youth having a primary care physician to support care coordination. System level recommendations include, but are not limited to, developing a written policy for the provision of HCT services, developing efficient and accredited health information systems to support the transfer of information and collaborative communication among sectors, and designated HCT champions within their pediatric and adult settings to facilitate and evaluate transition. It is important to acknowledge that since publishing current guidelines, the world has experienced an electronic revolution in health care amidst the COVID-19 pandemic. The prospect of using virtual appointments to increase the feasibility of recommended HCT practices (eg, scheduling joint appointments between pediatric and adult health care professionals or multidisciplinary teams) is not included in previous guidelines but should be considered.

DISCUSSION

A recognition of the differences between pediatric and adult health care by patients, families, and health care professionals is key to a successful transition. Pediatric health care professionals should use this knowledge to better prepare patients and families to help avoid shock/limit stress at the time of transfer. Adult health care professionals should be able to acknowledge differences in pediatric care to increase sensitivity to patient experiences and to guide future treatment goals/referrals. In relation to IBD treatment, Nardone and colleagues[18] identified seven key differences between pediatric and adult care: (1) multidisciplinary teams versus autonomously practicing physicians and/or nurse specialists; (2) family- versus patient-centered; (3) collaborative versus autonomous decision making; (4) access to resources; (5) age-specific areas for treatment/concerns; (6) unconscious versus conscious sedation during medical procedures; and (7) independence required during hospitalization. Most of these distinctions, except for possibly the need for medical procedures and period of hospitalization, often apply to all GIDs. A major distinction between pediatric and adult care that is important but not explicitly captured in the model by Nardone and colleagues[18] is the transition from a developmental approach to care (ie, focusing on developmental issues and adjusting policies to meet patient needs) to a more consistent, one-size-fits-all approach (ie, consistent policies and expectations for many adults across their lifespan). As a result, the specific needs of young people are often overlooked in the delivery of care as they are viewed simply as "adults" and, thus, are expected to be autonomous and are responsible for their own care.[60] Given that government officials, insurance providers, and policy makers within health care institutions abide by this philosophy toward health care delivery, we recognize that one's access to coverage for medications and policies for sedation and hospitalization are mandated based on the age of the individual. Therefore, these domains could also be viewed as age-specific concerns and areas for treatment. Taking into consideration the relatedness between these domains of care, we reconceptualized the differences between pediatric and adult care in this article within four main distinctions: (1) multidisciplinary versus mono-disciplinary (predominately medical) care; (2) family versus patient-centered; (3) collaborative versus autonomous; and (4) developmental versus consistent approaches to care (**Fig. 2**). **Table 1** provides

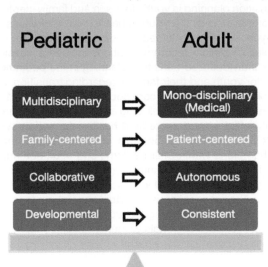

Fig. 2. Key distinctions between pediatric and adult care that should be taken into consideration when planning for HCT. These domains are presented on a weighted scale to emphasize the importance of adjusting these characteristics of care based on the individual needs of the patient, considering both systemic barriers and aspects of transition readiness.

Table 1
A list of recommendations for pediatric and adult gastroenterologists for addressing primary differences between pediatric and adult care

Pediatric Gastroenterology	Adult Gastroenterology
Multidisciplinary care → Medical care	
• Manage expectations by informing youth/families about the lack of integrated health care in adult clinics.	• Use nurse coordinators and/or mental health experts to facilitate transition.
• Discuss the use of mental health services across the lifespan and encourage youth to initiate conversations about referrals, as needed, with adult health care professionals.	• Offer longer appointment times for newly transferred patients.
	• Implement a greater emphasis on addressing psychosocial difficulties associated with GIDs in adulthood.
• Comprehensive transition risk assessments (eg, transition readiness, disease knowledge) before transfer to determine and communicate the potential need for alternate supports in adulthood (eg, mental health services). Additional factors such as mental health (eg, anxiety, depression), social skills, educational attainment, self-efficacy, exposure to role models, school attendance, family involvement, social integration, and socioeconomic barriers can impact transition readiness and response to transfer. These factors should be assessed, addressed, and communicated to the adult physician/team by a mental health professional before transfer.	○ Support patients in accessing mental health services through referral and regular follow-up.
	○ Seek funding opportunities for hiring a psychologist or social worker with a subspeciality in GIDs.
• Patients at risk of transition failure should have additional transition clinic visits before transfer and/or follow-up with the pediatric team.	
Family-centered → Patient-centered	
• Combine patient- and family-centered approaches in pediatric clinics by acknowledging the impact on the youth's condition on the family and the family's role in providing support while also respecting the patient's perspective and engaging them in a developmentally supportive manner.	• Recognize that sociocultural considerations and physical and/or cognitive disabilities of the patient are important for determining the extent to which family-related factors are essential to the patient's care.
• Provide opportunities for patients, when developmentally appropriate, to be seen in clinic on their own for at least part of the visit.	
• Describe the role of the family in the transition process as well as in adult care.	

(continued on next page)

Table 1
(continued)

Pediatric Gastroenterology	Adult Gastroenterology
• Discuss ways to provide formal (eg, GI support associations) and informal peer support (eg, peer mentor, peers within the youth's life) to the youth and family during each stage of the youth's life.	• Involve caregivers in the initial appointment but encourages patients to attend independently in subsequent sessions to reinforce autonomy.
Collaborative or caregiver-directed decision-making → Autonomous decision-making	• Recognition that HCT may be more complex and generally more difficult for youth with sociodemographic challenges, comorbidities, and physical and/or cognitive disabilities. For more complex cases, support caregiver involvement in the transition process and identify areas for extended support.
• Facilitate autonomous decision-making at the early adolescent stage (10–12 year old) through gradual education. This may include, but is not limited to, the following activities:	• Cultural awareness as well as cognitive and mental health assessments are needed to determine appropriate levels of caregiver involvement in adulthood.
1. Self-advocacy skills:	
• Educate and review information about diagnosis and transition process.	
• Explain the youth's rights and responsibilities and different roles involved in care.	
• Identify ways for the youth to stay informed and encourage questions/feedback.	
2. Independent Behaviors:	
• Find a method for youth to remember and track medications and appointments on their own.	
• Encourage self-reporting.	
• Teach ways of coping with anxiety, stress, or uncertainty.	
• Assess for knowledge in dealing with own care needs (eg, booking appointments, refilling prescriptions.)	
3. Knowledge and planning:	
• Learn medication names/doses.	
• Describe tests/procedures and reasons for them.	
• Increase knowledge and planning regarding sexual health, family history, social supports, education/work opportunities, and physical health and lifestyle choices (eg, active living, substance use, planning for trips).	

- Assess developmental age and cognitive ability of the patient to inform the level of support needed in all levels of transition planning.
- Information about multi-system issues, comorbidities, and physical and or cognitive disabilities information should be communicated to adult health care professionals.

Developmental → Consistent

- Often focused on pubertal development/growth.
- Explore the early onset of issues that are typically discussed in adulthood and/or prepare youth for initiating conversations with their adult health care professionals if/when these issues become relevant.
- Often focused on surveillance, occupational functioning, sexual functioning, fertility, and pregnancy.
- Ensure challenges with pubertal development/growth are resolved.

Examples of developmental changes in treatment and access to services are provided in the following domains: (1) *sedation*, (2) *hospitalization*, and (3) *coverage*.

Sedation (unconscious → conscious)

- Provide patients with coping strategies (eg, deep breathing) to manage anxiety before and after medical procedures. Mastery of coping skills early in development can improve readiness for procedures in adulthood.
- Introduce the possibly of conscious sedation in adulthood at the late transition phase.
- Provide patients with coping strategies (eg, deep breathing) to manage anxiety before and after medical procedures.
- Ensure patients are informed about the rationale and procedures for conscious sedation.

Hospitalization (overnight → visiting hours)

- When appropriate, encourage adolescents to stay in the hospital overnight alone.
- Consider the use of technology (ie, video calling) to offer connections with loved ones during hospitalization.

Coverage (covered → uncovered)

- During late adolescence (16–18 year old), discuss with youth further plans for insurance coverage. This may include provincial/federal aids, post-
- At first appointment, ensure that the young person has a plan for coverage and provide guidance as needed.

(continued on next page)

Table 1
(continued)

Pediatric Gastroenterology	Adult Gastroenterology
secondary health plans, extended caregiver insurance plans, or employment benefits.	• When possible, provide prescriptions covered within the patient's health plan.

General Recommendations for Pediatric and Adult Gastroenterology

• Written transition plans, developed at least 3 y before the transfer of care and updated annually, should be a part of each patient's health care record and include: dates, services, health education goals, identification of adult services, and health care professionals; goals for social leisure, education, vocation, finances, living arrangements; and sexual health and assessment of risk behaviors.

• Offer one conjoined appointment with both the pediatric and adult physician or overlapping of separate appointments with pediatric and adult physicians with the goal of patients being able to meet their adult physician at least once before their last visit with their pediatric health care professionals.

• At all stages of the transition process and planning, consider the engagement of community groups and condition-specific organizations where youth and their caregivers look for support and guidance. Community connections improve awareness and engagement

• Digital technologies should be considered for increasing the feasibility and access to conjoined appointments and/or allied health care professionals (eg, video conferencing software) as well as to provide more interactive and engaging options for education, behavioral interventions, and self-management skill building (eg, videos, computer-based activities).

• Access to a family physician in addition to specialized care can help to facilitate continuity of care, coordination of care, and access to health services within the community. Family physicians who see the entire family as patients can also have greater awareness of the family context and can provide more individualized support around overcoming sociodemographic challenges.

recommendations for supporting transition based on these four distinctions by integrating recommendations from current guidelines, available literature, and the clinical experiences of the authors.

SUMMARY

In conclusion, there is a wide range of HCT practices, but our understanding of what works best for patients with GID in North America and resources for implementing good HCT practices are limited. Without standard HCT policies/programs and appropriate resources, physicians, nurses, and allied health care professionals must ultimately rely on their own clinical judgment, advocacy skills, and trial-and-error guided by the extant literature.

CLINICS CARE POINTS

The following four clinical care points summarize the essential components of "good" health care transition (HCT) practices that we urge health care professionals to implement in their work with adolescents and young people with chronic gastrointestinal disorders (GID):

- Assess for *transition readiness* to determine the optimal timing of transfer and the types of support needed before, during, and after. This includes, but is not limited to, assessing for disease-specific knowledge, self-management skills, cognitive maturity, comfort with new health care professionals, and independence from caregivers.

- Equip patients with sufficient *knowledge* about their condition and its impact on past, present, and future functioning (eg, verbal and written information summary of medical records; educational resources such as brochures and websites) as well as the differences between pediatric and adult care.

- Develop an organized transition plan aimed at fostering *self-management skills and independence* in a developmentally appropriate, patient-centered manner. This transition plan is best developed collaboratively with patients and their families as early as 10 to 12 year old, documented in writing, and reviewed annually. Planning for access to medical care across the lifespan is vital (eg, insurance coverage, and transportation).

- Implement a well-organized and comprehensive *transfer of documents*, medical history, and treatment regimens between pediatric/adult care physicians, nurses, and allied health care professionals (ie, summary letter; sharing electronic medical records; phone meetings between professionals; and joint or overlapping appointments).

The best way to accomplish the above-mentioned clinical care points is to ensure patients have access to uninterrupted, coordinated, developmentally appropriate, and responsive *multidisciplinary care*. Within this team-based approach, the inclusion of mental health professionals, such as social workers and psychologists, can help to support youth and caregivers in developing the knowledge-base and skills needed to facilitate transition and to address the unique psychosocial challenges associated with being an emerging adult with a GID (eg, low self-esteem, poor self-efficacy skills, and building coping strategies). Nurse coordinators can support in providing information to clients and families, coordinating care between health professionals, facilitating the transfer of files, and assisting with accessing services within the community. In addition, involving other health professionals, such as dieticians, naturopathic doctors, physiotherapists, and exercise therapists, as needed, can help to provide holistic care to clients as they transition. Although there are clear financial and logistical barriers to offering integrated care in adulthood, low-cost HCT practices for adult physicians include conducting formal assessments or check-ins to uncover psychosocial needs, providing psychoeducation about allied health professions in the context of patients' symptoms, encouraging self-advocacy skills, and establishing multidisciplinary professional networks to facilitate regular referrals and follow-ups.

DISCLOSURE

The authors have nothing to disclose.

REFERENCES

1. Hyams JS, Di Lorenzo C, Saps M, et al. Childhood Functional Gastrointestinal Disorders: Child/Adolescent. Gastroenterology 2016;150(6):1456–68.e2.
2. Rasquin A, Di Lorenzo C, Forbes D, et al. Childhood Functional Gastrointestinal Disorders: Child/Adolescent. Gastroenterology 2006;130(5):1527–37.
3. Maddux MH, Deacy AD, Colombo JM. Organic Gastrointestinal Disorders. In: Carter B, Kullgren K, editors. Clinical handbook of psychological consultation in pediatric medical settings. Springer Nature; 2020. p. 195–210.
4. Lewis ML, Palsson OS, Whitehead WE, et al. Prevalence of Functional Gastrointestinal Disorders in Children and Adolescents. J Pediatr 2016;177:39–43.e3.
5. Abramson O, Durant M, Mow W, et al. Incidence, Prevalence, and Time Trends of Pediatric Inflammatory Bowel Disease in Northern California, 1996 to 2006. J Pediatr 2010;157(2):233–9.e1.
6. Baldassano RN, Piccoli DA. Inflammatory bowel disease in pediatric and adolescent patients. Gastroenterol Clin North Am 1999;28(2):445–58.
7. Rosen MJ, Dhawan A, Saeed SA. Inflammatory Bowel Disease in Children and Adolescents. JAMA Pediatr 2015;169(11):1053–60.
8. Carroll MW, Kuenzig ME, Mack DR, et al. The Impact of Inflammatory Bowel Disease in Canada 2018: Children and Adolescents with IBD. J Can Assoc Gastroenterol 2019;2(Supplement_1):S49–67.
9. Greenley RN, Hommel KA, Nebel J, et al. A Meta-analytic Review of the Psychosocial Adjustment of Youth with Inflammatory Bowel Disease. J Pediatr Psychol 2010;35(8):857–69.
10. Mackner LM, Greenley RN, Szigethy E, et al. Psychosocial Issues in Pediatric Inflammatory Bowel Disease: Report of the North American Society for Pediatric Gastroenterology, Hepatology, and Nutrition. J Pediatr Gastroenterol Nutr 2013; 56(4):449–58.
11. Mackner LM, Bickmeier RM, Crandall WV. Academic Achievement, Attendance, and School-Related Quality of Life in Pediatric Inflammatory Bowel Disease. J Dev Behav Pediatr 2012;33(2):106–11.
12. Engström I. Mental health and psychological functioning in children and adolescents with inflammatory bowel disease: a comparison with children having other chronic illnesses and with healthy children. J Child Psychol Psychiatry 1992; 33(3):563–82.
13. Ross SC, Strachan J, Russell RK, et al. Psychosocial Functioning and Health-related Quality of Life in Paediatric Inflammatory Bowel Disease. J Pediatr Gastroenterol Nutr 2011;53(5):480–8.
14. Robins PM, Smith SM, Glutting JJ, et al. A Randomized Controlled Trial of a Cognitive-Behavioral Family Intervention for Pediatric Recurrent Abdominal Pain. J Pediatr Psychol 2005;30(5):397–408.
15. Whitehead WE, Palsson O, Jones KR. Systematic review of the comorbidity of irritable bowel syndrome with other disorders: What are the causes and implications? Gastroenterology 2002;122(4):1140–56.
16. Chitkara DK, van Tilburg MAL, Blois-Martin N, et al. Early life risk factors that contribute to irritable bowel syndrome in adults: a systematic review. Am J Gastroenterol 2008;103(3). https://doi.org/10.1111/j.1572-0241.2007.01722.x.

17. Hardin AP, Hackell JM, COMMITTEE ON PRACTICE AND AMBULATORY MEDI-CINE. Age Limit of Pediatrics. Pediatrics 2017;140(3):e20172151.
18. Nardone OM, Iacucci M, Ghosh S, et al. Can a transition clinic bridge the gap between paediatric and adult inflammatory bowel disease care models? Dig Liver Dis 2020;52(5):516–27.
19. Arnett JJ. Conceptions of the Transition to Adulthood: Perspectives From Adolescence Through Midlife. J Adult Development 2001;8(2):133–43.
20. Arnett JJ. Emerging Adulthood: Understanding the New Way of Coming of Age. In: Arnett J, Tanner J, editors. Emerging adults in America: coming of age in the 21st century. American Psychological Association; 2006. p. 3–19.
21. Benson JE, Elder GH. Young Adult Identities and Their Pathways: A Developmental and Life Course Model. Dev Psychol 2011;47(6):1646–57.
22. Alazri M, Heywood P, Neal RD, et al. Continuity of Care. Sultan Qaboos Univ Med J 2007;7(3):197–206.
23. Blum RWM, Garell D, Hodgman CH, et al. Transition from child-centered to adult health-care systems for adolescents with chronic conditions: A position paper of the Society for Adolescent Medicine. J Adolesc Health 1993;14(7):570–6.
24. Bert F, Camussi E, Gili R, et al. Transitional care: A new model of care from young age to adulthood. Health Policy 2020;124(10):1121–8.
25. Stollon N, Zhong Y, Ferris M, et al. Chronological age when health care transition skills are mastered in adolescents/young adults with inflammatory bowel disease. World J Gastroenterol 2017;23(18):3349–55.
26. Lotstein DS, Inkelas M, Hays RD, et al. Access to Care for Youth with Special Health Care Needs in the Transition to Adulthood. J Adolesc Health 2008;43(1):23–9.
27. Cooley WC, Sagerman PJ, American Academy of Pediatrics AA of FP. Supporting the Health Care Transition From Adolescence to Adulthood in the Medical Home. Pediatrics 2011;128(1):182–200.
28. Philpott JR, Kurowski JA. Challenges in Transitional Care in Inflammatory Bowel Disease: A Review of the Current Literature in Transition Readiness and Outcomes. Inflamm Bowel Dis 2019;25(1):45–55.
29. Annunziato RA, Emre S, Shneider B, et al. Adherence and medical outcomes in pediatric liver transplant recipients who transition to adult services. Pediatr Transplant 2007;11(6):608–14.
30. Cadario F, Prodam F, Bellone S, et al. Transition process of patients with type 1 diabetes (T1DM) from paediatric to the adult health care service: a hospital-based approach. Clin Endocrinol 2009;71(3):346–50.
31. Zhao X, Bjerre LM, Nguyen GC, et al. Health Services Use during Transition from Pediatric to Adult Care for Inflammatory Bowel Disease: A Population-Based Study Using Health Administrative Data. J Pediatr 2018;203:280–7.e4.
32. Stinson JN, Stevens BJ, Feldman BM, et al. Construct validity of a multidimensional electronic pain diary for adolescents with arthritis. Pain 2008;136(3):281–92.
33. Gray WN, Holbrook E, Morgan PJ, et al. Transition Readiness Skills Acquisition in Adolescents and Young Adults with Inflammatory Bowel Disease: Findings from Integrating Assessment into Clinical Practice. Inflamm Bowel Dis 2015;21(5):1125–31.
34. Benchimol EI, Walters TD, Kaufman M, et al. Assessment of knowledge in adolescents with inflammatory bowel disease using a novel transition tool. Inflamm Bowel Dis 2011;17(5):1131–7.

35. Fishman LN, Barendse RM, Hait E, et al. Self-Management of Older Adolescents with Inflammatory Bowel Disease: A Pilot Study of Behavior and Knowledge as Prelude to Transition. Clin Pediatr (Phila) 2010;49(12):1129–33.

36. Sebastian S, Jenkins H, McCartney S, et al. The requirements and barriers to successful transition of adolescents with inflammatory bowel disease: Differing perceptions from a survey of adult and paediatric gastroenterologists. J Crohn's Colitis 2012;6(8):830–44.

37. Elli L, Maieron R, Martelossi S, et al. Transition of gastroenterological patients from paediatric to adult care: A position statement by the Italian Societies of Gastroenterology. Dig Liver Dis 2015;47(9):734–40.

38. Eluri S, Book WM, Kodroff E, et al. Lack of Knowledge and Low Readiness for Health care Transition in Eosinophilic Esophagitis and Eosinophilic Gastroenteritis. J Pediatr Gastroenterol Nutr 2017;65(1):53–7.

39. Gray WN, Maddux MH. Current Transition Practices in Pediatric IBD: Findings from a National Survey of Pediatric Providers. Inflamm Bowel Dis 2016;22(2):372–9.

40. Jawaid N, Jeyalingam T, Nguyen G, et al. Paediatric to Adult Transition of Care in IBD: Understanding the Current Standard of Care Among Canadian Adult Academic Gastroenterologists. J Can Assoc Gastroenterol 2020;3(6):266–73.

41. Ballou S, Keefer L. Psychological Interventions for Irritable Bowel Syndrome and Inflammatory Bowel Diseases. Clin Translational Gastroenterol 2017;8(1):e214.

42. Dovey T. A biopsychosocial framework to understand children and young people with gastrointestinal problems. In: Martin C, Dovey T, editors. Paediatric gastrointestinal disorders. London, UK: CRC Press; 2014.

43. Bradford A. Introduction to the Special Issue: Advances in Psychogastroenterology. J Clin Psychol Med Settings 2020;27(3):429–31.

44. Keefer L, Palsson OS, Pandolfino JS. Best Practice Update: Incorporating Psychogastroenterology Into Management of Digestive Disorders. Gastroenterology 2018;154(5):1249–57.

45. van Tilburg MAL. Psychogastroenterology: A Cure, Band-Aid, or Prevention? Children 2020;7(9):121.

46. Schurman JV, Friesen CA. Integrative treatment approaches: family satisfaction with a multidisciplinary paediatric Abdominal Pain Clinic. Int J Integr Care 2010;10:e51.

47. Varty M, Popejoy LL. A Systematic Review of Transition Readiness in Youth with Chronic Disease. West J Nurs Res 2020;42(7):554–66.

48. Colver A, Longwell S. New understanding of adolescent brain development: relevance to transitional health care for young people with long term conditions. Arch Dis Child 2013;98(11):902–7.

49. Leung Y, Heyman M, Mahadevan U. Transitioning the Adolescent Inflammatory Bowel Disease Patient: Guidelines for the Adult and Pediatric Gastroenterologist. Inflamm Bowel Dis 2011;17(10):2169–73.

50. Levy RL, Whitehead WE, Walker LS, et al. Increased Somatic Complaints and Health-Care Utilization in Children: Effects of Parent IBS Status and Parent Response to Gastrointestinal Symptoms. Official J Am Coll Gastroenterol ACG. 2004;99(12):2442–51.

51. Peterson CC, Palermo TM. Parental Reinforcement of Recurrent Pain: The Moderating Impact of Child Depression and Anxiety on Functional Disability. J Pediatr Psychol 2004;29(5):331–41.

52. Reed-Knight B, Blount RL, Gilleland J. The transition of health care responsibility from parents to youth diagnosed with chronic illness: A developmental systems perspective. Fam Syst Health 2014;32(2):219.
53. Laursen B, Hartl AC. Understanding loneliness during adolescence: Developmental changes that increase the risk of perceived social isolation. J Adolescence 2013;36(6):1261–8.
54. Cole R, Ashok D, Razack A, et al. Evaluation of Outcomes in Adolescent Inflammatory Bowel Disease Patients Following Transfer From Pediatric to Adult Health Care Services: Case for Transition. J Adolesc Health 2015;57(2):212–7.
55. Colver A, McConachie H, Le Couteur A, et al. A longitudinal, observational study of the features of transitional health care associated with better outcomes for young people with long-term conditions. BMC Med 2018;16(1):111.
56. Schütz L, Radke M, Menzel S, et al. Long-term implications of structured transition of adolescents with inflammatory bowel disease into adult health care: a retrospective study. BMC Gastroenterol 2019;19(1):128.
57. Canadian Association of Pediatric Health Centres (CAPHC). A guideline for transition from Paediatric to adult health care for youth with special health care needs: a national approach 2016. Available at: http://ken.caphc.org/xwiki/bin/view/Transitioning+from+Paediatric+to+Adult+Care/A+Guideline+for +Transition+from+Paediatric+to+Adult+Care. Accessed November 20, 2021.
58. Pinzon JL, Jacobson K, Reiss J. Say Goodbye and Say Hello: The Transition from Pediatric to Adult Gastroenterology. Can J Gastroenterol 2004;18(12):735–42.
59. Paone MC, Wigle M, Saewyc E. The ON TRAC Model for Transitional Care of Adolescents. Prog Transplant 2006;16(4):291–302.
60. Mulvale G, Nguyen T, Miatello A, et al. Lost in transition or translation? Care philosophies and transitions between child and youth and adult mental health services: a systematic review. J Ment Health (Abingdon, England) 2016;28:1–10.

Working with Trauma in the Gastroenterology Setting

Christina H. Jagielski, PhD, MPH*, Kimberly N. Harer, MD, ScM

KEYWORDS

- Trauma-informed care • Psychological trauma • Medical trauma • Abuse
- Iatrogenic harm

KEY POINTS

- History of trauma is common among patients with gastrointestinal complaints.
- Trauma can have a significant influence on an individual's physical and mental health, as well as one's experience with the medical system.
- Previous traumatic experiences can place patients at increased risk of retraumatization in the gastroenterology setting.
- Gastroenterologists and other gastrointestinal (GI) providers should be informed about the role of trauma in the GI setting in order to better provide trauma-informed approaches that can reduce risk of retraumatization, improve patient–provider interactions, and improve patient treatment and satisfaction.

INTRODUCTION

A history of trauma is a commonly overlooked and underappreciated facet of gastroenterology patients' medical history. According to the National Comorbidity Study, 61% of men and 51% of women have experienced at least one traumatic event.[1] Studies during the past 3 decades have revealed patients with gastrointestinal (GI) complaints, including irritable bowel syndrome (IBS), report higher rates of physical, emotional, and sexual abuse compared with healthy controls.[2–6] In a study of IBS patients, 60% of IBS patients reported a history of physical abuse, 55% emotional abuse, and 31% sexual trauma.[2] Although much of trauma-related research has been completed among IBS patients, a study of inflammatory bowel disease (IBD) patients by Taft and colleagues found 32% of patients with IBD met criteria for posttraumatic stress (PTS) symptoms and were more likely than IBS patients to attribute their PTS to their disease.[7]

Division of Gastroenterology and Hepatology, University of Michigan/Michigan Medicine, 1500 East Medical Center Drive, 3912, SPC 5362, Ann Arbor 48109 - 5362, USA
* Corresponding author. University of Michigan,1500 East Medical Center Drive, 3912, SPC 5362, Ann Arbor 48109 - 5362.
E-mail address: cjagiels@med.umich.edu
Twitter: @DrJagielski (C.H.J.)

Gastroenterol Clin N Am 51 (2022) 867–883
https://doi.org/10.1016/j.gtc.2022.07.012
0889-8553/22/© 2022 Elsevier Inc. All rights reserved.

Patients with a history of trauma are at risk of retraumatization when seeking medical care, including undergoing gastroenterological examinations and invasive procedures. Due to the higher prevalence of previous psychological trauma among GI patients, gastroenterology providers and staff need to have an understanding of prior trauma and the risk of retraumatization in the gastroenterology setting. In this review, we will provide a brief summary on what trauma is, discuss the impact of trauma on individuals, and provide strategies to improve trauma informed care (TIC) in the gastroenterology setting.

WHAT IS TRAUMA?

The Substance Abuse and Mental Health Services Administration states "Trauma results from an event, series of events or set of circumstances that is experienced by an individual as physically or emotionally harmful or threatening and has lasting adverse effects on the individuals functioning and physical, social, emotional, or spiritual well-being."[8] Trauma can overwhelm an individual's or community's resources to cope and can ignite the "fight, flight, or freeze" response, which can produce fear and a sense of vulnerability and helplessness.[8] An individual may experience trauma directly, witness a traumatic event occurring to others (eg, witnessing domestic violence as a child, observing a car accident), or hear about the details of the event that happened to someone they know. Trauma can be caused by human interactions or from nature. Although trauma is commonly thought of as being experienced by an individual, it is important to understand that trauma can generate a wide path of impact and involve families, communities, cultures, or across generations.

TYPES OF TRAUMA

Understanding the various types of trauma individuals may experience is imperative to understanding how a history of trauma may affect the presentation and care of gastroenterology patients. **Fig. 1** describes the most common categories of trauma.[8]

FACTORS THAT INFLUENCE TRAUMA

Not everyone who is involved in a traumatic event develops long-term effects. Numerous factors may influence whether an individual experiences an event as traumatic, how well they cope with the trauma, and what long-lasting effects of the trauma the person may experience. For example, a common factor that influences these outcomes is if the trauma was associated with an isolated versus repeated event. Individuals who undergo repeated or sustained traumas (eg, repeated sexual abuse, domestic violence, or chronic poverty) are more likely to experience traumatic stress reactions and other negative effects compared with those who experienced an isolated traumatic event.[8,9] Support following a traumatic event is also important. People who experience individual trauma are more likely to keep the trauma a secret, further reducing the likelihood of them receiving comfort, validation, or acceptance from others. Perceived shame and subsequent isolation can occur and inhibit individuals from seeking support. A lack of support may promote a distorted perception of responsibility for the traumatic event, resulting in a struggle with causation. For example, a sexual assault victim may feel responsible for the assault. These events can further promote feelings of isolation, and repeated trauma experiences enhance feelings of victimization.[8] This distorted perception of responsibility may be exacerbated in the GI setting, particularly for patients with disorders of gut–brain interaction, such as irritable bowel syndrome, who are commonly given the message "It is all in your

Trauma Categories

Interpersonal Trauma
Occurs between people, often those who know each other such as spouses or between parents and children. Examples of interpersonal trauma include physical and emotional abuse or neglect; sexual abuse or assault; intimate partner violence (IPV), also known as domestic violence; and elder abuse. IPV may involve aspects of actual or threatened physical, emotional, sexual abuse.

Adverse Childhood Trauma
Adverse childhood experiences including physical and emotional abuse, sexual abuse, growing up in a home with a substance abuse-dependent parent, a parent who is incarcerated, mentally ill, or a household member with suicidal ideation, witnessing spousal abuse between parents, divorce or separation.

Group Trauma
Impacts a particular group, such as first responders or military groups, that are at increased risk of losing multiple members.

Community or Culture Trauma
A wide range of violence or harm that impacts the sense of safety within a community (neighborhoods, schools, towns, reservations). Includes physical or sexual assaults, hate crimes, robberies, workplace or gang related violence, or shootings. Includes school shootings.

Mass Trauma
Results from disasters that affect large numbers of people directly or indirectly. The initial event causes destruction and the consequences of that event may cause additional stressful events that requires survivors to further adjust, as well as putting increased demands on first responders or disaster relief agencies. Examples include hurricanes or other natural disasters.

Political Terror and War
Political terror and war threatens the existence beliefs, wellbeing, or livelihood of a community. The overall goal of perpetrators is to maximize the uncertainty, anxiety, and fear of a large community with long lasting effects.

Historical Trauma
Historical Trauma results from events that affect an entire culture, intense enough that trauma influences future generations of the culture beyond those that experienced the trauma directly (for example the enslavement of African Americans, forced assimilation and relocation of American Indians, the violence and suffering suffered by the Jews and others during World Ward II, and other genocides)

System Oriented Trauma (retraumatization)
Triggering events that make an individual feel as though they are undergoing another trauma or re-experiencing a trauma. Patients may also experience primary trauma through systems such as a medical system.

Fig. 1. Categories of trauma.

head," a message that can portray a perception the provider thinks the patient caused their symptoms.

Survivors of group trauma are more likely to experience repeated trauma and may be encouraged to keep discussion of the trauma within the group out of concern that outsiders would not understand, which can reduce support following the trauma. Some individuals who experience repeated group trauma may also "shut down emotionally or repress traumatic experiences"[8] in order to complete the mission and may avoid seeking help or discourage others from seeking help out of concern that it will bring shame or break confidentiality of the group. Survivors of mass trauma often receive an outpouring of initial support and may feel less isolated due to experiencing the trauma with a large group of others; however, the attention and support may decline as time passes, quickly leaving survivors to cope on their own.[8] **Fig. 2** depicts additional factors that may influence how one experiences a traumatic event.

Additional factors that may influence how one experiences a traumatic event include whether or not the person has time to process the trauma. Individuals with a history of multiple, sequential traumatic experiences may not get time to process or make sense of the experiences. Others may have time to process but be unable to do so secondary

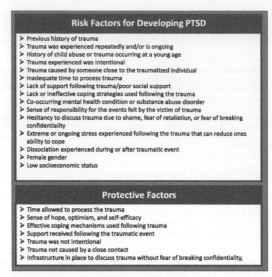

Fig. 2. Risk and protective factors for developing PTSD.

to a lack of a supportive environment to process within.[8] Another factor to consider is the relationship of the victim with the perpetrator and whether the act was intentional. Survivors often struggle to make sense of traumatic events caused by people close to them, such as a family member or partner. They may blame themselves as an act of making sense of the event or try to find ways to "make things right." Individuals with history of cooccurring mental health conditions or substance abuse are also at an increased risk of developing PTS following traumatic experiences.[8] Finally, an individual's method of coping with trauma is less important than how their coping response allows them to continue functioning in life, regulating their emotions, continue to engage meaningful relationships, and maintain self-esteem and well-being.[8]

IMPACT OF TRAUMA

Trauma has a significant influence on the nervous system and physical responses to everyday events. These manifestations may be seen in GI clinic when patients seek care for the physical responses, or these responses may affect how individuals interact with their GI care team. It is important to understand how the impact of trauma effects an individual's perceptions, interactions, and trust with health-care team members. **Fig. 3** outlines some common trauma symptoms.

Physiologic Arousal and Hypervigilance

A history of trauma is associated with high levels of physiologic arousal, alterations of the hypothalamic-pituitary axis and altered resting state neural networks related to increased anxiety.[10,11] Trauma may result in increased hypervigilance involving ongoing anxiety, and fear and panic in situations where these responses are not necessary.[8] Although these processes may be helpful in situations that are actually physically threatening, the ongoing nature of these processes while in nontraumatic circumstances can lead to negative behaviors and health effects. Responses to trauma are highly variable in both intensity and duration, with responses varying from mild to debilitating and short to long-lasting.

Trauma Symptoms
Somatic Symptoms
Hypervigilance
Belief System Changes
Emotional Dysregulation
Avoidance
Decreased Activity Level
Interpersonal Instability
Re-experiencing and Dissociation
Altered Attention, Consciousness, or Memory
Shame
System Oriented Trauma (retraumatization)

Fig. 3. Symptoms of trauma.

Emotional, Cognitive, and Behavioral Responses

Trauma reactions can be seen in multiple domains. Delayed emotional reactions include irritability and hostility, depression, fear of trauma recurrence, mood swings and instability, grief, shame, feelings of fragility or vulnerability, and emotional detachment from anything requiring emotional reaction. Delayed physical reactions include sleep disruption and nightmares, somatization, high cortisol levels, changes in appetite, increased susceptibility to infections, and hyperarousal. Cognitive reactions include intrusive memories, self-blame, preoccupation with the traumatic event, difficulty with decision-making, and suicidal ideation. Behavioral reactions include avoidance, relationship disturbances, decreased activity level, increased high-risk behaviors including alcohol and drugs, and withdrawal.[8]

Physical Responses

Many patients' primary responses to trauma are physical, meaning that medical providers may be the first to notice a potential influence of trauma. This is particularly true in the gastroenterology setting because a history of trauma has been associated with gastrointestinal symptoms and pain. Patients with a history of trauma report increased pain,[12] risk of pelvic floor problems,[13] and heightened gastroenterology procedure-related discomfort.[14–16] Patients with a history of trauma report worse GI-specific quality of life (QOL) compared with those without a trauma history. Although QOL scores improved following evidence-based GI behavioral treatments including cognitive behavioral therapy and gut-directed hypnosis, following treatment, patients with a history of trauma still reported significantly lower IBS QOL compared with those without a history of trauma.[17]

History of trauma is also associated with non-GI diseases. The Adverse Childhood Experience (ACE) study showed a graded relationship with number of ACEs to risk of ischemic heart disease, cancer, chronic lung disease, skeletal fractures, and liver disease.[18] ACEs are also associated with increased risk of obesity,[19] asthma and stroke,[20] autoimmune diseases,[21] and headaches.[22] ACEs are also associated with increased risk of alcohol abuse,[23] and other drug use,[24] depression,[25,26] and suicide.[27] In addition, patients with a history of substance abuse and history of trauma have worse treatment outcomes than those without a history of trauma.[28,29]

Somatization

Somatization, a focus on bodily symptoms as an expression of emotional distress, is common among patients with a history of trauma. Experiencing this manifestation of trauma can be influenced by cultural beliefs, particularly within cultures where expression of physical complaints is more accepted than expression of emotion. Although patients are often not aware of the tendency toward somatization and may be resistant to the role that emotional distress plays in GI symptoms, it is important for clinicians to avoid the initial assumption that physical complaints are related to emotional distress without proper medical workup.[8] In fact, if providers make biased assumptions that all of a patient's symptoms are explained through the lens of mood, anxiety, or even previous history of trauma, this may not only lead to ineffective treatments but may also contribute to retraumatization for patients who think their symptoms are not believed.

Dissociation

Dissociation is "a mental process that severs connections among a person's thoughts, memories, feelings, actions, and/or sense of identity."[8] Dissociation can serve as a protective element that prevents an individual from experiencing the full weight of a traumatic experience. Although this can be protective and healthy during the initial traumatic experience, patients with a history of PTS can experience ongoing dissociation as a coping response to deal with stress, which can be disruptive. Signs of dissociation include, fixed or "glazed" eyes, sudden flattening of affect, long periods of silence, monotonous voice, responses not congruent with the present context or situation, and excessive intellectualization.[30] Providers should monitor for signs of dissociation during sensitive procedures, examinations, or in situations where stressful content is being discussed as dissociation can have a significant influence on patient–provider interactions.

Posttraumatic Stress Disorder

Posttraumatic stress disorder (PTSD) involves ongoing symptoms following the experience of a traumatic event such as exposure to actual or threatened death, serious injury, or sexual violence. The estimated lifetime prevalence of PTSD in the United States is 6.8%.[31] In order to meet criteria for PTSD, an individual must experience symptoms in the following domains: intrusive symptoms (intrusive distressing memories of the event, dreams, flashbacks), persistent avoidance of stimuli associated with the traumatic event, negative alterations in cognition and mood, and alterations in arousal and reactivity.[32] Patients with a history of PTSD may be more at risk of increased anxiety in the medical setting, leading to increased likelihood of canceled appointments or procedures.

Complex Posttraumatic Stress Disorder

It is important to remember survivors of traumatic experiences often have experienced more than one type of trauma. Complex posttraumatic stress disorder (C-PTSD) was originally proposed in 1992 by Herman[33] and was recently added to the World Health Organization's (WHO) International Classification of Diseases revision (ICD-11). Herman defined C-PTSD as complex behavioral conditions in survivors of prolonged or multiple traumas. In addition to symptoms of PTSD, C-PTSD involves affect dysregulation, negative self-concept and relational difficulties. According to the National Health Service, C-PTSD tends to be more severe if traumatic events happened earlier in life, trauma was caused by a parent or caregiver, the person experienced trauma for an extended period of time, the person experienced the trauma alone, and/or the person was still in contact with the person responsible for the trauma.[34]

Symptoms of C-PTSD include feelings of shame or guilt, difficulty regulating emotions, periods of losing attention or concentration, dissociation, physical symptoms such as headaches, dizziness, chest pain, stomachaches, social isolation, relationship difficulties, destructive and risky behavior such as self-harm, alcohol or drug abuse, and suicidal behavior.[34] Of note, the DSM-5 has not included C-PTSD as a separate diagnosis, and there is an ongoing discussion on whether it is a distinct condition separate from simple PTSD and borderline personality disorder.[35]

MEDICAL TRAUMA AND THE RISK OF RETRAUMATIZATION

The medical setting itself has the potential to be an environment for psychological trauma. Medical trauma is defined as trauma occurring from direct contact with the medical setting. This type of trauma develops through a complex interaction between the patient, medical staff, medical environment, and the diagnostic or procedural experience, which can all have powerful psychological impacts due to the patient's unique interpretation of the events and interactions.[36]

Regarding the prevalence of medical trauma, a meta-analysis demonstrated the prevalence of PTSD was 10.2% across all medical populations when using a clinician-administered PTSD scale and 21.6% based on self-report questionnaire.[37] Specifically focusing on the GI population, a study by Taft and colleagues demonstrated 25% to 35% of IBD patients met criteria for moderate-to-severe symptoms of IBD-related PTS.[38] Predictors of PTS severity for patients with IBD included hospitalization experience, undergoing ileostomy surgery, symptom severity, age at onset, and ICU stays.[7] A qualitative study of patients living with IBD described additional factors that contributed to GI-related medical trauma including uncertainty related to IBD (when symptoms would occur and severity), poor information quality and exchange (eg, when a physician was in a hurry, stoic, or cold), receiving results of a colonoscopy without explanation (including seeing images of their colon), prolonged delays in diagnosis, and procedures such as the placement of a nasogastric tube, and surgeries such as those resulting in an ostomy, the surgeon not respecting patient preferences, and semantics of how the surgeon described a patient's health status.[39]

Primary Versus Secondary Medical Trauma

Medical trauma can be primary (the initial trauma occurring due to the medical setting itself) or secondary (retraumatization due to triggering aspects of the medical experience). Examples of primary trauma include being awake during a painful endoscopic procedure, traumatizing interaction(s) with health-care staff, or trauma due to being hospitalized during the COVID-19 pandemic when patients were not allowed to have a family member or advocate visit them for days or even weeks.

GI patients are at high risk for secondary trauma, and it is important for gastroenterology providers and staff to be aware of system factors that can lead to retraumatization (described in **Fig. 4**).[8]

Gastroenterology often involves discussion of private topics and examination of sensitive body areas in the clinic and endoscopy settings. Examples include discussion of manual disimpaction, rectal examinations, anorectal manometry, and colonoscopy. Patients with GI complaints are at risk of primary or secondary medical trauma. Knowledge of risk factors for retraumatization and having a trauma-informed plan for providers and staff can reduce the risk of additional iatrogenic psychological trauma, improve patient–provider communication, and improve patient care. Strategies for reducing risk of retraumatization are described later in this article.

Contributing Factors to Medical Re-traumatization

> Failing to screen for prior history of trauma
> Lack of understanding of how trauma impacts a patient's life
> Challenging or discounting reports of abuse or other trauma
> Use of isolation or physical restraints
> Use of a confrontational approach
> Labeling patient behavior or feelings as pathological
> Failing to provide security and safety
> Minimizing, discrediting, or ignoring patient responses
> Disrupting patient provider relationships by changing provider schedules or the provider no longer providing care
> Obtaining specimens/performing examinations in a non-private area
> Having patient undress in the presence of others

Fig. 4. Contributing factors to medical re-traumatization.

Impact of Previous Trauma on the Medical Setting

History of trauma has been shown to influence future health-care utilization in several ways. It is associated with increased hospitalizations, longer hospital stays, increased mental health visits,[40,41] and increased health-care costs.[42] A history of trauma is associated with lower odds of having health insurance or having a primary care provider.[43] A graded relationship between higher numbers of ACEs and increased cancellations or no-show appointments has also been demonstrated.[44]

A Canadian study of nearly 10,000 participants showed an association between childhood abuse and increased number of health problems, pain, disability, and frequent emergency department and health-care visits.[45] Having an understanding of how prior history of trauma can lead to both increased and decreased use of health care can help to reduce miscommunications between patient and provider. For example, increased medical visits due to unresolved GI complaints may stem from a feeling of not being taken seriously and can lead patients to continue to seek care until they feel their complaints have been taken seriously. Alternatively, patients may enact avoidance behaviors due to stress associated with the medical environment, which may lead to frequent cancellations or no-show appointments. These behaviors may result in providers labeling a patient as "difficult" or "noncompliant" when the patient's behaviors or interaction with the medical system may be explained through previous negative or stressful experiences. In the following section, we discuss how a trauma-informed approach can assist providers with identifying factors that may interfere with medical care and provide tips to improve patient–provider interactions and overall patient care.

Trauma Informed Care

TIC has been a significant area of research and clinical practice for the past 2 decades.[46,47] An important aspect of trauma is it often involves a hierarchical relationship between a known person or family member and a situation where the patient was disempowered. This can negatively influence a patient's core beliefs and perception of reality.[47] Because the relationship with medical providers can also be viewed as hierarchical, this places patients at risk for additional negative interactions in the medical system.

TIC is defined as "a holistic approach to health care that fosters understanding and thoughtful responses to individuals who have experienced trauma in their lives, thus supporting their resilience and self-efficacy."[48] Although there are many perspectives on what makes for TIC, the TIC approach incorporates at least 3 elements: (1) realizing the prevalence of trauma; (2) recognizing how trauma affects all individuals involved with the program, organization, or system, including its own workforce; and (3) responding by putting this knowledge into practice.[8] TIC requires all staff within a practice (receptionist, intake personale, direct care staff, supervisors, administrators, peer supports) to recognize that an individual's experience of trauma can greatly influence their receptivity to services; engagement with services; interactions with staff and clients; and responsiveness to program guidelines, practice, and interventions.[8]

TIC can help reduce the risk of retraumatization, improve patient–provider communication, decrease risks associated with misunderstanding patient reactions, and underestimating the need for referral for the evaluation and treatment of trauma. TIC may improve cost-effectiveness in services that are appropriately matched to the client and reduce risk of adverse effects.[8]

CONSIDERATIONS FOR GASTROENTEROLOGISTS PROVIDING TRAUMA INFORMED CARE
Screening

Gastroenterology examinations and procedures often require patients to expose sensitive areas, as well as undergoing uncomfortable touching of these areas. As such, providers should be prepared to assess for history of trauma to reduce the risk of retraumatization. Patients may be reluctant to disclose a history of trauma unprompted, possibly due to self-blame, shame, or fear of not being believed.[49] Patients may deny history of trauma at first but they may open up later when they develop more comfort with the provider.[50] Providers should be aware that some trauma survivors may be aware that something is wrong but they are unable to explain it to their provider due to history of dissociation.[50] Because of this, patients may have difficulty clearly describing physical and emotional symptoms, which can influence the provider's ability to make an accurate diagnosis.[50]

There is limited research regarding screening for trauma in gastroenterology; however, in a Dutch study, 54% of patients with a history of sexual trauma stated they wish their providers had inquired about history of trauma before colonoscopy.[16] In a small pilot study at a large academic gastroenterology practice, 54% of providers stated they routinely screened for trauma and 77% of gastroenterologists stated they rarely/never screened for trauma before a colonoscopy.[51]

Research from primary care demonstrates that patients were receptive to trauma screening.[52] Provider responses that were calm, accepting, and empathetic were deemed most helpful.[50] Factors that facilitated patient disclosure of trauma include providing assurance of privacy and confidentiality,[53] screening while patient was still fully clothed,[54] and not hurrying the history interview.[50] In a study of female sexual abuse survivors, patients stated that breaches of confidentiality resulted in "intense feelings of betrayal reminiscent of abuse."[53] The most common reason for not disclosing childhood sexual abuse was feeling a health-care provider would not believe them or be sensitive to the impact of abuse on their health care experience.[49] Feelings of shame, guilt, and stigma associated with physical and sexual abuse act as barriers to disclosure. Providing nonjudgmental and calm responses to disclosure is beneficial when taking a trauma history.[50,55,56] Male Childhood Sexual Abuse (CSA) survivors reported difficulty being cared for by male providers and were more likely to disclose to female providers.[56]

Fig. 5 outlines key points for screening for trauma.[8]

Patient-Centered Communication

Due to their trauma history, patients often feel powerless. Using communication that fosters resilience and empowerment with partnership and mutual collaboration can help to improve the patient–provider relationship.[50,57] Female Intimate Partner Violence survivors reported valuing providers openly discussing abuse and medical issues, being emotionally available, easy to contact and willing to take additional time during visits.[58]

Consent

Obtaining consent before beginning examinations or treatments, as well as periods of transition between different steps and procedures is an important aspect of TIC.[59] Female childhood sexual abuse survivors reported the importance of verbal consent helped with comfort and feeling in control.[50,59,60] Examples include asking a patient for permission to lift the patient's gown/clothing to attach electrocardiogram leads, asking permission to perform a physical examination, and asking for specific permission to perform sensitive or invasive examination component independently of permission to perform a general examination.

Creating a Sense of Safety

Sensitive procedures such as colonoscopies may cause flashbacks and distress for individuals with a history of trauma.[50] To prevent retraumatization, the procedure and sedation plan should be explained clearly. Patients may also benefit from bringing an advocate to chaperone their appointment. In the gastroenterology setting, feelings of safety may be impaired due to limited privacy or personal space, being interviewed in a room that feels too isolating or confining, undergoing physical examination by a medical professional of the same sex as the perpetrator of abuse, or being directed not to talk about the distressing experiences as a means of deescalating a traumatic stress reaction.[8] These behaviors should be avoided to prevent the risk of retraumatization.

Trauma Screening Key Points	Example Phrases and Actions
Provide context for why you are asking about trauma	"Many patients with a history of GI symptoms have experienced difficult life events such as abuse or other forms of trauma. Have you ever experienced any such events?"
Inquire about how history of trauma has impacted the patient's medical care.	"How have your prior experiences affected your healthcare and interactions with healthcare providers?"
Approach the patient in a matter of fact, yet supportive manner.	"I understand talking about your past experiences is very personal, and may be difficult or uncomfortable to talk about. However, understanding your past experiences helps me provide you with the best health care."
Be mindful of the patients' personal space	Cultural factors as well as the patient's level of distress may impact preference for personal space. Sitting neither too far, nor too close the patient can assist with comfort. Allow privacy when changing into exam gowns. Ask the patient permission to exam the patient (particularly sensitive areas such as the chest, neck, buttocks, or genital area)
Be mindful of tone and volume of voice.	A soothing and quiet demeanor is often helpful for patients who have experienced trauma.
Be aware of your own emotional reactions to hearing about trauma.	Asking or hearing about trauma can be distressing for a provider. Patients may have inaccurate interpretations to providers reactions. Do not allow discomfort prevent asking the patient about a history of trauma.
Elicit only the information that is necessary to provide medical care and to determine whether additional mental health support may be needed.	Asking about a history of trauma is often appropriate and recommended, particularly prior to performing invasive gastrointestinal testing. However, it is likely not necessary or appropriate for gastroenterology providers or staff to receive the full description of a patient's traumatic experience. This may add unnecessary distress for the patient.
Shift the control to the patient.	" You have right to refuse to answer any questions. You also have the option to be interviewed by a provider of the gender for which you are most comfortable. We can also talk about this at a later date if you choose. Choosing any of these options will not affect your health care. You are in control of how and when this discussion occurs."
Allow the patient time to adjust and cope if they become emotionally distressed by the conversation.	Providers may wish to provide grounding techniques such as breathing or having the patient identify sensory aspects of the room to help them return to the present (e.g. identifying what they can see, hear, or touch).
Avoid phrases that imply judgement.	Avoid phrases such as "it was God's will" or "everything happens for a reason."
Be mindful that trauma may be ongoing.	In the event of abuse, providers should inquire as to whether abuse, such as IPV, child abuse or elder abuse is ongoing. If so, providers should be prepared to report in mandatory reporting situations or have access to referral information for immediate support such as local resources for domestic violence.

Fig. 5. Key points for screening for trauma in the GI setting.

Respecting Patient Perspectives on Addressing Trauma

It is important to remember that patients are at different points in trauma healing. Many patients with a history of trauma may not think trauma is an ongoing factor for them and think they have already dealt with the impact of their personal trauma. Others may avoid approaching trauma, often out of concern that they cannot handle the symptoms that emerge from reexperiencing the traumatic memories. Others may gain a sense of control and empowerment, as well as understanding, by processing the traumatic experience.[8]

Minimizing Distress and Maximizing Autonomy

Having knowledge of the aforementioned trauma-related symptoms can assist providers in supporting their patients during health-care visits.[49,61,62] Patients who experience dissociation may need written information regarding examination results or instructions for follow-up care.[63] Physical therapists working with female sexual abuse survivors have used verbal techniques to help patients maintain focus because engagement is critical for providing care.[64] This directly applies to GI patients with pelvic floor dyssynergia who require biofeedback therapy. Another example of managing dissociation is illustrated by oncology nurses who taught a female CSA survivor to remain present during procedures.[65] Providers are encouraged to be flexible in order to reduce patient distress. Additional provider behaviors can include checking with patients regarding their comfort[59,60] and allowing for breaks or stopping procedures when the patient is overwhelmed.[50,59,62,64] Reeves and colleagues encourages a "constant analysis of the health benefit versus the emotional costs of continuing health care procedures."[66] Providers should evaluate whether it is appropriate to skip certain procedures that may not be necessary or appropriate for the patient at that time point due to trauma-related distress, or the provider should be open to modify their approach to improve patient comfort.[50] For example, determining if a physical examination is truly necessary at that time or whether invasive testing or procedures can be delayed. Providing adequate sedation or pain management during procedures is important because trauma patients can experience increased sensitization to pain.[15,63] Patients may also feel more comfortable if they are allowed to wear more clothes during examinations.[50,54] This may include allowing patients to wear a medical gown and pants for procedures that do not require access to that area, such as esophagogastroduodenoscopy. Patients with a history of IBD reported that feeling respected by nurses, feeling listened to by physicians, receiving adequate pain and anxiety control, and having a quiet room improved their hospitalization experience.[67]

Providing Care in Diverse Settings

Some populations and cultures are more likely to experience trauma, including those that face military action or political violence.[8] Other examples of culture-based traumatic experiences include being the recipient of racism and fear of or separation from a parent due to deportation. Culture influences both whether events are perceived as traumatic and how an individual interprets and assigns meaning to the trauma. Some traumatic experiences may have greater influence on a culture because it represents something significant for that culture or disrupts cultural practices or ways of life.[8] Culture also determines what is considered an acceptable response to trauma, including expression of distress, what is determined to be a legitimate concern and what warrants pursuit of receipt of help.

All providers carry their own personal and cultural perspectives, and it is critical that providers be mindful of their own beliefs, traditions, and biases in order to better understand the patient's needs through the trauma-informed lens.[68] Cultural humility "entails admitting that cultural experience is something one cannot fully analyze or understand but can seek to appreciate and respect."[68,69] Ranjbar and colleagues, has made suggestions on how to incorporate cultural humility into the medical setting. One suggestion includes avoidance of propagating stereotypes based on gender, race, ethnicity, religion, or other aspects of culture. An example of this includes asking, rather than making assumptions about, the patient's preference or comfort with physical distance or eye contact.

Secondary Trauma to Staff

Health providers with a personal history of trauma need to be aware of their own reactions to patient experiences and seek support from colleagues if the strain becomes challenging for their own well-being or ability to provide care.[70] The provision of peer support, supervision, consultation, and access to personal therapy can assist with reducing the negative influence of trauma on staff. This is particularly relevant to gastroenterology staff members who screen patients for trauma or assist in managing patients experiencing retraumatization.

Referral to Trauma-Informed Providers

Multidisciplinary care, including social work and psychotherapists may help with providing more comprehensive care.[66] Gastroenterologists should be aware of the resources available within their institution and in the community to offer patients who express openness or desire for additional services. It is imperative to understand the expertise of different mental health specialties to appropriately triage and navigate patient referrals to the appropriate psychological provider. For example, patients who have active PTS, report ongoing impact of trauma, or have had insufficient opportunity to process their traumatic experience(s) typically should be referred to a trauma-oriented provider. These are mental health providers with specialized training in the treatment of trauma. Patients whose primary concerns are in the treatment of depression, anxiety, panic, and other mental health conditions as well as general life stressors may benefit from working with a general mental health provider. Patients with active GI symptoms may benefit from working with a GI-specific psychologist or mental health provider to address the complexity of gut–brain dysregulation, introduce gut–brain psychotherapies (eg, GI-specific cognitive behavioral therapy, gut-directed hypnosis), and assist patients who are coping with the negative impacts of GI symptoms on QOL. Although most GI psychologists do not specialize in the treatment of trauma, GI-specific psychotherapies have been shown to be effective in improving GI-QOL in patients with a history of trauma.[17]

SUMMARY

Patients with a history of GI complaints report a high prevalence of previous psychological trauma. In addition, due to the sensitive nature of GI procedures, examinations, and treatments, GI patients are at risk of both primary and secondary medical trauma in the GI setting. The sensitive nature of discussing trauma, as well as lack of training and resources, often prevents many providers from asking about patient's prior trauma history. The lack of screening secondary to insufficient training and provider apprehension can unintentionally increase the risk of retraumatization. The development of a trauma informed approach in gastroenterology may assist in improving patient care and safety, reduce risk of retraumatization, and improve efficacy of treatments. Despite significant evidence on the role of trauma and GI, little is known about current practices of gastroenterologists in the United States. Gathering a better understanding of provider practices may assist with training needs to assist with improving TIC.

CLINICAL PEARLS

- Trauma can result from a broad range of traumatic experiences, affect both individuals and groups, and occur as an isolated event or recurrent events.
- Gastroenterology patients are more likely to have a history of trauma compared with healthy controls.
- Gastroenterology patients are at high risk for retraumatization secondary to the sensitive and invasive nature of GI examinations and testing (eg, rectal examinations, endoscopy, anorectal manometry).
- Patient interpretations of traumatic experiences can influence patient–provider interactions. A history of trauma may influence patient's disclosure of trauma to providers, perception of responsibility or self-blame for GI conditions, reaction to provider messaging about GI symptoms, and response or willingness to complete sensitive physical examinations or medical procedures.
- Trauma may present as hesitancy to complete or schedule clinic visits or testing, which often results in mislabeling patients as "noncompliant." Providers should consider trauma as a driver of these behaviors.
- The development of a trauma-informed approach in gastroenterology may assist in improving patient care and safety, reduce risk of retraumatization, and improve the efficacy of treatments.

DISCLOSURE

The authors have nothing to disclose.

REFERENCES

1. Kessler RC, Sonnega A, Bromet E, et al. Posttraumatic stress disorder in the National Comorbidity Survey. Arch Gen Psychiatry 1995;52(12):1048–60.
2. Bradford K, Shih W, Videlock EJ, et al. Association between early adverse life events and irritable bowel syndrome. Clin Gastroenterol Hepatol 2012;10(4): 385–90, e1-3.
3. Drossman DA, Leserman J, Nachman G, et al. Sexual and physical abuse in women with functional or organic gastrointestinal disorders. Ann Intern Med 1990;113(11):828–33.
4. Halland M, Almazar A, Lee R, et al. A case-control study of childhood trauma in the development of irritable bowel syndrome. Neurogastroenterology Motil 2014; 26(7):990–8.
5. Heitkemper MM, Cain KC, Burr RL, et al. Is childhood abuse or neglect associated with symptom reports and physiological measures in women with irritable bowel syndrome? Biol Res Nurs 2011;13(4):399–408.
6. Ju T, Naliboff BD, Shih W, et al. Risk and Protective Factors Related to Early Adverse Life Events in Irritable Bowel Syndrome. J Clin Gastroenterol 2018. https://doi.org/10.1097/mcg.0000000000001153.
7. Taft TH, Bedell A, Craven MR, et al. Initial Assessment of Post-traumatic Stress in a US Cohort of Inflammatory Bowel Disease Patients. Inflamm Bowel Dis 2019; 25(9):1577–85.

8. Center for Substance Abuse Treatment (US). Trauma-Informed Care in Behavioral Health Services. Rockville (MD): Substance Abuse and Mental Health Services Administration (US); 2014. Report No.: (SMA) 14-4816.

9. Suliman S, Mkabile SG, Fincham DS, et al. Cumulative effect of multiple trauma on symptoms of posttraumatic stress disorder, anxiety, and depression in adolescents. Compr Psychiatry 2009;50(2):121–7.

10. Brown VM, LaBar KS, Haswell CC, et al. Altered resting-state functional connectivity of basolateral and centromedial amygdala complexes in posttraumatic stress disorder. Neuropsychopharmacology 2014;39(2):351–9. In press.

11. Keeshin BR, Cronholm PF, Strawn JR. Physiologic changes associated with violence and abuse exposure: an examination of related medical conditions. Trauma Violence Abuse 2012;13(1):41–56. In press.

12. Drossman DA, Li Z, Leserman J, et al. Health status by gastrointestinal diagnosis and abuse history. Gastroenterology 1996;110(4):999–1007.

13. Postma R, Bicanic I, van der Vaart H, et al. Pelvic floor muscle problems mediate sexual problems in young adult rape victims. J Sex Med 2013;10(8):1978–87.

14. Borum ML, Igiehon E, Shafa S. Sexual abuse history in patients. Gastroenterol Nurs 2009;32(3):222–3.

15. Davy E. The endoscopy patient with a history of sexual abuse: strategies for compassionate care. Gastroenterol Nurs 2006;29(3):221–5.

16. Nicolai MP, Keller JJ, de Vries L, et al. The impact of sexual abuse in patients undergoing colonoscopy. PLoS One 2014;9(1):e85034.

17. Jagielski CH, Chey WD, Riehl ME. Influence of trauma on clinical outcomes, quality of life and healthcare resource utilization following psychogastroenterology intervention. J Psychosom Res 2021;146:110481.

18. Felitti VJ, Anda RF, Nordenberg D, et al. Relationship of childhood abuse and household dysfunction to many of the leading causes of death in adults. The Adverse Childhood Experiences (ACE) Study. Am J Prev Med 1998;14(4): 245–58.

19. Merrick MT, Ford DC, Ports KA, et al. Prevalence of Adverse Childhood Experiences From the 2011-2014 Behavioral Risk Factor Surveillance System in 23 States. JAMA Pediatr 2018;172(11):1038–44.

20. Gilbert LK, Breiding MJ, Merrick MT, et al. Childhood adversity and adult chronic disease: an update from ten states and the District of Columbia, 2010. Am J Prev Med 2015;48(3):345–9.

21. Dube SR, Fairweather D, Pearson WS, et al. Cumulative childhood stress and autoimmune diseases in adults. Psychosom Med 2009;71(2):243–50.

22. Anda R, Tietjen G, Schulman E, et al. Adverse childhood experiences and frequent headaches in adults. Headache 2010;50(9):1473–81.

23. Dube SR, Anda RF, Felitti VJ, et al. Adverse childhood experiences and personal alcohol abuse as an adult. Addict Behav 2002;27(5):713–25.

24. Dube SR, Felitti VJ, Dong M, et al. Childhood abuse, neglect, and household dysfunction and the risk of illicit drug use: the adverse childhood experiences study. Pediatrics 2003;111(3):564–72.

25. Anda RF, Whitfield CL, Felitti VJ, et al. Adverse childhood experiences, alcoholic parents, and later risk of alcoholism and depression. Psychiatr Serv 2002;53(8): 1001–9.

26. Chapman DP, Whitfield CL, Felitti VJ, et al. Adverse childhood experiences and the risk of depressive disorders in adulthood. J Affect Disord 2004;82(2):217–25.

27. Dube SR, Anda RF, Felitti VJ, et al. Childhood abuse, household dysfunction, and the risk of attempted suicide throughout the life span: findings from the Adverse Childhood Experiences Study. JAMA 2001;286(24):3089–96.

28. Driessen M, Schulte S, Luedecke C, et al. Trauma and PTSD in patients with alcohol, drug, or dual dependence: a multi-center study. Alcohol Clin Exp Res 2008;32(3):481–8.

29. Najavits LM, Harned MS, Gallop RJ, et al. Six-month treatment outcomes of cocaine-dependent patients with and without PTSD in a multisite national trial. J Stud Alcohol Drugs 2007;68(3):353–61.

30. Briere J. Therapy for adults molested as children: beyond survival. 2nd ed. Springer; 1996.

31. Harvard Medical School. National Comorbidity Survey. https://www.hcp.med.harvard.edu/ncs/index.php. [Accessed 2 May 2022].

32. American Psychiatric Association, Diagnostic and statistical manual of mental disorders, 5th ed. 2013.The, American Psychiatric Association is the publisher.

33. Herman JL. Complex PTSD: A syndrome in survivors of prolonged and repeated trauma. J Trauma Stress 1992;5(3):377–91.

34. Service NH. Complex PTSD - Post-traumatic stress disorder. Available at: https://www.nhs.uk/mental-health/conditions/post-traumatic-stress-disorder-ptsd/complex/.

35. Cloitre M, Garvert DW, Weiss B, et al. Distinguishing PTSD, Complex PTSD, and Borderline Personality Disorder: A latent class analysis. Eur J Psychotraumatol 2014. https://doi.org/10.3402/ejpt.v5.25097.

36. Hall MF, Hall SE. Managing the psychological impact of medical trauma; A guide for mental health and health care professionals. Springer; 2016.

37. Cyr S, Guo X, Marcil MJ, et al. Posttraumatic stress disorder prevalence in medical populations: A systematic review and meta-analysis. Gen Hosp Psychiatry 2021;69:81–93.

38. Taft TH, Quinton S, Jedel S, et al. Posttraumatic Stress in Patients With Inflammatory Bowel Disease: Prevalence and Relationships to Patient-Reported Outcomes. Inflamm Bowel Dis 2022;28(5):710–9.

39. Pothemont K, Quinton S, Jayoushe M, et al. Patient Perspectives on Medical Trauma Related to Inflammatory Bowel Disease. J Clin Psychol Med Settings 2021. https://doi.org/10.1007/s10880-021-09805-0.

40. Cannon EA, Bonomi AE, Anderson ML, et al. Adult health and relationship outcomes among women with abuse experiences during childhood. Violence Vict 2010;25(3):291–305.

41. Kartha A, Brower V, Saitz R, et al. The impact of trauma exposure and post-traumatic stress disorder on healthcare utilization among primary care patients. Med Care 2008;46(4):388–93.

42. Brignone E, Gundlapalli AV, Blais RK, et al. Increased Health Care Utilization and Costs Among Veterans With a Positive Screen for Military Sexual Trauma. Med Care 2017;55(Suppl 9 Suppl 2):S70–7.

43. Alcala HE, Valdez-Dadia A, von Ehrenstein OS. Adverse childhood experiences and access and utilization of health care. J Public Health (Oxf) 2018;40(4):684–92.

44. Koball AM, Rasmussen C, Olson-Dorff D, et al. The relationship between adverse childhood experiences, healthcare utilization, cost of care and medical comorbidities. Child Abuse Negl 2019;90:120–6.

45. Chartier MJ, Walker JR, Naimark B. Separate and cumulative effects of adverse childhood experiences in predicting adult health and health care utilization. Child Abuse Negl 2010;34(6):454–64.
46. Elliott DE, Bjelajac P, Fallot RD, et al. Trauma-informed or trauma-denied: Principles and implementation of trauma-informed services for women. J Community Psychol 2005;33:461–77.
47. Harris M, Fallot RD. Envisioning a trauma-informed service system: a vital paradigm shift. New Dir Ment Health Serv Spring 2001;89:3–22.
48. Hopper EK, Bassuk EL, Olivet J. Shelter from the storm: trauma-informed care in homelessness services settings. Open Health Serv Policy J 2010;3:80–100.
49. McGregor K, Glover M, Gautam J, et al. Working sensitively with child sexual abuse survivors: what female child sexual abuse survivors want from health professionals. Women Health 2010;50(8):737–55.
50. Roberts SJ. The sequelae of childhood sexual abuse: a primary care focus for adult female survivors. Nurse Pract 1996;21(12 Pt 1):42, 45, 49-52.
51. Jagielski CH, Riehl ME, Chey WC. How often do gastroenterologists's screen for psychological trauma? Identifying an unmet need. Dig Dis Week 2019. Presentation at Digestive Diseases Week, San Diego, CA.
52. Kalmakis KA, Shafer MB, Chandler GE, et al. Screening for childhood adversity among adult primary care patients. J Am Assoc Nurse Pract 2018;30(4):193–200.
53. van Loon AM, Koch T, Kralik D. Care for female survivors of child sexual abuse in emergency departments. Accid Emerg Nurs 2004;12(4):208–14.
54. Robohm JS, Buttenheim M. The gynecological care experience of adult survivors of childhood sexual abuse: a preliminary investigation. Women Health 1996; 24(3):59–75.
55. Stalker CA, Russell BD, Teram E, et al. Providing dental care to survivors of childhood sexual abuse: treatment considerations for the practitioner. J Am Dent Assoc 2005;136(9):1277–81.
56. Teram E, Stalker C, Hovey A, et al. Towards malecentric communication: sensitizing health professionals to the realities of male childhood sexual abuse survivors. Issues Ment Health Nurs 2006;27(5):499–517.
57. Raja S, Hasnain M, Hoersch M, et al. Trauma informed care in medicine: current knowledge and future research directions. Fam Community Health 2015;38(3): 216–26.
58. Battaglia TA, Finley E, Liebschutz JM. Survivors of intimate partner violence speak out: trust in the patient-provider relationship. J Gen Intern Med 2003; 18(8):617–23.
59. Coles J, Jones K. Universal Precautions": perinatal touch and examination after childhood sexual abuse. Birth 2009;36(3):230–6.
60. Muzik M, Ads M, Bonham C, et al. Perspectives on trauma-informed care from mothers with a history of childhood maltreatment: a qualitative study. Child Abuse Neglect 2013;37(12):1215–24.
61. Cadman L, Waller J, Ashdown-Barr L, et al. Barriers to cervical screening in women who have experienced sexual abuse: an exploratory study. J Fam Plann Reprod Health Care 2012;38(4):214–20.
62. Seng JS, Hassinger JA. Relationship strategies and interdisciplinary collaboration. Improving maternity care with survivors of childhood sexual abuse. J Nurse Midwifery 1998;43(4):287–95.
63. Draucker CB, Spradlin D. Women sexually abused as children: implications for orthopaedic nursing care. Orthop Nurs 2001;20(6):41–8.

64. Dunleavy K, Kubo Slowik A. Emergence of delayed posttraumatic stress disorder symptoms related to sexual trauma: patient-centered and trauma-cognizant management by physical therapists. Phys Ther 2012;92(2):339–51.
65. Wygant C, Hui D, Bruera E. Childhood sexual abuse in advanced cancer patients in the palliative care setting. J Pain Symptom Manage 2011;42(2):290–5.
66. Reeves E. A synthesis of the literature on trauma-informed care. Issues Ment Health Nurs 2015;36(9):698–709.
67. Taft TH. Prevalence, impact and risk factors for PTSD in IBD. 2022.
68. Ranjbar N, Erb M, Mohammad O, et al. Trauma-Informed Care and Cultural Humility in the Mental Health Care of People From Minoritized Communities. Focus (Am Psychiatr Publ) 2020;18(1):8–15.
69. Tervalon M, Murray-Garcia J. Cultural humility versus cultural competence: a critical distinction in defining physician training outcomes in multicultural education. J Health Care Poor Underserved 1998;9(2):117–25.
70. Roberts SJ, Chandler GE, Kalmakis K. A model for trauma-informed primary care. J Am Assoc Nurse Pract 2019;31(2):139–44.

Sociocultural Considerations for Food-Related Quality of Life in Inflammatory Bowel Disease

Tina Aswani-Omprakash, BS, BA^{a,b},
Neha D. Shah, MPH, RD, CNSC, CHES[b,c,d],*

KEYWORDS

- Inflammatory bowel disease • IBD • Sociocultural • Food culture
- Diet-related disparities • Food avoidance • Restrictive eating
- Food-related quality of life

KEY POINTS

- Food-related quality of life (FRQoL) involves the influence of diet, eating patterns, and food-related anxiety on quality of life.
- Food avoidance and restrictive eating has been identified as a contributor to reduced FRQoL in inflammatory bowel disease (IBD).
- Sociocultural influences on FRQoL in IBD may include food culture, diet acculturation, diet-related disparities, food insecurity, and diet quality.

INTRODUCTION

The prevalence of gastrointestinal (GI) disorders has been increasing globally and within minority groups migrating to Western countries from countries that have lower prevalence.[1] The varying environmental, cultural, and religious factors between minority groups may influence the physical and psychosocial lived experience, thus quality of life (QoL) and health-related quality of life (HRQoL), of minority groups living with GI disorders. The severity of symptoms has been shown to be associated with reduced HRQoL in GI disorders.[2–4] Symptoms may include nausea, vomiting, altered bowel habits, gas, bloating, and/or cramping.

When aspects of QoL and mental health are combined with diet, food-related quality of life (FRQoL) emerges as a factoring concept in the nutrition and psychosocial

^a Mount Sinai Icahn School of Medicine, New York, NY 10029, USA; ^b South Asian IBD Alliance, New York, NY 10021, USA; ^c Colitis and Crohn's Disease Center, University of California, San Francisco, CA 94115, USA; ^d Neha Shah Nutrition, San Francisco, CA 94105, USA
* Corresponding author. Colitis and Crohn's Disease Center, University of California, 1701 Divisadero Street Suite 120, San Francisco, CA 94115.
E-mail address: neha.shah@ucsf.edu
Twitter: @ownyourcrohns (T.A.-O.); @nehagastrord (N.D.S.)

Gastroenterol Clin N Am 51 (2022) 885–895
https://doi.org/10.1016/j.gtc.2022.07.013
0889-8553/22/© 2022 Elsevier Inc. All rights reserved.

evaluations of the patient suffering from GI disorders. FRQoL is the evaluation of how diet, eating patterns, and food-related anxiety influence the QoL of the patient.[5] Patients may implement restrictive food patterns as an effort to alleviate symptoms. Food avoidance and restriction may consequently result in nutritional consequences of unintentional weight loss, nutrient deficiencies, and sarcopenia. Disordered eating may also arise when food avoidance and restriction is prolonged voluntarily by the patient.

In the context of inflammatory bowel disease (IBD), which encompasses Crohn disease (CD) and ulcerative colitis (UC) as a part of immune-mediated continuum of inflammatory diseases, the QoL and HRQoL are found to be significantly reduced in IBD in both children and adults.[6] IBD can include a gamut of GI symptoms such as abdominal pain, rectal bleeding, weight loss, anemia, altered bowel habits, gas, bloating, and cramping. It can result in significant illness via complications of strictures, fistulas, sepsis, and bowel cancers. The QoL is found to be less in those with active disease compared with those in remission and in those with CD compared with those with UC.[7] A lack of social support and lower economic status has been found with greater psychological distress in IBD as well.[8]

Poor FRQoL has been found to be associated with restrictive eating in IBD.[9] A prevalence of food avoidance (28%–89%) and restrictive eating (41%–93%) was identified in patients with IBD.[10] Risk factors associated with loss of FRQoL were associated more so with women, a diagnosis of CD, a presence of active disease, symptom severity, significant misinformation around diet, and worries of having GI symptoms with diet.[11]

The prevalence of pediatric and adult IBD in the United States is estimated to be 77.0 and 478.4 per 100,000 individuals in 2016, respectively.[10] More recent data estimate the prevalence in the United States of IBD to be approximately 3.1 million (1.3% of its population) with a substantially increased prevalence of IBD in non-White races and ethnicities.[12,13] Given that population demographics are changing rapidly, and the United States will soon become a nation of minorities as the majority,[13] sociocultural influences of diet acculturation, food insecurity, and diet-related disparities also become factoring concepts with regard to QoL, HRQoL and thus, potentially FRQoL.[13]

The influence of these elements in IBD on FRQoL beyond food avoidance and restrictive eating is not well-known. The purpose of this review is to primarily discuss current evidence for FRQoL as well as its sociocultural influences in patients with IBD. The perspective of the lived patient experience will be included along with a discussion of future directions for the provision of research and cultural competency.

SOCIOCULTURAL CONCEPTS FOR FOOD CULTURE

An introductory discussion of sociocultural concepts because it relates to food culture is imperative to the subsequent discussions of FRQoL (**Fig. 1**).

The term sociocultural has evolved from the concepts behind sociocultural theory. As part of this theory, culture gives humans the tools to adapt intellectually into the culture in which they live.[14] Food is a constituent of that; humans adapt to the food they grew up with as a part of their culture.

Diet Acculturation

Acculturation of diet may occur with migration and refers to the "*process that occurs when members of a minority group adopt the eating patterns/food choices of the host country.*"[15] Along with adoption of a new way of eating, immigrants may continue some traditional practices of their own food culture as well.

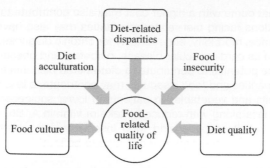

Fig. 1. Sociocultural influences to consider for food-related quality of life.

Food is also often a means of expressing and retaining one's identity.[16] That is, people are able to connect to one another in their own culture via food, which creates a sociocultural dynamic around food becoming a vehicle of socialization and human connection. Food culture thereby comprises the sociocultural aspect of eating and includes the *"beliefs, values, and attitudes"* a community may accept around food, acknowledging that practices may vary within communities and religions in the same country. Acceptance of food choices within a culture are determined by biologic cues of taste and smell, repetitive exposure of foods, level of social support, and availability of resources.[17] Food culture may also dictate how food practices are passed through generations from parents to their children. Gender and social roles are defined within a food culture. Expansion of the concept of food culture may also encompass the infrastructure of the food system within a community, which may involve food acquirement, distribution, finances, and eating environment.

Food Insecurity

Food insecurity refers to *"the household-level condition of limited or uncertain access to adequate and nutritious food,"* and 11.1% of American households have experienced food insecurity in 2018.[18] The populations that may experience food insecurity are the young, racial/ethnic minorities and those who have less household income. The treatment and management of a GI diagnosis using diet can be challenging in the presence of food insecurity.

Affordability determines the level of access to foods of nutritional value that are recommended for a diagnosis. Food insecurity is associated with an increase in visits to the emergency room, hospital admissions, and costs; moreover, food insecurity is largely correlated with poor HRQoL. There is also an association found between food insecurity and risk for depression and anxiety.[19,20] Screening for depression and anxiety is indicated with identification of food insecurity.

Diet-Related Disparities

Disparities related to diet can be referred to as *"differences in dietary intake, dietary behaviors, and dietary patterns in different segments of the population, resulting in poorer dietary quality and inferior health outcomes for certain groups and an unequal burden in terms of disease incidence, morbidity, mortality, survival, and quality of life."*[21] The demographics, socioeconomic status, psychosocial, environmental, and cultural characteristics of specific populations influence dietary intake and its related behaviors, which may also contribute to diet-related disparities. Income is a primary socioeconomic contributor to diet-related disparities.[21] The inadequate access to nutritious foods that come with a higher cost may also contribute to diet-related disparities.[22] Populations facing diet-related disparities may also have higher rates of prevalence, incidence, morbidity, and mortality for chronic diagnoses related to alterations in diet, such as cardiovascular disease, diabetes, and obesity. Diet acculturation is also with the potential to contribute to diet-related disparities.[21]

Diet-related disparities and food insecurity may contribute to less diet quality.[23] Dietary intake of fruits and vegetables in patients of lower socioeconomic status has been found to be less along with reduced intake of vitamin A, B6, calcium, magnesium, and zinc in adults experiencing food insecurity.[24] In children experiencing food insecurity, only fruit consumption was found to be less.

INFLAMMATORY BOWEL DISEASE AND FOOD-RELATED QUALITY OF LIFE

The following discussions will review FRQoL and its sociocultural influences in the realm of IBD.

Sociocultural and Food-related Quality of Life

Diet has been identified as an environmental risk factor. Risk for IBD may arise as immigrants that have migrated to a new country undergo a change in lifestyle and environment in their new country. Adoption of the Western diet that is higher in animal protein, saturated fats, processed foods, and lower in fruits, especially in fruits and vegetables, has been implicated in the development of IBD.[25] There are limited studies on how the change in food culture in setting of diet acculturation may influence FRQoL in IBD. A cross-sectional study of 58 adult Hispanic immigrants (29 with IBD after immigration and 29 controls) in the United States found the rates for diet acculturation were similar between those with IBD and in the controls.[26] The patients with IBD here were found to have a greater intake of non-whole grains and less intake from fruits and vegetables in comparison to the controls.

Food insecurity and lack of social support were found in adults with IBD in one study. There is an estimate of 3.1 million adults with IBD living in the United States, in which 12% of the patients reported to experience food insecurity and minimal social support.[27] The results further showed that 19% of patients were concerned that food would run out before being able to buy more and 16% of patients reported that food did run out before obtaining money to buy more. Overall, 1 in 8 patients with IBD has food insecurity and minimal social support. IBD patients found to have food insecurity were significantly more likely to have financial adversity with medical bills. There is, however, no increased use of the emergency room.

Nutrient inadequacies have been associated with loss of FRQoL. A multi-center study of 1576 pediatric and adult patients (aged older than 16 years) evaluated the association between nutrient intake and FRQoL.[28] Questionnaires were distributed to patients to evaluate FRQoL, QoL, distress, fatigue, anxiety, and depression. The European Prospective Investigation into Cancer Food Frequency Questionnaire was used to collect intake data from diet. The results showed that FRQoL was correlated with recurrent active disease and reduced intake of dietary fiber, calcium, phosphorus, and magnesium. Additional studies are warranted to gain understanding of how nutrient adequacies can also arise in the setting of food insecurity and diet-related disparities.

Symptoms and Food-related Quality of Life

Several studies have evaluated FRQoL in adult and pediatric patients with IBD with the FRQoL-29 questionnaire that has been validated for its use in adults with IBD.[29] In a study of 175 adult patients (80 with irritable bowel syndrome [IBS] and 95 with IBD) showed that symptom severity was the highest predictor for FRQoL in both patient populations.[5] A study of 108 adult patients with IBD completed multiple questionnaires with the FRQoL-29, Harvey Bradshaw Index, Simple Clinical Colitis Activity Index, Nine-Item Avoidant/Restrictive Food Intake Disorder Screen, and the Depression Anxiety Stress Scale-21.[9] The results showed that patients with IBD exhibiting restrictive eating and have active disease were found to have reduced FRQoL. Regardless of the severity of active disease, patients with UC had less FRQoL than patients with CD. The patients with less disease activity and history of prior surgery for IBD were found to have a higher FRQoL. A prospective and cross-sectional single-center study had 60 children and adolescents with CD complete the FRQoL-29 questionnaire to evaluate FRQoL.[30] The results showed that FRQoL was reduced in the patients with CD along with their siblings when compared with controls. Factors of age and nutrition risk were found to be correlated with less FRQoL.

The trial and error process of which foods may serve as triggers to symptoms was also found to reduce FRQoL.[31] Having minimal guidance and less knowledge of how to identify foods may trigger or not trigger symptoms served as a contributing factor to experiencing stress with foods, including lack of pleasure with meals and having fear with eating in social settings. The labor involved with grocery shopping and meal preparation to help plan for meals tailored to IBD also was associated with less FRQoL. Level of support from family for meals was found to vary, which led to eating in isolation for some. To learn of the level of support in diet, it would be beneficial to also learn of family dynamics within a food culture, especially of gender and social roles with diet.

Malnutrition and Food-related Quality of Life

Malnutrition in IBD is found in 65% to 75% in CD and 18% to 62% in UC and is correlated with an increase in rates of hospital admissions as well as duration of the hospital stay.[32] Malnutrition involves a constellation of symptoms of decreased nutritional intake, unintentional weight loss, loss of muscle and fat stores, and changes in functional capacity. Within inflammatory contributors, malnutrition can arise based on the segment(s) of the bowel that is (are) involved in active disease. Within social/environmental contributors, practices of restrictive eating as an effort to reduce symptoms or control inflammation can cause malnutrition.[33] Food insecurity can also contribute to malnutrition.[34,35] The early screening of malnutrition will allow timely implementation of interventions for its treatment and management. There are various tools in existence to aid in the identification of malnutrition, such as the Malnutrition Universal Screening Tool and the Subjective Global Assessment.

In IBD, malnutrition has been shown to correlate with a decrease in QoL. In a cross-sectional study of 68 adult patients with CD and 35 adult patients with UC showed that mild-to-moderate malnutrition was present in 17 patients.[36] The Subjective Global Assessment screening tool was used to identify malnutrition, and the RAND 36-item Health Survey was used to assess QoL. In another study, 78 inpatients with IBD were recruited to complete questionnaires with the IBD Questionnaire, Perceived Social Support Scale, Hospital Anxiety and Depression Scale, Perceived Stress Scale, Crohn's Disease Activity Index, and the Nutritional Risk Screening 2002.[37] Out of the 78 patients, 76 patients had anxiety, 71 patients had depression, and 46 patients were identified to be at risk for malnutrition. The presence of active disease was associated with the risk of malnutrition as well as anxiety, depression, and reduced QoL. Food avoidance also contributed to malnutrition and food-related anxiety.

FOOD-RELATED QUALITY OF LIFE AND OTHER GASTROINTESTINAL DISORDERS

In brief, the following discussions will highlight FRQoL and its sociocultural influences in the realm of other GI disorders.

Celiac Disease

Celiac disease (CeD) is an immune dysregulation that results in damage to the lining of the small bowel because of gluten consumption.[38] Gluten is a storage grain protein found in wheat, barley, rye, and malt. In review of the results from the 2009 to 2012 National Health and Nutrition Examination Survey, non-Hispanic whites were more likely to have CeD compared with other races.[39] The gluten-free (GF) diet is the lifetime treatment of CeD.

There are varying impacts of the GF diet on HRQoL in adolescents and adults. In adolescents, the taste of GF products may not be as appealing and may result in not making substitutions for gluten, leading to restrictive eating.[40] Navigating the GF diet while dining out and traveling with friends is shown to be a burden. In adults, adherence to the GF diet along with symptom control has been shown to improve QoL[41]; however, high attentiveness to the diet with very strict adherence has also been shown to increase anxiety and reduce QoL.[42] Food insecurity with GF products is known because cost and access to GF products may vary within regions. In a study that compared cost and availability of GF products to gluten-containing products in the United States, it was shown that the cost of GF products was 183% more than the gluten-containing products.[43] Patients experiencing food insecurity had lower adherence to the GF diet and, overall, were shown to have reduced HRQoL. Other sociocultural influences on FRQoL are not known in CeD.

Gastroparesis

Gastroparesis is delayed gastric emptying of contents from the stomach into the small intestine without a mechanical obstruction present.[44] In review of data from the National Institutes of Health Gastroparesis Consortium, the prevalence of diabetic gastroparesis is greater in non-Hispanic blacks and Hispanics than non-Hispanic whites. With regard to symptoms, non-Hispanic blacks had more vomiting than Hispanic patients. Further studies are needed because there are less data on FRQoL as well as its sociocultural influences. These data include patients living with gastroparesis who report social isolation in conjunction with intolerance and changes with diet.[45] A study on evaluating stigma experiences in patients with gastroparesis showed that questions asked of why only small portions are eaten and comments for diet-related unsolicited advice contributed to psychological distress.[46]

Irritable Bowel Syndrome

IBS is a disorder of gut–brain interaction, which is associated with recurrent abdominal pain and alterations between diarrhea and constipation as well as mixed components of both as determined by the Rome IV criteria.[47] The prevalence of IBS based on Rome IV criteria was found to be similar among the United States, Canada, and the United Kingdom at 4.4% to 4.8%.[48] Food avoidance and restriction is known to reduce FRQoL in IBS,[49] as well as there is a reduced QoL and higher symptom severity with more self-reported food intolerances.[50] With a highlight, the 3-phase low-FODMAP diet has been shown to promote symptom reduction in IBS and, in turn, increase QoL.[51,52] Sociocultural influences on FRQoL are not known in IBS.

PERSPECTIVE OF THE LIVED EXPERIENCE

As a patient who has had multiple colorectal surgeries to treat her CD, patient advocate and coauthor of this article, Tina Aswani-Omprakash, shares her lived experience with sociocultural aspects that contributed to the loss of her FRQoL. From being in recurrent active disease to frequent changes in medications to undergoing a colectomy, j-pouch, fistula repair, and stoma creation, Aswani-Omprakash has faced the highs and lows of the psychosocial impact and food-related anxiety in living with virulent IBD. This in addition to subsequent diagnoses of IBS, gastroparesis, and small intestinal bacterial overgrowth (SIBO), Aswani-Omprakash has faced significant challenges in managing her diet in the setting of having multiple diagnoses. This has led to many mental health challenges around food, which is something she has had to navigate to regain FRQoL.

As a practicing lacto-vegetarian, Aswani-Omprakash was often told to "at least eat eggs or fish for protein" without further consideration for her diet or for her religious beliefs within Hinduism. After undergoing the initial surgery, she was told to consume foods such as bread, applesauce, bananas, and rice, none of which really encompassed the cultural foods she was used to eating such as roti (Indian bread), vegetable curries, and dal (lentil). There was also minimal guidance on how to reintroduce fiber after having her colon removed, which left her navigating her food-related anxiety along with her food choices on her own.

Throughout the years, she thought she was not a part of her culture because of not being able to eat many of the spicy, fried, or sweet dishes that are enjoyed during many celebrations. During religious rituals, she was not able to eat prasad (food offering) to pay reverence. At weddings, she was not able to enjoy the mélange of foods and was often asked multiple questions around why she is not eating or enjoying herself at the weddings. Not being able to partake in religious or cultural events with friends and family has left her feeling like she stands out like a sore thumb and that she has offended those around her by not accepting their offerings for food. These experiences have taken away from her the ability to feel like she too can have the same richness of cultural experience as her friends and family.

In addition to the above challenges, she again developed obstructive and constipation-related symptoms in the setting of SIBO after having had so many surgeries. She desperately self-restricted carbohydrates that were deemed fermentable in hopes to reduce the symptoms. Her diet, already limited to begin with as a vegetarian, now has further limitations. She eventually underwent another surgery malnourished to remove multiple sites of bowel obstruction and scar tissue. There were significant concerns on what her recovery would entail after surgery.

Now a few months out of surgery, Aswani-Omprakash describes feeling scared about reintroducing carbohydrates. She is not only afraid of eating sandwiches that contain bread, she is also afraid of eating pastas and even legumes that may potentially ferment in her small bowel. Reintroducing these foods has been a challenge and every time she experienced symptoms, she is set back for several weeks emotionally and physically. She describes it as a crippling cycle to reintroduce foods, have symptoms, and then develop fears around those foods again, which was enough to self-restrict again.

Moreover, Aswani-Omprakash faced significant socioeconomic barriers to care that led to financial hardship. A day before her initial surgery, she received a telephone call from her Human Resources department informing her that she has been terminated from her job which led her to urgently apply for Consolidated Omnibus Budget Reconciliation Act (COBRA) health insurance and overall, care for herself financially during and after surgery. As a 24-year-old woman, she had to pay several hundred dollars a month for health insurance along with copays, coinsurance, and deductibles. In addition, she was responsible to cover fees toward intravenous parenteral nutrition because she was not able to eat in sufficient amounts through diet just yet. Once she tapered off parenteral nutrition, she also paid for enteral nutrition formulas around the clock as she began to slowly reintroduce foods back into the diet. This was in addition to the household payments she helped her mother with and to cover the cost of the car trips, tolls, and parking garages she had to pay at clinic visits for specialized care twice a week on average. Aswani-Omprakash describes this experience as back-breaking, from trying to get through surgery physically and emotionally. She thought she could not afford to eat healthy in the setting of trying to meet the financial demands of her care.

Nevertheless, Aswani-Omprakash endured through the many challenges and has come out on the other side managing all of her chronic digestive ailments with the help of her multidisciplinary specialists and regaining FRQoL and, therefore, overall QoL with the guidance of her GI dietitian and her psychologist.

FUTURE DIRECTIONS

Overall, there are limited studies here on how sociocultural influences affect FRQoL. In addition to diet acculturation, another consideration to factor in for FRQoL is that changes in food culture may arise with the use of therapeutic diets, which may affect the adherence to diets. As food insecurity is a social/environmental contributor to malnutrition, learning of its extent is needed to identify resources to improve access and adherence to diet to reduce malnutrition. Sociocultural considerations overall warrant additional studies and resources to evaluate influences on FRQoL, which include changes in food culture, process of diet acculturation, existence of food insecurity, presence of diet-related disparities, and level of diet quality.

It is imperative to learn of sociocultural influences as part of a clinical, nutrition, and psychosocial evaluation of a patient to aid in developing culturally competent interventions to optimize FRQoL, especially of various races and ethnicities. Perhaps, the most salient improvement of FRQoL involves a multidisciplinary team of physicians, nurses, dietitians, psychologists, and social workers to implement clinical guidelines and interventions in a way to best help the patient. A partnership between the patient and the various providers of the team must be in place to help bring discussions forward on how to balance disease management along with sociocultural influences on diet and FRQoL.

CLINICS CARE POINTS

- Patients with IBD have reported food insecurity and minimal social support.
- Diet inadequacies have been correlated with reduced FRQoL.
- Further studies are indicated to identify the presence of sociocultural influences on FRQoL in IBD to also help determine culturally competent interventions, especially in racial and ethnic groups.

DISCLOSURE

T. Aswani-Omprakash: Consultant for AbbVie, Arena Pharmaceuticals, Boehringer Ingelheim, Genentech-Roche, Hollister, Inc., Janssen, Takeda. N.D. Shah: Consultant for GI on Demand (American College of Gastroenterology and Gastro Girl).

REFERENCES

1. Ahmed S, Newton PD, Ojo O, et al. Experiences of Ethnic Minority Patients Who Are Living with a Primary Bowel Condition or Bowel-Related Symptoms of Other Chronic Diseases: A Systematic Review. BMC Gastroenterol 2021;1(1):322. Published online.
2. Varni JW, Shulman RJ, Self MM, et al. Gastrointestinal symptoms predictors of health-related quality of life in patients with inflammatory bowel disease. J Pediatr Gastroenterol Nutr 2016;63(6):e186–92.
3. Parkman HP, Wilson LA, Yates KP, et al. Factors that contribute to the impairment of quality of life in gastroparesis. Neurogastroenterol Motil 2021;33(8):e14087.
4. Varni JW, Shulman RJ, Self MM, et al. Gastrointestinal symptoms predictors of health-related quality of life in pediatric patients with functional gastrointestinal disorders. Qual Life Res 2017;26(4):1015–25.
5. Guadagnoli L, Mutlu EA, Doerfler B, et al. Food-related quality of life in patients with inflammatory bowel disease and irritable bowel syndrome. Qual Life Res 2019;28(8):2195–205.
6. Knowles SR, Graff LA, Wilding H, et al. Quality of life in inflammatory bowel disease: a systematic review and meta-analyses—part I. Inflamm Bowel Dis 2018; 24(4):742–51.
7. Knowles SR, Keefer L, Wilding H, et al. Quality of life in inflammatory bowel disease: a systematic review and meta-analyses—part II. Inflamm Bowel Dis 2018; 24(5):966–76.
8. Slonim-Nevo V, Sarid O, Friger M, et al. Effect of social support on psychological distress and disease activity in inflammatory bowel disease patients. Inflamm Bowel Dis 2018;24(7):1389–400.
9. Day AS, Yao CK, Costello SP, et al. Food-related quality of life in adults with inflammatory bowel disease is associated with restrictive eating behaviour, disease activity and surgery: a prospective multi-centre observational study. J Hum Nutr Diet 2021;35(1):234–44. Published online.
10. Ye Y, Manne S, Treem WR, et al. Prevalence of inflammatory bowel disease in pediatric and adult populations: recent estimates from large national databases in the United States, 2007–2016. Inflamm Bowel Dis 2020;26(4):619–25.
11. Day AS, Yao CK, Costello SP, et al. Food avoidance, restrictive eating behaviour and association with quality of life in adults with inflammatory bowel disease: A systematic scoping review. Appetite 2021;167:105650.
12. Xu F, Dahlhamer JM, Zammitti EP, et al. Health-risk behaviors and chronic conditions among adults with inflammatory bowel disease—United States, 2015 and 2016. Morbidity Mortality Weekly Rep 2018;67(6):190.
13. Barnes EL, Loftus EV Jr, Kappelman MD. Effects of race and ethnicity on diagnosis and management of inflammatory bowel diseases. Gastroenterology 2021;160(3):677–89.
14. Daneshfar S, Moharami M. Dynamic assessment in Vygotsky's sociocultural theory: Origins and main concepts. J Lang Teach Res 2018;9(3):600–7.
15. Satia-Abouta J, Patterson RE, Neuhouser ML, et al. Dietary acculturation: applications to nutrition research and dietetics. J Am Diet Assoc 2002;102(8):1105–18.
16. Almerico GM. Food and identity: Food studies, cultural, and personal identity. J Int Business Cult Stud 2014;8:1.
17. Monterrosa EC, Frongillo EA, Drewnowski A, et al. Sociocultural influences on food choices and implications for sustainable healthy diets. Food Nutr Bull 2020;41(2_suppl):59S–73S.

18. Hanmer J, DeWalt DA, Berkowitz SA. Association between food insecurity and health-related quality of life: a nationally representative survey. J Gen Intern Med 2021;36(6):1638–47.
19. Hadley C, Patil CL. Seasonal changes in household food insecurity and symptoms of anxiety and depression. Am J Phys Anthropol 2008;135(2):225–32.
20. Arenas DJ, Thomas A, Wang J, et al. A systematic review and meta-analysis of depression, anxiety, and sleep disorders in US adults with food insecurity. J Gen Intern Med 2019;34(12):2874–82.
21. Satia JA. Diet-related disparities: understanding the problem and accelerating solutions. J Am Diet Assoc 2009;109(4):610.
22. Darmon N, Drewnowski A. Contribution of food prices and diet cost to socioeconomic disparities in diet quality and health: a systematic review and analysis. Nutr Rev 2015;73(10):643–60.
23. Leung CW, Tester JM. The association between food insecurity and diet quality varies by race/ethnicity: an analysis of national health and nutrition examination survey 2011-2014 results. J Acad Nutr Diet 2019;119(10):1676–86.
24. Hanson KL, Connor LM. Food insecurity and dietary quality in US adults and children: a systematic review. Am J Clin Nutr 2014;100(2):684–92.
25. Hou JK, Abraham B, El-Serag H. Dietary intake and risk of developing inflammatory bowel disease: a systematic review of the literature. Official J Am Coll Gastroenterol ACG. 2011;106(4):563–73.
26. Damas OM, Estes D, Avalos D, et al. Hispanics coming to the US adopt US cultural behaviors and eat less healthy: implications for development of inflammatory bowel disease. Dig Dis Sci 2018;63(11):3058–66.
27. Nguyen NH, Khera R, Ohno-Machado L, et al. Prevalence and Effects of Food Insecurity and Social Support on Financial Toxicity in and Healthcare Use by Patients With Inflammatory Bowel Diseases. Clin Gastroenterol Hepatol 2021;19(7):1377–86.
28. Whelan K, Murrells T, Morgan M, et al. Food-related quality of life is impaired in inflammatory bowel disease and associated with reduced intake of key nutrients. Am J Clin Nutr 2021;113(4):832–44.
29. Hughes LD, King L, Morgan M, et al. Food-related quality of life in inflammatory bowel disease: development and validation of a questionnaire. J Crohn's Colitis 2016;10(2):194–201.
30. Brown SC, Whelan K, Frampton C, et al. Food-Related Quality of Life in Children and Adolescents With Crohn's Disease. Inflamm Bowel Dis 2022;izac010. Published online.
31. Czuber-Dochan W, Morgan M, Hughes LD, et al. Perceptions and psychosocial impact of food, nutrition, eating and drinking in people with inflammatory bowel disease: A qualitative investigation of food-related quality of life. J Hum Nutr Diet 2020;33(1):115–27.
32. Nguyen GC, Munsell M, Harris ML. Nationwide prevalence and prognostic significance of clinically diagnosable protein-calorie malnutrition in hospitalized inflammatory bowel disease patients. Inflamm Bowel Dis 2008;14(8):1105–11.
33. Casanova MJ, Chaparro M, Molina B, et al. Prevalence of malnutrition and nutritional characteristics of patients with inflammatory bowel disease. J Crohn's Colitis 2017;11(12):1430–9.
34. Steiner G, Geissler B, Schernhammer ES. Hunger and obesity as symptoms of non-sustainable food systems and malnutrition. Appl Sci 2019;9(6):1062.
35. Borras AM, Mohamed FA. Health inequities and the shifting paradigms of food security, food insecurity, and food sovereignty. Int J Health Serv 2020;50(3):299–313.

36. Pulley J, Todd A, Flatley C, et al. Malnutrition and quality of life among adult in-flammatory bowel disease patients. JGH Open 2020;4(3):454–60.
37. Cao Q, Huang YH, Jiang M, et al. The prevalence and risk factors of psycholog-ical disorders, malnutrition and quality of life in IBD patients. Scand J Gastroen-terol 2019;54(12):1458–66.
38. Rubio-Tapia A, Hill ID, Kelly CP, et al. American College of Gastroenterology clin-ical guideline: diagnosis and management of celiac disease. Am J Gastroenterol 2013;108(5):656.
39. Mardini HE, Westgate P, Grigorian AY. Racial differences in the prevalence of ce-liac disease in the US population: National Health and Nutrition Examination Sur-vey (NHANES) 2009–2012. Dig Dis Sci 2015;60(6):1738–42.
40. Cadenhead JW, Wolf RL, Lebwohl B, et al. Diminished quality of life among ado-lescents with coeliac disease using maladaptive eating behaviours to manage a gluten-free diet: a cross-sectional, mixed-methods study. J Hum Nutr Diet 2019; 32(3):311–20.
41. Casellas F, Rodrigo L, Lucendo AJ, et al. Benefit on health-related quality of life of adherence to gluten-free diet in adult patients with celiac disease. Revista Espa-ñola de Enfermedades Digestivas. 2015;107(4):196–201.
42. Wolf RL, Lebwohl B, Lee AR, et al. Hypervigilance to a gluten-free diet and decreased quality of life in teenagers and adults with celiac disease. Dig Dis Sci 2018;63(6):1438–48.
43. Lee AR, Wolf RL, Lebwohl B, et al. Persistent economic burden of the gluten free diet. Nutrients 2019;11(2):399.
44. Camilleri M, Parkman HP, Shafi MA, et al. Clinical guideline: management of gas-troparesis. Am J Gastroenterol 2013;108(1):18.
45. Bennell J, Taylor C. A loss of social eating: the experience of individuals living with gastroparesis. J Clin Nurs 2013;22(19–20):2812–21.
46. Taft TH, Craven MR, Adler EP, et al. Stigma experiences of patients living with gastroparesis. Neurogastroenterol Motil 2022;34(4):e14223.
47. Lacy BE, Pimentel M, Brenner DM, et al. ACG clinical guideline: management of irritable bowel syndrome. Official J Am Coll Gastroenterol ACG. 2021;116(1): 17–44.
48. Palsson OS, Whitehead W, Törnblom H, et al. Prevalence of Rome IV functional bowel disorders among adults in the United States, Canada, and the United Kingdom. Gastroenterology 2020;158(5):1262–73.
49. Melchior C, Algera J, Colomier E, et al. Food avoidance and restriction in irritable bowel syndrome: relevance for symptoms, quality of life and nutrient intake. Clin Gastroenterol Hepatol 2022;20(6):1290–8.
50. Böhn L, Störsrud S, Törnblom H, et al. Self-reported food-related gastrointes-tinal symptoms in IBS are common and associated with more severe symptoms and reduced quality of life. Official J Am Coll Gastroenterol ACG 2013;108(5): 634–41.
51. Eswaran S, Chey WD, Jackson K, et al. A diet low in fermentable oligo-, di-, and monosaccharides and polyols improves quality of life and reduces activity impair-ment in patients with irritable bowel syndrome and diarrhea. Clin Gastroenterol Hepatol 2017;15(12):1890–9.
52. Kortlever TL, Ten Bokkel Huinink S, Offereins M, et al. Low-FODMAP diet is asso-ciated with improved quality of life in IBS patients—a prospective observational study. Nutr Clin Pract 2019;34(4):623–30.

UNITED STATES POSTAL SERVICE ®

Statement of Ownership, Management, and Circulation
(All Periodicals Publications Except Requester Publications)

1. Publication Title	2. Publication Number	3. Filing Date
GASTROENTEROLOGY CLINICS OF NORTH AMERICA	000 – 279	9/18/22

4. Issue Frequency	5. Number of Issues Published Annually	6. Annual Subscription Price
MAR, JUN, SEP, DEC	4	$368.00

7. Complete Mailing Address of Known Office of Publication (Not printer) (Street, city, county, state, and ZIP+4®)

ELSEVIER INC.
230 Park Avenue, Suite 800
New York, NY 10169

Contact Person
Malathi Samayan

Telephone (Include area code)
91-44-4299-4507

8. Complete Mailing Address of Headquarters or General Business Office of Publisher (Not printer)

ELSEVIER INC.
230 Park Avenue, Suite 800
New York, NY 10169

9. Full Names and Complete Mailing Addresses of Publisher, Editor, and Managing Editor (Do not leave blank)

Publisher (Name and complete mailing address)
DOLORES MELONI, ELSEVIER INC.
1600 JOHN F KENNEDY BLVD. SUITE 1800
PHILADELPHIA, PA 19103-2899

Editor (Name and complete mailing address)
KERRY HOLLAND, ELSEVIER INC.
1600 JOHN F KENNEDY BLVD. SUITE 1800
PHILADELPHIA, PA 19103-2899

Managing Editor (Name and complete mailing address)
PATRICK MANLEY, ELSEVIER INC.
1600 JOHN F KENNEDY BLVD. SUITE 1800
PHILADELPHIA, PA 19103-2899

10. Owner (Do not leave blank. If the publication is owned by a corporation, give the name and address of the corporation immediately followed by the names and addresses of all stockholders owning or holding 1 percent or more of the total amount of stock. If not owned by a corporation, give the names and addresses of the individual owners. If owned by a partnership or other unincorporated firm, give its name and address as well as those of each individual owner. If the publication is published by a nonprofit organization, give its name and address.)

Full Name	Complete Mailing Address
WHOLLY OWNED SUBSIDARY OF REED/ELSEVIER, US HOLDINGS	1600 JOHN F KENNEDY BLVD. SUITE 1800 PHILADELPHIA, PA 19103-2899

11. Known Bondholders, Mortgagees, and Other Security Holders Owning or Holding 1 Percent or More of Total Amount of Bonds, Mortgages, or Other Securities. If none, check box ☐ None

Full Name	Complete Mailing Address
N/A	

12. Tax Status (For completion by nonprofit organizations authorized to mail at nonprofit rates) (Check one)
The purpose, function, and nonprofit status of this organization and the exempt status for federal income tax purposes:
☒ Has Not Changed During Preceding 12 Months
☐ Has Changed During Preceding 12 Months (Publisher must submit explanation of change with this statement)

PS Form 3526, July 2014 [Page 1 of 4 (see instructions page 4)]   PSN: 7530-01-000-9931   PRIVACY NOTICE: See our privacy policy on www.usps.com.

13. Publication Title		14. Issue Date for Circulation Data Below
GASTROENTEROLOGY CLINICS OF NORTH AMERICA		JUNE 2022

15. Extent and Nature of Circulation			Average No. Copies Each Issue During Preceding 12 Months	No. Copies of Single Issue Published Nearest to Filing Date
a. Total Number of Copies (Net press run)			213	172
b. Paid Circulation (By Mail and Outside the Mail)	(1)	Mailed Outside-County Paid Subscriptions Stated on PS Form 3541 (Include paid distribution above nominal rate, advertiser's proof copies, and exchange copies)	82	66
	(2)	Mailed In-County Paid Subscriptions Stated on PS Form 3541 (Include paid distribution above nominal rate, advertiser's proof copies, and exchange copies)	0	0
	(3)	Paid Distribution Outside the Mails Including Sales Through Dealers and Carriers, Street Vendors, Counter Sales, and Other Paid Distribution Outside USPS®	69	60
	(4)	Paid Distribution by Other Classes of Mail Through the USPS (e.g., First-Class Mail®)	0	0
c. Total Paid Distribution (Sum of 15b (1), (2), (3), and (4))			151	126
d. Free or Nominal Rate Distribution (By Mail and Outside the Mail)	(1)	Free or Nominal Rate Outside-County Copies Included on PS Form 3541	45	33
	(2)	Free or Nominal Rate In-County Copies Included on PS Form 3541	0	0
	(3)	Free or Nominal Rate Copies Mailed at Other Classes Through the USPS (e.g., First-Class Mail)	0	0
	(4)	Free or Nominal Rate Distribution Outside the Mail (Carriers or other means)	0	0
e. Total Free or Nominal Rate Distribution (Sum of 15d (1), (2), (3) and (4))			45	33
f. Total Distribution (Sum of 15c and 15e)			196	159
g. Copies not Distributed (See Instructions to Publishers #4 (page #3))			17	13
h. Total (Sum of 15f and g)			213	172
i. Percent Paid (15c divided by 15f times 100)			77.04%	79.24%

* If you are claiming electronic copies, go to line 16 on page 3. If you are not claiming electronic copies, skip to line 17 on page 3.

PS Form 3526, July 2014 (Page 2 of 4)

16. Electronic Copy Circulation		Average No. Copies Each Issue During Preceding 12 Months	No. Copies of Single Issue Published Nearest to Filing Date
a. Paid Electronic Copies	▶		
b. Total Paid Print Copies (Line 15c) + Paid Electronic Copies (Line 16a)	▶		
c. Total Print Distribution (Line 15f) + Paid Electronic Copies (Line 16a)	▶		
d. Percent Paid (Both Print & Electronic Copies) (16b divided by 16c × 100)	▶		

☒ I certify that 50% of all my distributed copies (electronic and print) are paid above a nominal price.

17. Publication of Statement of Ownership
☒ If the publication is a general publication, publication of this statement is required. Will be printed   ☐ Publication not required.
in the DECEMBER 2022 issue of this publication.

18. Signature and Title of Editor, Publisher, Business Manager, or Owner

Malathi Samayan - Distribution Controller

Malathi Samayan   Date 9/18/22

I certify that all information furnished on this form is true and complete. I understand that anyone who furnishes false or misleading information on this form or who omits material or information requested on the form may be subject to criminal sanctions (including fines and imprisonment) and/or civil sanctions (including civil penalties).

PS Form 3526, July 2014 (Page 3 of 4)   PRIVACY NOTICE: See our privacy policy on www.usps.com.

Moving?

Make sure your subscription moves with you!

To notify us of your new address, find your **Clinics Account Number** (located on your mailing label above your name), and contact customer service at:

Email: journalscustomerservice-usa@elsevier.com

800-654-2452 (subscribers in the U.S. & Canada)
314-447-8871 (subscribers outside of the U.S. & Canada)

Fax number: 314-447-8029

Elsevier Health Sciences Division
Subscription Customer Service
3251 Riverport Lane
Maryland Heights, MO 63043

*To ensure uninterrupted delivery of your subscription, please notify us at least 4 weeks in advance of move.